Assessment of Communication Disorders in Adults

Assessment of Communication Disorders in Adults

M. N. Hegde, PhD
Don Freed, PhD

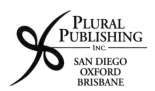
PLURAL
PUBLISHING
INC.

SAN DIEGO
OXFORD
BRISBANE

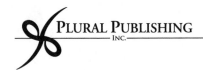

PLURAL PUBLISHING
INC.

5521 Ruffin Road
San Diego, CA 92123

e-mail: info@pluralpublishing.com
Web site: http://www.pluralpublishing.com

49 Bath Street
Abingdon, Oxfordshire OX14 1EA
United Kingdom

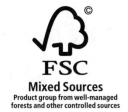

FSC
Mixed Sources
Product group from well-managed
forests and other controlled sources

Cert no. SW-COC-002283
www.fsc.org
© 1996 Forest Stewardship Council

Library of Congress Cataloging-in-Publication Data

Hegde, M. N. (Mahabalagiri N.), 1941-
  Assessment of communication disorders in adults / M. N. Hegde and Don Freed.
     p. ; cm.
  Includes bibliographical references and index.
  ISBN-13: 978-1-59756-414-4 (alk. paper)
  ISBN-10: 1-59756-414-1 (alk. paper)
  1. Communicative disorders--Diagnosis. I. Freed, Donald B. II. Title.
  [DNLM: 1. Communication Disorders--diagnosis. 2. Adult. WL 340.2]
  RC423.H38268 2010
  616.85'5--dc22
                                                2010053115

Contents

Preface

This book, *Assessment of Communication Disorders in Adults* together with the previously published *Assessment of Communication Disorders in Children* (Hegde & Pomaville, 2008), provides a comprehensive set of resources and protocols for assessing both adults and children with communication disorders. The two books share the same clinical philosophy: Clinicians need both scholarly information on disorders of communication and practical protocols for assessing them. Clinicians often do not find both scholarly information and ready-to-use assessment protocols in the same source. Our aim in writing this book is to address this limitation and provide the clinicians both a knowledge base of disorders and a set of practical protocols that they can readily individualize and use in assessing clients with communication disorders.

Clinicians generally tend to specialize in assessing and treating either children or adults with communication disorders. It was thought, therefore, that two comprehensive books, each addressing communication disorders either in children or in adults would be preferable to most clinicians. Furthermore, a single book on assessing all disorders of communication in all age groups would not be practical or manageable, unless it is designed to offer only somewhat superficial background information and brief descriptions of assessment procedures. To make both the background information and practical procedures adequate for assessment, we have designed separate books for children and adults.

This book and its companion volume, *Assessment of Communication Disorders in Children* (Hegde & Pomaville, 2008), share a common organizational structure. In both the books, two chapters are devoted to each disorder—one for background information and the other for assessment protocols. The first chapter on each disorder gives the definitions and descriptions of a disorder and offers a review of the basic and clinical research on that disorder. The second chapter provides practical assessment protocols that are ready to be individualized and used in assessment sessions.

The current volume is organized into eight parts. Part I, *Foundations of Assessment*, has two chapters that address common assessment procedures. Chapter 1 gives an overview of the basic assessment procedures essential for evaluating and diagnosing all disorders of communication in adults. It describes such essential procedures as the written case history, the initial clinical interview, hearing screening, orofacial examination, diadochokinetic evaluation, speech and language samples, standardized tests, postassessment counseling, and assessment reports. The second chapter provides a set of common protocols used in assessing all disorders. The chapter includes a case history protocol, protocol and instructions for conducting an orofacial examination, diadochokinetic assessment, hearing screening, and an outline for assessment reports.

The rest of the book, divided into seven parts, is devoted to assessing specific disorders of communication. Description of motor speech disorders (apraxia of speech and dysarthria) and their assessment protocols are offered in Part II. Aphasia and its assessment protocols may be found in Part III. Subsequent parts describe the right hemisphere syndrome (Part IV), dementia (Part V), traumatic brain injury (VI), fluency disorders (Part VII), and voice disorders (Part VIII).

Within each part, a specific disorder is described in an initial chapter. Each descriptive chapter includes a review of the epidemiology, causation and classification, associated clinical conditions, assessment issues and procedures, differential diagnostic information, and analysis and integration of assessment results relative to a specific disorder. Each resource chapter concludes with a section on postassessment counseling in which the clinician discusses the assessment results with the clients, their caregivers, or both. The section also includes questions clients and their family members typically ask. The answers are written in a dialogue format that the student and the beginning clinician can model after.

The second chapter that follows in each section provides disorder-specific assessment protocols. The protocols written for each disorder offer more than the typical resources clinicians can find in the literature. These protocols are *practical, detailed, and precisely written procedures* that clinicians can follow in making a complete and valid assessment. An additional feature useful to clinicians is that the protocols may be individualized on the CD and printed out for clinical use. In addition, the common and the standard assessment protocols given in Chapter 2 may be combined with specialized protocols given in the respective chapters on motor speech disorders, aphasia, right-hemisphere syndrome, traumatic brain injury, dementia, fluency disorders, and voice disorders. Please see the next section on how to create client-specific and personalized assessment packages.

We would also like to thank Sandy Doyle and Stephanie Meissner for their excellent editorial support, Angie Singh and her team for the fine production of this book, and Madeline Woodard for her outstanding marketing efforts.

Creating Client-Specific Assessment Packages with Protocols on the CD

A unique feature of this book is a combination of scholarly resources and ready-to-use assessment protocols. The protocols are modular pieces that can be combined to create client-specific packages for assessing all adult clients with any disorder of communication.

What are Assessment Protocols?

Assessment protocols are detailed forms that include the methods of assessing clients with communication disorders. Each form describes a specific diagnostic task (e.g., clinical interview, orofacial examination, assessment of naming difficulties, measurement of dysfluencies, or assessment of vocally abusive behaviors). A protocol is not just a description of the task to be completed; it is a set of procedures the clinician can follow to complete the diagnostic task. The advantages of the protocols include the following:

Protocols save clinicians their assessment preparation time. With minor modifications, the clinician can use them in collecting assessment data.

Protocols are similar to criterion-referenced measures. Although not standardized, they provide standard methods of assessing skills that clinicians typically use. In some ways, they are better than standardized test measures because the procedures can be appropriately modified to suit individual clients. Such modifications are unacceptable in the administration of standardized tests.

Results of protocols logically lead to treatment targets. Compared to the scores on a standardized test, the results of each protocol suggest more valid treatment targets for the assessed client. Instead of deriving a score for each skill, the protocols show all the items assessed; the clinician can readily see the items the client fails or rates relatively low. Unlike on a standardized test, most skills are assessed with multiple items on a protocol. In most cases, the clinician can estimate the performance level or even a percent correct response rate and select treatment targets based on this estimate. For example, if a client with aphasia fails 80% of the naming items presented, then the clinician may conclude that naming is a valid treatment target for that client. The clinician would be free to use other acceptable levels of performance (e.g., 70% or 90% accuracy). Therefore, the emphasis in protocols is the existing skill level, not a score to be compared with norms. Treatment targets are readily generated from the existing skills levels in given clients.

These assessment protocols are neither prescriptive nor rigid. They are flexible forms that may be modified, as described in the next section.

Creating Client-Specific Assessment Packages

Clinicians know that each client needs a slightly different package of assessment procedures. Even the common assessment procedures (e.g., the case history and the orofacial examination) may need to be modified to suit individual clients. Therefore, these protocols were designed such that they can both be modified and then combined to create comprehensive as well as client-specific assessment packages. The clinician may put together such packages by:

Modifying all protocols provided on the CD. Because they are formatted in the simple MS Word format, the clinician can modify all common and disorder-specific protocols given on the CD. After entering the name and other personal information on each protocol, the clinician can change, add, or delete questions or items on any protocol. Because assessment is an individualized and dynamic process, we do not expect the clinician to photocopy the protocols given in the book. We expect that they would use the protocols on the CD to modify them so that they are relevant to their individual clients.

Selecting the protocols that are essential for assessing a specific client. In addition to all common protocols, the clinician can select any of the other protocols. For example, in assessing a client with Broca's aphasia, the clinician may select all the (modified) common protocols, aphasia protocols, and perhaps specific motor speech disorder protocols to put together a comprehensive package for that client. In assessing a client with cluttering, protocols for cluttering as well as stuttering may be selected and combined with the common protocols. In essence, needed protocols may be efficiently assembled for clients with multiple disorders of communication.

Printing the modified and combined package of protocols. All protocols are printable from the CD. The clinician can print the selected and modified set of protocols to take to the assessment session a complete package of assessment materials.

Making further modifications during assessment. Because the protocols are assessment of skill levels, the clinician can further modify assessment items during the session. For example, in assessing a client with aphasia, the clinician may substitute names of the client's family members on the naming assessment protocol. Such additional modifications in the assessment session may be essential in evaluating clients with varied ethnocultural backgrounds.

We would like to see clinicians freely individualize these protocols for their use in assessing their adult clients. We believe that these practical and timesaving protocols help select the most appropriate means of assessing adults with communication disorders. Furthermore, the clinician can efficiently write an assessment report using the outline given on the CD.

PART I

Foundations of Assessment

CHAPTER 1

Assessment of Adults: An Overview

- Written Case History
- The Initial Clinical Interview
- Hearing Screening
- Orofacial Examination
- Diadochokinetic Tasks
- Speech-Language Sample
- Standardized Assessment Instruments
- Assessment of Functional Communication
- Assessment of Communication Quality of Life
- Postassessment Counseling
- Analysis and Integration of Assessment Results
- Assessment Report

Assessment of communication disorders in clients of any age precedes diagnosis and treatment. The terms *assessment* and *evaluation* generally mean the same. Both terms refer to a set of activities designed *to determine the value of something*. In clinical practice, assessment is done to diagnose a communication disorder, make predictive statements about prognosis, and to recommend treatment. In exceptional cases, an assessment may reveal no clinically significant problem or a potential problem that needs to be reevaluated later.

If assessment is a series of activities, *diagnosis* may be one of the end products. Ideally, *diagnosis* is the specification of a cause of a disorder or disease. In practice, and especially when causes are unclear or unknown, diagnosis helps determine whether a clinical problem exists, and if it does, its defining characteristics. In some cases, a diagnosis may be tentative, subject to later revision based on additional assessment. Pointing out specific or potential causes could be be helpful in treatment planning.

Assessment of communication disorders in adults is multifaceted. It is no longer sufficient to consider assessment purely in terms of *linguistic deficiencies* or *deviations* a client might experience. Communication impairments go beyond purely linguistic or verbal behavior deficits. These deficits arise in the context of a genetic, environmental, social, and ethnocultural history of individuals. Furthermore, an individual client's unique physiological, behavioral, familial, and specific learning history also affect communication, its disorder, and the client's treatment and rehabilitation. To the extent practical, such variables need to be considered in assessment and treatment planning.

Another aspect of assessment that has gained much clinical attention is not only the causal and background factors related to the disorder, but also the consequences of the disorder. Clinicians have a strong reason to understand the negative consequences that follow a disorder of communication, for it is those consequences that the clinician needs to modify or eliminate if possible. In planning effective treatment, the clinician needs to find out ways the disorder has affected a client's social participation, occupational choices, everyday living, personal and family interaction, and the overall quality of life.

Assessment of communication disorders in adults is further complicated by causal or coexisting neurological and neurodegenerative diseases that are relatively less common in children who exhibit speech-language difficulties. Although a failure to learn verbal behavior skills defines certain disorders of communication in children, it is the loss or impairment of learned verbal behaviors that defines most disorders in adults. There are, of course, exceptions. A disorder that originated during the early childhood years, such as stuttering and cluttering, may persist into adulthood in some individuals and be a lifelong problem. Children, too, can lose verbal skills they have learned up to the point of brain injuries they may sustain. Nonetheless, assessment of several forms of communication disorders in adults must be made in the context of neurological and neurodegenerative diseases. The effects of such diseases on the current communication skills, potential improvement in skills (prognosis), and the intensity of treatment to be offered, needs to be considered in assessment.

In assessing each type of communication disorder, the clinician uses certain common procedures as well as some that are unique to the disorder being evaluated. Pairs of subsequent chapters in the book address a particular disorder and the unique aspects of its assessment. In this chapter, we describe procedures that are common to assessing all adult disorders of communication, which include:

- A written case history
- Interview of the client and the caregivers
- Hearing screening
- Orofacial and diadochokinetic examination
- Speech-language samples
- Standardized test administration
- Assessment of functional communication
- Assessment of communication quality of life
- Assessment report

Written Case History

Most clinics keep a printed case history form that they mail to clients seeking clinical services. It is a questionnaire the client or a caregiver fills out and sends back to the clinic. A sample *Adult Case History Protocol* is given in Chapter 2. The case history form asks questions and provides space for the client to respond. The questions usually relate the reason for seeking services, the onset and the nature of the communication disorder, the general health status of the client, the family background, the client's education and occupational information, and so forth. Studying the information on the case history, the clinician can frame questions for the interview. The typical case history includes different sections that seek information necessary to understand the client.

The Client Identifying Information

The top section of a case history provides space for the client to write his or her name, date of birth, age, address, and phone number. Space may allow for a caregiver's name and telephone number. The name and telephone number of the client's physician and the source of referral also may be written in this section of the case history.

It is essential that either the client or the caregiver provides accurate identifying information, referral sources, and the physician's phone number. Speech-language pathologists (SLPs) need to send their assessment report to the referring processionals and the client's physician, when these are different individuals. Keeping in touch with the client's physician and the referring professional is important to have needed follow-up examinations of the client. It is also important to maintain a professional relationship that helps build a referral source.

Information on Prior Professional Services

Some clients will have received services from other professionals, including speech-language pathologists. It is important to understand all prior services the client will have received for the disorder of communication, as well as for the associated medical condition. On the case history form, the client may list prior services, but it will be the clinician's responsibility to contact the professionals to get their service reports on the client. Before contacting other professionals for their reports, the SLP should always get the written permission from the client.

It will be essential to get reports from audiologists who may have assessed and prescribed a hearing aid for the client. If the client has had a stroke, tumor, or traumatic brain injury, a neurologist's or other medical professional's report would be valuable in understanding the kinds of communication disorder the client exhibits. Medical reports will be similarly valuable in cases of neurodegenerative diseases that cause dementia and associated disorders of communication. An otorhinolaryngologist's report will be essential to assess and treat clients with voice disorders.

Reports on prior assessment and treatment of communication disorders are essential to understand the client's past and current speech-language skills and deficits. The SLP who knows what past treatments succeeded or failed can more appropriately tailor the treatment to the client.

The clinician can explore prior services with the client during the interview, regardless of whether reports have been obtained before the assessment session. This may be the time to get the client's permission to contact other professionals for their reports.

Client's Description of the Problem

Clients and caregivers may describe the communication problem in their own words. It is important to know how the client and the caregivers view the difficulty and how they characterize it. Depending on the level of knowledge they have about the disorder, the descriptions given by clients and others may be more or less specific.

If the written description is vague, the clinician will have to spend more time during the interview to get more specific information. People often say that they have difficulty talking or they cannot talk as well as they did before. Such descriptions may apply to any disorder of communication. It will be the clinician's responsibility to direct the discussion during the interview to the specific kinds of difficulties that help define the problem for the clinician as well as for the client and the family.

Medical History

Relevant medical history of the client is a part of the case history form. This section is especially important in assessing communication disorders in adults because of their common association of neurological and neurodegenerative diseases in this population. Prior illnesses, accidents, or hospitalizations may be reported in this section. On many case history forms, a printed list of diseases may provide a chance for the clients to place a check mark against the ones they have had.

Some medical conditions, such vocal nodules, strokes, and traumatic brain injury, will be especially relevant to the disorder of communication being evaluated. During the interview, it is the clinician's responsibility to get more details from the client and the caregivers on all associated medical conditions.

The Client's Family or Other Living Arrangement

It is important to know whether an adult or an elderly client lives alone, is a resident in an extended healthcare facility, or lives with one or more family members. Some clients may be assessed relatively soon after the onset of the problem, and such clients may be in a hospital or a rehabilitation facility. This is generally true of individuals with aphasia, motor speech disorders, traumatic brain injury, and right hemisphere syndrome. The same individuals also may be assessed after they are discharged from the medical facility in a free-standing speech-language and hearing clinic. Clients with fluency disorder are generally assessed in speech-language and hearing clinics.

Regardless of where the client lives, it is important to assess his or her daily living activities. How does the client spend time? Is the client able to independently attend to his or her daily activities? How much help does the client need to manage the various activities? If the client lives with a family member, the clinician is more likely to get detailed information on daily living activities as well as the general family background. The degree of impairment compared to premorbid motor and communication skills will be better assessed with the help of a family member, especially the spouse of the client. Gauging family support for treatment and generalization and maintenance of treated skills is also an aspect of assessment.

Verbal and Cultural Background

The case history form should allow space for the clients and their caregivers to describe their verbal (linguistic) as well as their cultural background. While most forms do not include questions about the ethnic background of clients, they do include questions about the bilingual status of clients and their families. Ethnocultural differences may be handled during the interview.

Bilingual clients may specify the language they usually speak, read, and write. They might suggest which language is the primary (stronger) language. Whether the second language is spoken by all in the family, and which of the two languages is routinely spoken at home will be of interest to the clinician. This information will have an effect on the assessment procedures. The clinician who does not know the client's stronger primary language will have to find an interpreter, select appropriate assessment tools, and make other changes. The relative strengths and weaknesses of the two languages, their effects on assessment and treatment may then be discussed more fully during the interview.

Educational and Occupational Background

The level of education the client has achieved is an important piece of information entered on a case history form. Education of spouses or other primary caregivers might also be important to be noted on the form. The level of education may suggest appropriate reading and writing materials to be used during assessment. Assessment procedures tailored to the client's education also may produce data that can be more readily used in treatment planning. The family education level might suggest effective ways in which the clinician can help them to provide support for maintaining the client's treatment gains at home.

With adult clients, the occupational history assumes a particular significance. Some clients may have been retired, but premorbidly, they may have maintained activities and hobbies that required certain kinds of speaking, reading, writing, and motoric skills. It is important to assess the extent to which such skills are now impaired and whether the client's activities and hobbies are negatively affected.

Other adult clients might still be holding a job to which they plan to return. Whether this is a realistic plan is something the clinician may need to assess, although this assessment is periodic in the course of treatment. Whether the client will return to the former position may depend on the degree of recovery (with or without treatment) of the skills that are essential to perform the job-related tasks. In all cases, however, it will be desirable to include hobby- or job-related communication and literacy skills in the client's treatment plan. Therefore, it is essential to gain information on the client's activities, hobbies, and job-related skills through the case history and the clinical interview.

Limitations of Case History Information

The case history is a good means of collecting information from the clients and their caregivers. It helps the clinician understand the communication problem from their standpoint. Nonetheless, the reliability and validity of case history information may be variable across clients and their caregivers.

The client and the family members may have differing views of the client's problem, and they may make conflicting claims about the client's limitations in performing everyday activities. Either party may over- or underestimate the communication problem and its effects on the quality of life. In some cases, they may guess requested information, and their guesses may or may not be valid. In other cases, the respondents may not understand all the questions, may interpret them differently, or may be variable in wording their answers.

Such limitations do not negate the value of a case history. Good clinicians interpret the answers carefully. During the interview, the clinician will tactfully explore the different meanings and interpretations of the client and the caregivers.

The Initial Clinical Interview

The clinical interview may be considered an extension of the case history. The advantage of the interview is that it is interactive; the clinician and the informants may go back and forth to make sure that they both understand each other. The interview offers a good opportunity for the clinician to get any vague or potentially inaccurate information on the case history form clarified or corrected.

The clinical interview serves a few significant purposes. First, the interview is more than just asking questions; it is an opportunity to get acquainted with the client and his or her caregivers. The interview is the beginning of a working relationship that develops as the client schedules additional services to the client. Second, the interview is designed to overcome some of the limitations of the case history. For instance, the client, the caregivers, and the clinician, by talking over what is written on the case history, may come to certain conclusions or consensus about the disorder that were hard to arrive at, based just on the written information. Obviously, any misunderstanding or misinterpretation of the case history questions will be cleared. Another limitation of the case history the clinician may overcome during the interview is to get more details on selected aspects of the client's communication difficulty. The clinician may concentrate on the client's premorbid skills, expectations about returning to a previous job, his or her understanding of treatment or rehabilitation, and so forth. Third, the interview is a forum to not only ask questions, but also answer them. Clients and their caregivers are likely to come to the assessment situation with many questions they need answers for. It is the responsibility of the clinician to answer those questions.

To establish a good working relationship with the client and the caregivers, the clinician should conduct the interview in a supporting manner. The clinician should avoid rapid-fire questioning. The clinician should not only expect answers, but also invite comments, thoughts, and feelings related to the communication problem. The clinician should reflect on what the informants say and summarize their views. These actions will help assure the client and the caregivers that the clinician is a concerned and caring professional. By the time the interview is over and the clinician is ready to begin the assessment tasks, the client and the caregivers should feel at ease and comfortable in the clinical situation.

At the outset, the clinician introduces herself and engages the client and the informants in a brief duration of informal conversation. The clinician then gives a description of what lies ahead for the client and the approximate time it will take. The clinician will then say that she or he would like to go over the case history form, ask questions to get additional information, find out what they think is the problem, and answer any questions they may have about the assessment plan.

The interview will take more or less time, depending on the complexity and severity of the disorder being evaluated. A more completely filled-in case history form will save interview time. Informants who more readily and completely answer questions also will help finish the interview in less time.

The specific questions asked during the interview will depend on the disorder being assessed. Therefore, in their respective protocols chapters, a disorder-specific interview protocol is provided for apraxia of speech, dysarthria, aphasia, right hemisphere syndrome, dementia, traumatic brain injury, fluency disorders, and voice problems. In this chapter, we offer general guidelines on conducting a productive and supportive interview, as given in Hegde and Pomaville (2008), and modified to suit the adult clients:

1. **Be prepared for the interview.** Review the written case history ahead of time. Be clear about the areas you wish to explore during the interview. Develop a list of major questions that need to be asked. A structured, well-planned interview promotes a professional image and reduces clinician anxiety.

2. **Arrange for comfortable seating and lighting.** Conduct the interview in a physical environment that is comfortable, attractive, well lit, and free from distractions.

3. **Record your interview (audio or video).** Do not rely on your memory; take notes on critical information the interviewee offers. However, try not to take excessive written notes, as this tends to take attention away from the client and the informants, and may reduce the amount of information they provide. Limit your written notes to a few key points or items you want to explore further later during the interview.

4. **Treat the client with respect.** Clients with severe neurological disorders or neurodegenerative diseases with profoundly impaired communication may

have difficulty understanding questions or performing simple assessment tasks. Yet, they should be treated with respect. Do not address them by their first name until you have come to know then better and they indicate that they are fine with it.

5. **Take your time.** Do not rush the informants, limit their responses, complete their sentences, or interrupt their comments. Let them speak freely and redirect them only as needed. Give them a patient and sympathetic listening; but do not patronize or show excessive sympathy and concern that adults might dislike.

6. **Avoid certain kinds of questions.** Do not ask too many questions that can be answered with a simple "yes" or "no." Use open-ended questions.

7. **Do not talk too much.** Avoid talking too much yourself, and do not fall into stereotypical, repetitive responses.

8. **Limit the use of professional jargon, but do not talk down.** Use technical terms sparingly. Define or describe specialized terms in everyday language. Do not try to explain *grammatical difficulties* to a client's spouse who is a professor of linguistics.

9. **Do not put words in the informants' mouths.** Let the client and the caregivers describe the problem in their own terms. After they have done this, seek clarifications or details, and suggest the technical terms when it is helpful.

10. **Explore the conditions of onset.** Seek information about the client's physical symptoms and etiologic factors by exploring the conditions associated with the onset and development of the communication disorder. Conditions associated with onset of communication disorders in adults include various neurological or neurodegenerative diseases (leading to motor speech disorders, aphasia, dementia, right hemisphere syndrome), laryngeal diseases (leading to voice disorders), head injury (leading to intellectual and communication disorders), stress and a need to escape from stressful situations (leading to a form of aphonia), laryngeal trauma or vocal abuse (leading to dysphonias), and so forth. Stuttering in adults will have started in early childhood days and the conditions of onset may be unclear; but neurogenic stuttering will be of recent onset associated with neurological diseases.

11. **Find out what the client and the caregivers think and feel.** Address the client's and family members' feelings, dispositions, and beliefs regarding the communication problem, its origin, and potential remediation. Some of them may have strong beliefs about the causation of communication disorders and how to handle them.

12. **Take note of the client's strengths.** Do not concentrate solely on the impairments and weaknesses of the client. Being realistic, highlight the strengths to reassure the client and the family members. For instance, highlight the fact that a particular client with aphasia is young, well educated, and already has shown good physical recovery, and that these strengths suggest good prognosis for improved communication skills with sustained treatment.

13. **Rephrase questions at different times.** Ask the same question several ways during the interview to confirm that you are getting reliable and consistent responses.

14. **Repeat important points.** Throughout the interview, repeat the critical pieces of information you have learned from the client and the family. This will help them validate the information.

15. **Be sensitive to cultural differences.** Understand the cultural and language differences of the client and the family. If there are language barriers that could interfere with obtaining or sharing information, arrange for an interpreter's help.

16. **Summarize at the end.** At the end of the interview, summarize the key points to allow the informants to rephrase or correct your misunderstandings. Ask if they have any additional questions.

17. **Tell them what the next step will be.** Finish the interview by telling what will be done next and thanking them for their information.

Hearing Screening

Some older adults with a disorder of communication may have had their hearing assessed by an audiologist. Some may be hearing aid users. Other adults may not have had their hearing tested in recent times or not at all. Therefore, it is essential to screen the hearing of adult clients whose hearing has not been assessed. Using a well-maintained and calibrated audiometer, the clinician may screen the client's hearing at 20 dB for the frequencies of 500, 1000, 2000, and 4000 Hz. A referral to an audiologist may be made if the client fails the hearing screening. The form for recording the results of the hearing screening is included as part of the *Orofacial Examination and Hearing Screening Protocol* presented in Chapter 2.

Orofacial Examination

Speech-language pathologists routinely perform an orofacial examination of all clients they assess. This examination helps evaluate the structural adequacy of the oral mechanism for speech production. Structural inadequacies may impede speech production. In some cases, speech production may be negatively affected with no obvious structural deviation. In either case, the clinician needs to rule out both structural and functional problems in producing speech sounds. An orofacial examination is not only a means of observing deviations in the structures of speech production, but also any irregularities in the strength, range, coordination, and consistency of movements.

The detail and the depth of orofacial examination depend on the disorder the client presents. While it is performed on all clients, the examination is especially detailed in assessing clients with neuromotor disorders associated with their communication problems. Clients with apraxia of speech, dysarthria, and traumatic brain injury need in-depth examination of the orofacial structure and function, along with an assessment of their diadochokinetic rate, described in the next section. Clients who have aphasia due to frontal lesions also are good candidates for thorough orofacial and diadochokinetic assessments.

The clinician needs to assemble the following materials to complete an orofacial examination:

- Gloves
- Flashlight
- Tongue depressor
- Mirror
- Stopwatch or a clock with a second hand

To complete the assessment, the clinician may use the *Orofacial Examination and Hearing Screening Protocol* provided in Chapter 2. The chapter also contains *Instructions for Conducting the Orofacial Examination: Observations and Implications*.

Diadochokinetic Tasks

Diadochokinetic tasks are used to assess an individual's production of rapidly alternating speech sounds. Typically, these are divided in alternate motion rate (AMR) and sequential motion rate (SMR) tasks. It is important to observe the rate, accuracy, and consistency of the individual's speech production during these tasks, particularly as single syllables are combined to create longer or more complex utterances. Such an assessment is especially helpful in the differential diagnosis of dysarthria and apraxia of speech. For example, individuals with flaccid and spastic dysarthria usually demonstrate slow but *regular* AMRs. In contrast, individuals with ataxic dysarthria often produce slow and *irregular* AMRs. With apraxia of speech, errors are often inconsistent, and speech often breaks down as the length and complexity of the utterance increase. An individual may be able to produce the single-syllable phonemes in the AMRs but will be unable to produce the same phonemes in a multisyllable production (SMRs). In addition, sound-syllable transpositions, repetitions, or additions are more likely to occur. Groping and searching behaviors might also be observed if verbal apraxia is present (see *Apraxia of Speech Assessment Protocol* in Chapter 4).

Diadochokinetic syllable tasks usually consist of having the individual produce the following sounds continuously and as quickly as possible: /pʌ/, /tʌ/, /kʌ/, /pʌtə/, and /pʌtəkə/. These phonemes are selected because they require the use of different muscle groups. The phoneme /p/ requires labial activity, /t/ requires elevation of the tongue tip to the front of the oral cavity (alveolar ridge), and /k/ requires posterior tongue elevation to the back of the oral cavity (velum).

Speech-Language Sample

A naturalistic speech and language sample can be valuable in assessing various disorders of communication in adults. Speech-language samples are the best means of assessing syntactic structures, grammatic morphemes, conversational skills (including topic initiation, topic maintenance, and conversational repair strategies), production of speech sounds in connected speech, and speech dysfluencies. In assessing adult neurogenic communication disorders, however, extended conversational samples do not seem to play as major a role as they do in assessing child language disorders. Many tests of aphasia, for example, have subtests for narrative or discourse skills. Most include subtests of syntax and morphological features.

Unlike the young child client, the adult client in most cases is an informant; the adult talks about his or her difficulty. Adult clients with fluency and voice problems and many with aphasia and motor speech disorders can talk with the clinician to describe their problems, and give information on their educational, occupational, and family backgrounds. Exceptions are people with severe global aphasia, mutism, and those with dementia-related confusion. Obviously, a speech-language sample with clients who are mute is out of question, and it is nonproductive with clients who are severely globally aphasic. The language of a confused patient can be analyzed for impairments, however. Similarly, a severely paraphasic and neologistic (hence mostly meaningless) language sample of Wernicke's aphasia also can be analyzed. Therefore, clinicians can always consider the interview as a means of assessing conversational skills, syntactic and morphological features, vocal characteristics (including pitch, loudness, and quality), dysfluencies, and speech sound productions. Most clinicians assessing adult clients treat the interview as the speech-language sample. Clinicians then may supplement it with such specific tasks as story telling or retelling, picture description, sentence completion, and so forth. Most of these specific tasks are included in standardized tests designed to assess adult communication disorders, particularly neurogenic speech and language disorders. If those tests are not appropriate, the clinician can design client-specific story telling, narrative, monologue, and such other tasks to assess specific language skills. In assessing fluency disorders, some clinicians may prefer to record a conversational speech and a monologue. Guidelines to record these tasks are provided in Chapter 15.

Standardized Assessment Instruments

Speech-language pathologists routinely use standardized tests in assessing aphasia, apraxia of speech, dysarthrias, and traumatic brain injury. Several tests are available for assessing these disorders. Fewer tests are available for assessing dementia globally, although clinicians use task-specific tests (e.g., memory tests, IQ tests, other cognitive tests) to assess aspects of dementia. In assessing fluency disorders, standardized or criterion-referenced tests target emotions, attitudes, avoidance reactions, and to some extent, quality of life. In assessing voice disorders, standardized tests are uncommon.

Clinicians prefer standardized tests for their obvious advantages. Among others, they give a structure for assessment, their procedures are standard across clients, and each major assessment task may have a subtest. A client's performance may be compared against norms to determine if there is a deficiency. Tests may minimize variability of scores when different examiners administer them on the same client. Two or more clinicians can interpret the results on a client in the same or similar manner. In essence, standardized tests are convenient.

Selection of Standardized Tests

In spite of their significant advantages, standardized tests have their limitations that should be considered in selecting them for administration. From a practical standpoint, tests that allow for in-depth and comprehensive assessment are often too long. Some aphasia tests, for example, may take up to 6 hours to administer and an additional considerable time to analyze the results. Tests that are short enough to be practical may not assess as deeply as those that are long. Besides such practical problems, tests have other limitations that may be more or less magnified in the case of individual tests (Hegde & Pomaville, 2008). Therefore, clinicians should carefully consider the variables that affect the usefulness and applicability of tests before selecting them for administration.

Extensive discussion of the standardization process and advantages and disadvantages of tests may be readily found in other sources (Anastasi & Urbina, 1997; Hegde & Pomaville, 2008; Van Ornum, Dunlap, & Shore, 2008). Therefore, here we will summarize the guidelines for selecting standardized tests, adapted from Hegde and Pomaville (2008); asking and answering the following kinds of questions will evaluate tests for their suitability:

- **Are tests the sole source of information or are they supplementary?** Standardized tests should not be sole source of information. In most cases, they may provide only supplementary information. Test scores should be analyzed in the context of a detailed case history, clinical interview, observations of the client's caregivers, reports from other professionals, criterion-referenced assessment tools, informal questionnaires, speech and language samples, narrative and discourse samples, and so forth.

- **Who were included in the standardization sample?** Whether the client's age, social and educational level, ethnic and linguistic background were represented in the standardization sample is probably the most critical question to ask in administering standardized tests in a pluralistic society. Do not administer a test to a particular client if his or her general characteristics were not represented in the sample drawn for standardizing that test. Administer tests that have been standardized on large and representative national samples. If well-standardized tests are not available, use only such other means as clinical interview, client-specific tasks you design for assessing particular skills, criterion-referenced measures, conversational and discourse samples, and other nonstandardized methods of assessment. Note that all the assessment protocols provided in this book are task-specific and nonstandardized; they are akin to criterion-referenced assessment tools.

- **Is the test manual detailed and comprehensive?** The selected test should have a detailed test manual to administer and score the test items. It should report acceptable levels of reliability and validity and should adequately describe the normative sample.

- **Does the test sample skills adequately?** A test may sample a skill inadequately or superficially. An adequate test should give multiple opportunities to produce a skill (e.g., phonemes, grammatic morpheme, syntactic structures, requests, or responses to commands).

- **Are the normative data current?** Recently restandardized tests tend to be more representative of the ethnoculturally changing population than tests standardized in the past.

- **Is the test reliable?** Reliability is consistency of scores upon repeated administration on the same individuals. As described fully in Hegde and Pomaville (2008), a test may report different kinds of reliability (e.g., *test-retest, split-half, parallel-form, interobserver,* and *intraobserver*). A test that reports different kinds of reliability may be preferred to the one that reports only one kind. The degree of reliability is just as important; the correlation coefficient should be .90 or higher.

- **Is the test valid?** Validity is the extent to which the test measures what it claims to measure. As fully described elsewhere (Hegde & Pomaville, 2008), validity also is of different kinds (e.g., *content, construct, criterion, concurrent,* and *predictive*). Tests that report multiple kinds of validity may be preferred over those that report only one kind or otherwise weak validity.

- **Are the stimulus items appropriate for the client?** A test may contain either dated stimuli (e.g., an antique kitchen stove that current clients are unfamiliar with) or they may contain stimulus items that are unfamiliar to culturally diverse clients. A test that contains such stimulus items should be avoided.

- **Am I trained to administer the test?** Other than student clinicians who are being trained to administer tests, professionals should ask themselves whether they are competent in administering a test. If they have not received adequate training in administering a particular test, they should then select the one for which they are well trained. Clinicians should seek training in administering newer tests.

Once a test is selected and administered, the clinician is responsible to interpret the results fairly and validly. If for some reason, a test that is inadequately standardized on a particular ethnocultural group is administered to a member of that group, then it is even more critical to interpret the results cautiously, tentatively, or perhaps not at all. Similar approaches to interpreting test results are essential if specific items on an administered test are found to be dated or inappropriate. One should know that tests do not diagnose—the clinician does.

Available standardized tests are described in the *resources* chapter on each disorder. For instance, apraxia of speech tests are described in Chapter 3, dysarthria tests are described in Chapter 5, and aphasia tests are described in Chapter 7.

Assessment of Functional Communication

In some ways, functional communication assessment contrasts with traditional assessment that typically includes standardized tests and speech-language samples. Functional communication assessment is important, partly because the cost of treating nonfunctional skills may not be reimbursed by third parties (Frattali, 1998) and partly because functional communication *is* essential to daily living. Nonetheless, there is no standard definition of *functional communication*, and different views exist on the scope of the term.

In one sense, functional communication is *basic* communication. It is not the communication of a university professor who gives a lecture on neurolinguistic deep structures. Functional communication need not be verbal; any mode, including gestures and signs may be effective and functional. Most functional communication assessment tools (some are described in Chapter 7) generally target such basic communication skills as requests to fulfill basic needs (e.g., toileting, eating, drinking), managing daily activities (e.g., using the telephone, understanding traffic signals and signs, making a grocery list), basic social skills (e.g., greeting others, bidding goodbye), and so forth.

Another, related concept of functional communication is that it is communicative behaviors emitted in natural settings—whether the skills are basic or advanced. In the context of his or her impairments, what is adequately functional for one client may be inadequate for another (Frattali, 1998). For instance, for a retired man with global aphasia, basic communication of needs and management of daily living activities may be functional. But for a younger woman with traumatic brain injury, who is still holding her position as a teacher and wants to return to her job, and the prospects of returning are realistic, basic communication is not functional enough; she needs more than basic communication to perform her teaching job.

Standard assessment procedures adequately target more advanced functional skills. Assessment of discourse, narrative skills, syntactic and morphologic skills, abstract language production, and so forth target more advanced communication skills that are indeed functional for certain individuals. To the contrary, most published functional communication assessment tools target basic communication. Several well-known functional communication assessment tools are available; many are disorder specific; the earliest ones were related to stroke and aphasia. Sarno's (1969) *Functional Communication Profile*, designed for patients with aphasia, is the earliest assessment tool of its kind. Other instruments include *Communicative Abilities in Daily Living* (Holland, 1998), the *Communicative Effectiveness Index* (Lomas, Pickard, Bester, & Associates, 1989), the *Communication profile: A functional skills survey* (Payne, 1994), and the American Speech-Language-Hearing Association's *Functional Assessment of Communication Skills for Adults* (ASHA-FACS) (Frattali, Thompson, Holland, Wohl, & Ferketic, 1995).

ASHA FACS contains questions in four major domains: social communication (SC), communication of basic needs (BN), daily planning (DP), and reading/writing/number concepts (RWN). Examples of assessment domains include:

- Refers to family members by name (SC)
- Initiates communication with other people (SC)
- Expresses feelings (BN)
- Recognizes familiar faces (BN)
- Understands simple signs (RWN)
- Writes short messages (RWN)

We offer a *Functional Communication Assessment Protocol* in Chapter 2. It is also available on the CD. Accessing the protocol on the CD, clinicians can modify the protocol to suit the individual client, the disorder being evaluated, and the kinds of communication barriers the client faces. The protocol may be appropriate to use in evaluating clients with aphasia, apraxia of speech, dysarthria, dementia, right hemisphere syndrome, and traumatic brain injury. Generally speaking, functional communication assessment is not critical in clients with stuttering or a voice disorder. Exceptions might include clients neurogenic stuttering or severe spasmodic dysphonia, whose communication skills may be vastly compromised. Whether the clients with these disorders are able to manage basic, functional, and everyday communication may be of interest to the clinician.

Assessment of Communication Quality of Life

Similar to functional communication, quality of life (QOL) assessment is nontraditional and contrasts with the traditional assessment of disorders or impaired communication. Assessment of QOL is driven by the realization that diseases and disorders alter the way individuals lead their lives. Individuals with impaired communication and any associated medical conditions may be unable to do what they want to do. Physical and communication problems may restrict their daily activities, social participation, job performance, hobbies, vacation plans, and their general enjoyment of life. Consequently, individuals may feel less competent, depressed, and think of themselves in unfavorable terms ("low self-image"). Individuals may generally feel that their lives have changed for the worse, experience less enjoyment, and think that their quality of life has degraded.

The degree to which clients think that their QOL is degraded may partly depend on how they cope with their impairments. The same impairments may produce different reactions in different individuals. Some individuals cope better, find alternative ways of enjoying life, compensate for their impairments more effectively, and manage to maintain a more optimistic, even enthusiastic, outlook on their lives. Others who do not cope with their problems as well, may feel discouraged, even depressed, and take a more pessimistic view of their lives and future possibilities of enjoyment.

QOL assessment instruments usually are questionnaires. A well-known general QOL assessment questionnaire is the World Health Organization Quality of Life (WHOQOL-BREF) (2004). It asks such questions as:

- How would you rate your quality of life?
- How satisfied are you with your health?
- How much do you enjoy life?
- How safe do you feel in your daily life?

A QOL assessment questionnaire that is specific to communication problems is the *Quality of Communication Life Scale* (QCL) (Paul, Frattali, Holland, & Associates, 2004). Examples of items on this scale include:

- I like to talk to people.
- People understand me when I talk.
- I make my own decisions.
- In general, my quality of life is good.

We offer two options for assessing QOL of individuals with communication disorders. In Chapter 2 and on the CD, we have included a *Communication Quality of Life Assessment Protocol (CQOL)*. This QOL assessment protocol is most suitable to assess clients with aphasia, dysarthria, apraxia of speech, dementia, right hemisphere syndrome, traumatic brain injury, and neurogenic stuttering. These disorders affect not only communication, but also general health, daily living activities, finance and daily math skills, hobbies, and behavior health. Therefore, the CQOL includes questions about communication and general quality of life. Some of these assessment domains may not be especially relevant to people with stuttering, cluttering, and most voice disorders. Therefore, we also offer specific QOL assessment protocols for fluency disorders (Chapter 16) and voice disorders (Chapter 18).

Postassessment Counseling

The clinician ends the assessment session with a period of counseling. As in the initial interview, the clinician sits down with the client and the accompanying caregivers to discuss the findings of the assessment. Even though a complete analysis of the results will be made later, the clinician can answer a few basic questions from the knowledge gained during the assessment. The clinician can suggest additional assessment or make a tentative diagnosis, recommend treatment, and suggest prognosis. The clinician might recommend the client for other specialists, offer educational information on the disorder and its management, and answer the client's and caregivers questions.

The exchange between the clinician and the client and the caregivers during the postassessment counseling will be disorder specific. The clinician will discuss the findings related to the disorder. The type of diagnostic, prognostic, and treatment information presented to them will depend on the disorder. Therefore, the *protocols* chapters on apraxia of speech, dysarthria, aphasia, traumatic brain injury, dementia, fluency disorder, and voice disorders describe a typical dialogue between the clinician and the caregivers. The clinician should modify, reword, add, or skip statements as found appropriate to inform the client and his or her caregivers.

The client and the caregivers know they have a problem, and may even know the specific diagnosis (e.g., aphasia, stuttering, or voice disorder). In most cases, the clinician will not surprise them with the diagnosis. Nonetheless, the client and the caregivers may not be fully aware of the causes and consequences of the disorder. They may want to know why the disorder exists or why it is of a certain severity. Having told the clinician how the disorder has affected the life of the client and the caregivers, they may want to know what additional effects may be expected and when. Often, the client and the family may not have been fully informed about the associated medical condition (e.g., vocal fold pathology or neurodegenerative diseases). The clinician may discuss these conditions in the context of the client's communication problem.

Probably the most critical question the client and the caregivers may have for the clinician is whether there is a good chance of improvement with communication treatment and what kind of treatment will help them achieve their goal. Questions related to the duration and cost of treatment, and the kinds of support the client will need to sustain treatment at home, will be important as well.

The structure of postassessment counseling is similar to the initial clinical interview. The difference is that in the initial interview, the clinician is a sympathetic listener seeking facts, comments, information, thoughts, and feelings of the client and the caregivers relative to the client's problem. While still being a sympathetic listener, the clinician during the postassessment counseling informs, educates, supports, and reassures the client and the caregivers. It is also an opportunity to solidify a professional working relationship with the client and the caregivers.

Analysis and Integration of Assessment Results

Following the assessment session, the clinician makes a complete analysis of assessment results and integrates them with information obtained from various sources. A relatively firm and valid diagnosis depends on this analysis and integration.

An analysis of the information obtained from the case history and interview, reports from other specialists, clinical assessment results, any instrumental evaluations, results of standardized tests, functional communication assessment, and QOL measures will help understand the client, the family, and the client's communication problems, as well as associated conditions. The clinician may take the following steps to analyze and integrate the assessment data.

1. **The analysis should result in a profile of the client and the family.** Using the information obtained through the case history, interview, and assessment procedures, the clinician may draw a profile of the client and his or her family. The nature of the disorder, the conditions of its onset, the effects of the disorder on the client and the caregivers, the family dynamics, and the limitations and strengths of the client and the family members will be described in the profile. The client's educational and occupational history and the expectations about future employment will be part of this profile. The client's ethnocultural background that may affect how the disorder is viewed and how he or she view the treatment or rehabilitation options will be important to note. If the client is bilingual, it will be essential to describe the client's strengths and limitations in each of the two languages and how they affect treatment planning and implementation. The profile should include the client's reaction to his or her own impairments, interests, hobbies, special talents, or favorite activities.

2. **Different kinds of assessment results should be integrated.** The clinician will have information from case history, interview, speech and language samples, orofacial examination, hearing screening, standardized tests, alternative assessment procedures (e.g., client-specific or criterion-referenced protocols), clinical judgments or ratings, instrumental assessment (especially of voice disorders), functional communication, and quality-of-life assessments. An analysis of these sources of information, along with information obtained from other professionals, should help obtain a comprehensive and consistent clinical picture of the client. If there are discrepancies, the clinician needs to find out why.

3. **Reports from other specialists should be integrated.** Other professionals who have assessed or treated various diseases will contribute significantly to an understanding of the client's communication disorder. For example, it will be important to know whether the client has been diagnosed with a neurological disorder, a neurodegenerative disease including dementia, malignant or benign laryngeal growths, strokes, head injury, right hemisphere syndrome, and so forth. If the treatment has been offered in the past—whether medical or communicative—the clinician needs to know the procedures, their results, and the client's as well as the family members' evaluation of the results.

4. **A final diagnosis will be based on the integrated assessment information.** The final diagnosis may be more or less challenging, depending on the type of communication disorder, associated diseases, and phenotypical similarity to disorders of different etiologies. The clinician suggests whether the diagnosis is stable or is likely to change over time. For example, an initial diagnosis of a specific type of aphasia may change over time. A patient with head injury may recover from his or her initial coma.

5. **Recommendations follow the diagnosis.** Typically, treatment is recommended. The nature of treatment may be outlined to the client, the family members, and other caregivers. Various treatment options may be described.

6. **The diagnosis and related data may suggest a tentative prognosis.** A careful analysis of the assessment data, culminating in a diagnosis, typically suggests a prognosis. The clinician makes prognostic statements in probabilistic terms. The prognostic statements are conditional in the sense that the probability of a good prognosis may vary, depending on conditions of treatment, no treatment, more or less intensive treatment, the client's cooperation and motivation, the family support, and the nature of the associated diseases (e.g., curable, reversible, clinically manageable with residual effects, progressive).

Assessment Report

Writing a report is the final step in completing an assessment. Following the analysis and integration of assessment results, the clinician would write a diagnostic report. We have included an *Assessment Report Outline* in Chapter 2 to facilitate this task. The outline, though appropriate for most diagnostic reports, should be modified to fit the particular disorder and the client for whom the report is written. A copy of the report may be sent to the client, the caregivers, and the referring specialists.

The assessment result should help develop a treatment plan for the client. Most likely the client will be seen in the same facility for treatment. If so, the treatment plan will be more fully developed after a discussion with the client and the caregivers. If the client is being referred to another facility for treatment, the diagnostic report and treatment recommendations may be sent to that facility.

References

Anastasi, A., & Urbina, S. (1997). *Psychological testing* (7th ed.). Upper Saddle River, NJ: Prentice-Hall.

Frattali, C. M. (1998). Measuring modality-specific behaviors, functional abilities, and quality of life. In C. M. Frattali (Ed), *Measuring outcomes in speech-language pathology* (pp. 55–88). New York, NY: Thieme.

Frattali, C. M., Thompson, C. K., Holland, A. L., Wohl, C. B., & Ferketic, M. M. (1995). *Functional assessment of communication skills for adults* (ASHA FACS). Rockville, MD: American Speech-Language-Hearing Association.

Hegde, M. N., & Pomaville, F. (2008). *Assessment of communication disorders in children.* San Diego, CA: Plural.

Holland, A. L., Frattali, C. M., & Fromm, D. (1998). *Communication activities in daily living* (2nd ed.). Austin, TX: Pro-Ed.

Lomas, J., Pickard, L., Bester, S., & Associates (1989). The communicative effectiveness index: Clinical and research assessment of head injury outcome. *International Rehabilitation Medicine, 7,* 145–149.

Paul, D. R., Frattalli, C. M., Holland, A. L., & Associates (2004). *Quality of communication life scale.* Bethesda, MD: American Speech-Language-Hearing Association.

Payne, J. C. (1994). *Communication profile: A functional skills survey.* Tucson, AZ: Communication Skill Builders.

Sarno, M. T. (1969). *The functional communication profile: Manual of directions.* New York, NY: New York University Medical Center, Institute of Rehabilitation Medicine.

Van Ornum, W., Dunlap, L., & Shore, M. F. (2008). *Psychological testing across the life span.* Boston, MA: Upper Saddle River, NJ: Pearson Education.

World Health Organization Quality of Life (WHOQOL-BREF) (2004). Geneva, Switzerland: Author.

CHAPTER 2

Common
Assessment Protocols

- Adult Case History Protocol
- Instructions for Conducting the Orofacial Examination in Adults: Observations and Implications
- Orofacial Examination and Hearing Screening Protocol
- Diadochokinetic Assessment Protocol for Adults
- Functional Communication Assessment Protocol
- Communication Quality of Life Assessment Protocol
- Adult Assessment Report Outline

Several protocols are essential to assess communication disorders in all adult clients. A case history form, for example, is filled out by all adults who seek clinical services. During their assessment, all adult clients receive an orofacial examination, a diadochokinetic test, and a hearing screening. The end product of all assessment is a report on the findings, a diagnosis, and recommendations for treatment. Clinicians will find in this chapter a set of protocols that they need in assessing all of their adult clients.

These common protocols should be combined with specific protocols provided in chapters on various communication disorders. For example, the case history protocol should be combined with specific assessment protocols for aphasia or stuttering. The clinician can select specific protocols and combine them with the standard protocols to create a comprehensive assessment package. To efficiently prepare for assessment, the clinician may print the entire assessment package out of the provided CD.

Note: The *Functional Communication Assessment Protocol* and the *General Quality of Life Assessment Protocols* may be administered at the discretion of the clinician. When the assessment time is at a premium, functional assessment may be relatively less important in some cases. For instance, many adult clients with fluency or voice disorders may not have their basic and functional communication impaired. On the other hand, functional communication may be impaired in clients with severe forms of aphasia, apraxia of speech, dementia, dysarthria, traumatic brain injury, and right hemisphere syndrome. The *Functional Communication Assessment Protocol* is especially relevant to clients with those disorders. Similarly, the *General Quality of Life Assessment Protocol* is more relevant to clients whose communication skills are severely impaired. If warranted, the clinicians may administer either or both of the protocols to any client. Disorder-specific quality of life assessment protocols are provided for people who stutter and those with voice disorders.

Adult Case History Protocol

Today's Date _____

General Information

Name: _____   Date of Birth: _____

Gender: ☐ Male   ☐ Female

Address _____   E-mail _____

City _____   Zip _____

Phone: (Home) _____ (Cell) _____

Occupation: _____   Business Phone: _____

Employer: _____

Single: _____   Widowed: _____   Divorced: _____   Spouse's Name: _____

Spouse's Occupation: _____

Today's informant: _____

Names, ages, and gender of children: _____

_____

Referred By: _____   Phone: _____

Address: _____

Have you been tested and/or evaluated at this clinic before? _____

If yes, how long ago was your last visit?

_____

Names and relation of other persons living in home: _____

_____

What languages do you speak? _____

What is your primary language? _____

Highest grade completed or degree earned? _____

(continues)

Adult Case History Protocol (continued)

Describe your current speech or language problem: _____

_____

_____

What do you think caused the problem? _____

_____

_____

When was your problem first noticed? _____

_____

Who noticed your earliest problem? Yourself or someone else? _____

_____

What were the earliest signs (symptoms, difficulties) of your problem? _____

_____

How has the problem changed since it was first noticed? _____

_____

_____

How has your communication problem affected your personal, social, and occupational life?

_____

_____

List other speech-language specialists you have seen and describe their conclusions or recommendations: (Please provide copies of test reports/test results)

_____

_____

_____

List any other specialists (physicians, psychologists, neurologists, etc.) you have seen, and the specialists' conclusions or suggestions: (Please provide copies of reports/test results)

_____

_____

_____

Describe any other speech, language, learning, or hearing problems in your family:

_____

_____

_____

Medical History

General health is: ☐ good   ☐ fair   ☐ poor

Provide the approximate ages at which you experienced the following illness and conditions:

Adenoidectomy _____	Allergies _____	Asthma _____
Chicken pox_____	Colds _____	Convulsion _____
Croup _____	Diabetes _____	Draining ear _____
Ear infections_____	Dizziness _____	Epilepsy _____
Headaches _____	Encephalitis _____	German measles _____
Tonsillitis _____	Pneumonia _____	Tonsillectomy _____
Ulcers _____	Visual problems _____	Meningitis _____
Influenza _____	Hearing aids _____	Heart problems _____
Meningitis _____	Hearing loss_____	High fever _____
Numbness _____	Mastoiditis _____	Measles _____
Otosclerosis _____	Mumps _____	Noise exposure _____
Stroke _____	Brain injury_____	Brain tumors _____
Brain hemorrhage_____	Paralysis _____	Seizures _____
Alzheimer's disease _____	Parkinson's disease_____	Pick's disease _____
Huntington's disease _____	Other neurological diseases (specify) _____	

_____

_____

Vocal nodules_____   Laryngeal cancer _____

Other laryngeal diseases (specify) _____

_____

Do you smoke? _____ How much per day? _____

(continues)

Adult Case History Protocol (continued)

List all prescription and nonprescription medication used during the past year: _____

_____

_____

Describe any eating or swallowing difficulties you have experienced: _____

_____

_____

List any major accidents, illnesses, surgeries, or hospitalizations (include dates): _____

_____

_____

_____

Provide any additional information that you might believe to be helpful in the evaluation or remediation process:

_____

_____

_____

_____

Person completing the form: _____

Relationship to client: _____

Signed: _____ Date: _____

PLEASE ATTACH ANY REPORT YOU HAVE FROM ANOTHER AGENCY, SCHOOL, OR HEALTH CARE PROVIDER.

Instructions for Conducting the Orofacial Examination in Adults: Observations and Implications

1. Gather the materials needed to complete the orofacial examination and hearing screening:
   - Gloves
   - Flashlight
   - Tongue depressor
   - Mirror
   - Stopwatch or clock with a second hand
   - Food or drink items (optional)
   - Protocols: *Orofacial Examination and Hearing Screening*, this protocol, (optional), *Apraxia of Speech Assessment Protocol* or *Dysarthric Speech Assessment Protocol* (optional)

2. Position the client so his or her face and mouth are at eye level.

3. Observe general facial symmetry and the appearance of structures: eyes, nose, mouth, ears, hair/hairline, jaw, eyebrows, forehead, and chin. Note any irregularities or signs of asymmetry.

   Implications
   - Asymmetry, as indicated by drooping of one eye, cheek, or corner of the mouth may indicate neurologic involvement, unilateral facial paresis (weakness), or paralysis.
   - Structures that appear unusual, out of alignment with each other, or asymmetric may indicate craniofacial anomalies or be characteristic of certain syndromes or medical conditions.

4. Observe the client's breathing.

   Implications
   - *Clavicular breathing* (characterized by elevation of the shoulders with each breath) may be associated with excess tension in the neck and shoulders and may contribute to hyperfunction in the larynx and consequent voice problems.
   - *Irregular breathing patterns or inadequate respiration* may affect speech prosody or have a negative effect on vocal quality.
   - *Mouth breathing* is often associated with an open mouth posture and forward tongue carriage. In case of mouth breathing, the nasal patency should be checked to make sure nasal breathing is possible. If nasal breathing is absent or difficult, and the speech is hyponasal, the client should be referred to a medical evaluation to determine why.

5. Observe the client's lips at rest and note any irregularities such as scars or discolorations.

6. Observe labial strength and range of motion on the following tasks:
   - round/pucker the lip
   - elongate the lips (smile, showing me your teeth)
   - alternate pucker-smile-pucker-smile
   - open lips wide
   - close lips tightly and puff up cheeks (sustain intraoral pressure)
   - bite lower lip as if making an /f/ sound
   - say "puh-puh-puh"

   Implications
   - Labial weakness, as indicated by an inability to round/pucker the lips tightly, elongate the lips symmetrically, or close the lips tightly to sustain intraoral air pressure, may indicate neurologic involvement. If the lips pull to one side during elongation, then they will pull to the strong side, thus the opposite side is weak.
   - If the client is unable to sustain intraoral air pressure because air escapes through the lips, labial weakness is indicated. If air escapes through the nose, along with hypernasality or nasal emission, velopharyngeal insufficiency or incompetence is indicated. Administer the *Resonance and Velopharyngeal Function Assessment Protocol* found in Chapter 18.
   - Difficulty producing the /p/ sound also may indicate labial weakness or incoordination.
   - Sequencing or motor programming difficulties, as indicated by searching and groping behaviors, difficulty alternating the pucker-smile, or difficulty coordinating the movements needed to puff up the cheeks or bite the lower lip, may indicate the presence of apraxia.

7. Observe the surface appearance of the client's tongue. Note any irregularities, scars, or discolorations.

8. Observe lingual strength and range of motion as you ask the client to:
   - stick the tongue out as far as possible
   - push against a tongue blade (to assess strength)
   - elevate the tongue tip as if trying to touch your nose
   - tongue tip down, as if trying to touch the chin
   - tongue tip left
   - tongue tip right
   - alternate tongue to left and right sides

- put tongue inside cheek on right side and push cheek out (the clinician can push against the cheek to assess strength)
- put tongue inside cheek on left side and push cheek out (the clinician can push against the cheek to assess strength)
- place tongue tip on alveolar ridge, then draw tip back along hard palate

Implications

- ○ The following observations indicate lingual weakness or incoordination: an inability to protrude the tongue or push against the tongue blade, difficulty elevating or lowering the tongue tip, difficulty moving the tongue from side to side or pushing against the cheek. Tongue movement will be slow and possibly accompanied by lingual tremor. Range of motion will be reduced. If weakness is on one side (unilateral), then the tongue will deviate to the weak side upon protrusion, and the client will have trouble moving the tongue toward the strong side.

- ○ Inability to protrude the tongue beyond the lips and a heart-shaped tongue when protruded indicate a short lingual frenulum. This is known as *ankyloglossia* or "tongue tie," which may or may not affect articulation. Have the client attempt to produce several speech sounds requiring tongue elevation (e.g., /t/, /d/, /n/, /k/). If the client cannot contact the palate to produce these sounds, then the frenulum may need to be clipped by a physician.

- ○ Sequencing or motor programming difficulties, as indicated by searching and groping behaviors, difficulty alternating tongue movements, or difficulty coordinating the movements needed to put the tongue in the cheek or draw it back along the hard palate, may indicate the presence of apraxia.

9. Observe the general condition of the teeth and gums. Note any dental appliances or prostheses.

10. Observe the alignment or dental occlusion. Have the client open the mouth wide. Place a tongue blade alongside the teeth on one side and gently pull the cheek out to observe the teeth on that side. Have the client bite down so the upper and lower teeth are together. Compare the alignment of the upper first molar to the lower first molar. Repeat for the other side.

    - *Normal occlusion:* The lower first molar (mandibular) is one-half tooth ahead of the upper first molar (maxillary)
    - *Class I—Neutrocclusion:* The maxilla and mandible are in correct alignment, but individual teeth are misaligned, rotated, or jumbled
    - *Class II—Distocclusion:* The mandible is too far back in comparison to the maxilla (will appear as if jaw is underdeveloped or chin is receding)
    - *Class III—Mesiocclusion:* Mandible is too far forward in relation to the maxilla (midface may appear underdeveloped or jaw may appear overdeveloped)

11. Have the client bite down and observe the dental alignment from the front. Note any irregularities.

    - *Open bite:* While biting down, an open space (vertical space) remains between the upper and lower teeth—may be an anterior open bite or a lateral open bite

    - *Overbite:* While biting down, the upper anterior teeth overlap the bottom teeth excessively (more than one-third of the lower teeth are covered by the upper teeth)

    - *Overjet:* Horizontal projection of the upper incisors in front of the lower incisors ("buck teeth"), commonly associated with a Class II malocclusion

    - *Underbite:* The upper incisors rest behind the lower incisors, commonly associated with a Class III malocclusion

    Implications

    ○ Discoloration or cares may be the result of poor dental hygiene, poor nutrition, medications, or other medical conditions.

    ○ Poorly developed or misshapen teeth may be associated with various medical conditions or syndromes.

    ○ Poorly aligned or missing teeth can also be associated with various craniofacial anomalies or syndromes.

    ○ Severe malocclusion or dental alignment problems may interfere with articulation.

    ○ An openbite or overjet may be associated with a tongue thrust or forward tongue carriage.

12. Observe the soft palate, uvula, faucial arches, tonsils and pharyngeal area. Assess the velopharyngeal mechanism during the following tasks:

    - Have the client sustain "ah" for as long as possible. You should observe symmetric elevation of the uvula and medial movement of the faucial arches upon phonation.

    - Have the client say "ah-ah-ah" forcefully. You should see the uvula move up and down, symmetrically with phonation.

    - Have the client sustain /u/ while you alternately occlude and open the nostrils (pinch and release the nose gently). This is called the *alternate nose holding technique.* The quality of voice should not change as you occlude and releases the nose. Any change in quality is an indication of hypernasality. A protocol for a more detailed evaluation of velopharyngeal function is presented in the voice protocols, Chapter 18.

    Implications

    ○ Asymmetry of the faucial arches or deviation of the uvula to one side may indicate neurologic involvement. The arches will tend to "droop" on the weak side, and the uvula will deviate to the strong side upon elevation.

- ○ A change of vocal quality (hypernasality) during the alternate nose holding technique (described previously) may indicate VPI. Administer the *Resonance and Velopharyngeal Function Assessment Protocol* found in Chapter 18.
- ○ A weak or absent *gag reflex* may be associated with velopharyngeal weakness or neurologic impairment. For some children and adults, however, lack of a gag reflex is normal.
- ○ A hyperactive gag reflex may be associated with hypersensitivity requiring the clinician to try desensitizing the individual, or may prohibit use of a tongue blade in the mouth.

Note: Reproduced with adaptation from Hegde, M. N., & Pomaville, F. (2008). *Assessment of communication disorders in children: Resources and Protocols.* San Diego, CA: Plural Publishing. Reproduced with permission.

Orofacial Examination and Hearing Screening Protocol

Client's Name: _____ DOB: _____

Examiner: _____ Date of Exam: _____

☐ Facial Symmetry at Rest
Comments:

☐ Breathing
Comments:

> **SCORING KEY**
> + within normal limits
> − deviation noted
> **W** weakness noted
> **NR** No Response

Lips
Describe Lip Deviations or Indications of Weakness:

☐ Appearance at Rest
☐ Round Lips (pucker)
☐ Draw Corners Back (smile)
☐ Close Lips and Puff Cheeks
☐ Bite Lower Lip

Tongue
Describe Tongue Deviations or Indications of Weakness:

☐ Surface Appearance at Rest   Describe:
☐ Lingual Frenum
☐ Stick Out as Far as You Can   ☐ Push Against Tongue Blade to Assess Strength
☐ Tip Up   ☐ Tip Down
☐ Tip Right   ☐ Tip Left   ☐ Alternate Left to Right
☐ Push Against Inside of Each Cheek or Tongue Blade on Each Side to Assess Strength
☐ Place Tip on Alveolar Ridge   ☐ Draw Tip Back along Hard Palate

Dentition and Occlusion
☐ General Condition of Teeth   ☐ Describe:
☐ **Occlusion** Based on Lateral View of First Molars (Check below, as appropriate)
   ☐ Normal occlusion: mandibular first molar is one-half tooth ahead of maxillary first molar
   ☐ Class I, Neutrocclusion (maxilla and mandible are in correct occlusion, but individual teeth are misaligned, rotated or jumbled)
   ☐ Class II, Distocclusion (mandible is too far back in relation to maxilla)
   ☐ Class III, Mesiocclusion (mandible is too far forward in relation to maxilla)

☐ Alignment (Check below, as appropriate)
    ☐ Open bite   ☐ Overbite   ☐ Overjet   ☐ Underbite

Hard Palate

☐ General Appearance   ☐ Vault Height   ☐ Vault Width

Comments:

Soft Palate and Pharynx

☐ Appearance and Symmetry of Soft Palate at Rest
☐ Appearance of the Uvula   ☐ Bifid Uvula
☐ Appearance of Faucial Arches at Rest   ☐ Palatine Tonsils

Describe any deviations of the soft palate or faucial arches, at rest:

Velopharyngeal Mechanism

Assess the velopharyngeal mechanism during the tasks described below:

Have the client sustain "ah" for as long as possible.
Have the client say "ah – ah – ah."

☐ Vertical movement of the velum (up and back)   ☐ Symmetry of movement
☐ Medial movement of the lateral pharyngeal walls   ☐ Symmetry of movement

Have the client sustain /u/ while you alternate occluding and opening the nostrils.

Was there a change in vocal quality?   ☐ YES ☐ NO
Was hypernasality present?   ☐ YES ☐ NO

Comments:

(continues)

Orofacial Examination and Hearing Screening Protocol (continued)

Hearing Screening

	500 Hz	1000 Hz	2000 Hz	4000 Hz
Right Ear	_____	_____	_____	_____
Left Ear	_____	_____	_____	_____

Completed at _____ dB (loudness level)

☐ Passed.   ☐ Failed the hearing screening—audiologic evaluation recommended.

☐ Hearing Screening not completed. Why?

Comments on the Hearing Screening:

_____

Note: Reproduced with adaptation from Hegde, M. N., & Pomaville, F. (2008). *Assessment of communication disorders in children: Resources and Protocols.* San Diego, CA: Plural Publishing. Reproduced with permission.

Diadochokinetic Assessment Protocol for Adults

Patient Instructions: "Take a deep breath and say "puh, puh, puh" as quickly and evenly as you can." Demonstrate for the patient. Repeat the instructions for /tʌ/ and /kʌ/. Grade the patient's productions on the follow parameters:

	Yes	No	Severity
Is the production unrhythmic?	_____	_____	_____
Is the production excessively fast?	_____	_____	_____
Is the production excessively slow?	_____	_____	_____
Are consonant productions imprecise?	_____	_____	_____
Are there pitch changes?	_____	_____	_____
Is there a blurring of the syllables?	_____	_____	_____
Is there equal spacing between syllables?	_____	_____	_____
Is tremor evident?	_____	_____	_____
Is hypernasality present?	_____	_____	_____
Is nasal emission audible?	_____	_____	_____
Do the lips or jaw show reduced range of motion?	_____	_____	_____
Does loudness vary significantly?	_____	_____	_____

Severity ratings: 1 = no impairment, 2 = mild, 3 = moderate, 4 = severe.

Count the number of syllables produced during a 5-second interval:

	/pʌ/	/tʌ/	/kʌ/	/pʌtʌkʌ/
Trial 1				
Trial 2				
Trial 3				
Average				

Norm: Approximately 30 repetitions for a 5-second interval is average for adults; however, /kʌ/ can be slightly slower.

(continues)

Diadochokinetic Assessment Protocol for Adults (continued)

Sequential Motion Rate

Patient Instructions: "This time I want you to make those three sounds, 'puh,' 'tuh,' and 'kuh,' all together." Demonstrate for the patient. Record the number of productions in a 5-second trial above.

	Yes	No	Severity
a. Do the articulators move smoothly from syllable to syllable?	_____	_____	_____
b. Are substitutions, omissions, or transpositions evident?	_____	_____	_____

Describe error productions: _____

_____

Functional Communication Assessment Protocol

Name: _____ Age: _____ DOB: _____ Diagnosis _____

Clinician: _____ Date: _____ Respondent(s) _____

The clinician may have a caretaker fill out this form, or fill it out herself during assessment in consultation with the client and the caretakers.

	Observed since the illness				
	Always	Usually	Rarely	Never	N/A

Making Requests and demands:
  "May I have . . . "
  "I want . . . "
  "Give me . . . "
  "I like . . . "
  "I don't want . . . "
  "Don't do . . . "
  "Can you help me . . . "
  "Can you tell me . . . "
  "What is that . . . "
  "I don't understand . . . "
  "I don't like . . . "
  "What are you doing?"
  "Is dinner ready?"
  Just names the items (e.g., "water")
  Points to what is needed
  Gestures (e.g., *eating* or *drinking*)
  Says "yes" or "no" when communication choices are offered
  Nods or shakes head when communication choices are offered					

Describing bodily states
  Describes in a sentence (e.g., "I have a headache;" "I am hungry;" "I am angry")
  Describes in a word (e.g., "Headache," "Hungry," "Angry")
  Points to the body part or gestures					

(continues)

Functional Communication Assessment Protocol (continued)

	Observed since the illness				
	Always	Usually	Rarely	Never	N/A
Describing objects or events					
Describes in sentences					
Describes in phrases					
Utters a single word					
Points to objects and events					
Engaging in conversation					
Participates like before the illness					
Limited to a few short sentences					
Limited to a few phrases and words					
Answers questions with sentences					
Answers in phrases					
Limited to "yes" "no" responses					
Usually remains silent					
Usually leaves the room					
Naming persons					
Names colleagues					
Names the family members					
Names only a few persons					
Names none, but points to					
Neither names nor points to					
Naming household objects					
Names most familiar objects					
Names only a few objects					
Names none but points to					
Talking on the telephone					
Almost like before the illness					
Only to family members					
Only to old friends					
Only to doctors' offices					
Watching TV					
Watches and understands the shows					
Shows some frustration					
Does not understand the shows					
Stopped watching since the illness					

	Observed since the illness				
	Always	Usually	Rarely	Never	N/A
Telling or Reciting					
The time of the day					
The days of the week					
The months of the year					
Numbers up to _____					
Songs sung before					
Only hums					
Reading					
Books					
Magazines/newspapers					
Familiar signs (e.g., traffic)					
Recipes and follows them					
Directions and follows them					
Financial statements					
Writing					
Thank you notes					
Brief letters					
Grocery lists					
Messages for others					
Notes to self (e.g., *to do* lists)					
Checks					
Telephone numbers down					
Other (specify) _____					
_____					

Communication Quality of Life Assessment Protocol

Name: _____ Age: _____ DOB: _____

Clinician: _____ Date: _____ Respondent(s) _____

Give the following instructions:

"I would like to know how your communication difficulty has affected your life. I want you to tell me the level of your satisfaction with various aspects or activities of your life. For each item, I will ask, are you satisfied, somewhat satisfied, somewhat dissatisfied, or dissatisfied with your current health status. I will ask similar questions about other aspects of life."

A simple way to administer most of the listed items is to start with the item itself. For example:

- "Moving around in the house. Are you satisfied, somewhat satisfied, somewhat dissatisfied, or dissatisfied?"
- "Food preparation. Are you . . . ?"
- "Balancing the checkbook. Are you . . . ?"

	Satisfied	Somewhat satisfied	Somewhat dissatisfied	Dissatisfied	N/A
Basic communication Conversational skills					

General Health
    Your health status
    Moving around in the house
    Taking a walk
    Physical strength and stamina
    Rest and sleep					

Daily Activities
    Personal care
    Food preparation
    Washing and cleaning
    Keeping appointments
    Grocery shopping
    Personal shopping
    Telling time
    Using a calendar					

	Satisfied	Somewhat satisfied	Somewhat dissatisfied	Dissatisfied	N/A
Following map directions					
Taking care of pets					
Gardening					
Driving experience					
Recreational activities					
Others: _____					
_____					
_____					
Social Interactions					
Spending time with family					
Doing activities with family					
Spending time with friends					
Doing activities with friends					
Finances and daily math					
Reading financial statements					
Balancing the checkbook					
Using ATM machines					
Transacting at the bank					
Paying correct amount of cash					
Counting the change received					
Using the credit card					
Paying bills					
Writing checks					
Hobbies					
How you are maintaining your hobbies					
Specify: _____					
_____					
How you are performing some hobbies					
Specify: _____					
_____					
For having abandoned some hobbies					
Specify: _____					
_____					

(continues)

Communication Quality of Life Assessment Protocol (continued)

	Satisfied	Somewhat satisfied	Somewhat dissatisfied	Dissatisfied	N/A
Specialized Skills					
How you use computers					
How you use power tools					
How you use nonpower tools					
Other skills (specify)					
_____					
_____					
Occupational Outlook					
With the return to your previous position					
With your plan to return to your job					
With your inability to return to your job					
Behavioral Health					
Regarding your general mood					
With the level of your cheerfulness					
With your need for companionship					
Your optimistic outlook on life					
Your interest in daily activities					
Overall quality of life					

Adult Assessment Report Outline

Identifying Information

Client: Date of Birth:

Address: Diagnosis:

City/State/ZIP: Referred By:

Phone Number: Clinician:

Date of Report:

Background and Presenting Complaint

This information will be extracted from the Case History Form and the Interview.

Include in the first paragraph:

- The name, age, and gender of the client
- The place where the evaluation was completed
- The date of the evaluation
- Who accompanied the child and who served as the primary informant for the assessment
- The caregiver's presenting complaint or primary concern
- Information on any prior speech-language services

History

Onset and Development of the Disorder

This information will be extracted from the Case History Form and the Interview.

- Describe the time and conditions of the onset of the disorder for which help is being sought.
- Describe how the disorder has changed over time.
- Describe the client's reaction to his or her communication problem.
- Describe previous professional evaluation and treatment and the effects of previous clinical services.
- Describe services received from other professionals.
- Describe the effect of the disorder on the client's social, academic, and personal life.
- Take note of any associated clinical conditions.

(continues)

Adult Assessment Report Outline (continued)

Medical History

This information will be extracted from the Case History Form and the Interview.

This section may be more or less detailed, depending on the presence or absence of medical complications.

- Describe the client's illnesses, allergies, sensory deficits (e.g., hearing loss or visual problems), neuromotor problems (e.g., paralysis or paresis), and intellectual disabilities.
- Describe medical or surgical treatments the client may have received and the consequences of such treatments.
- Describe the client's current health.

Family, Social, and Occupational History

This information will be extracted from the Case History Form and the Interview.

This section should be as detailed as possible to understand the family constellation that influences treatment outcome.

- Describe the members of the family with whom the client lives.
- Take note of the spouse's education and occupation.
- Describe the language or languages spoken by the client and other family members; pay special attention to the client's bilingual status; ascertain the client's proficiency in the primary and secondary language.
- Describe the client's social and occupational environment and any effects the communication problem may have on it.

Observations and Assessment Results

Hearing Screening

Results will have been recorded on the Orofacial Examination and Hearing Screening Protocol included in Chapter 2.

- State whether the client passed or failed the hearing screening test.
- If the client failed the hearing screening test, note the need for a complete audiologic evaluation.

Orofacial Examination and Diadochokinetic Tasks

Results will have been recorded on the Orofacial Examination and Hearing Screening Protocol included in Chapter 2.

- Summarize your findings of the orofacial examination.

- State whether the orofacial structures are adequate for speech production.

- Summarize any deviations that might affect speech production.

- Suggest needed additional referrals (e.g., a neurologist, an otolaryngologist, an audiologist).

Speech Production

Results will have been recorded on protocols included in Chapter 4 (apraxia of speech) and Chapter 6 (dysarthria).

Note that this section will be detailed if the client has been assessed for motor speech disorders; if the client has been assessed for a fluency, voice, or a language disorder (e.g., aphasia), general comments about the his or her speech skills may be made in the report.

- Summarize the results of any standardized tests
  - include an inventory of phoneme errors
  - report any standardized scores
- Summarize the results of your speech sample analysis
  - list the phoneme errors
  - compare the results of standardized test results and speech sample analysis
  - state the percent intelligibility of speech
  - discuss factors contributing to intelligibility
  - comment on prosody, voice, and fluency as observed during spontaneous speech
- Write a summative statement about the existing and missing speech production skills that integrates observations based on standardized tests, language sample, and alternative procedures used.

Language

Results will have been recorded on protocols included in Chapter 8 (aphasia).

Note that this section will be detailed if the client has been assessed for a language disorder; if not, general comments about the client's language skills may be made in the report.

- Summarize results of standardized language tests
  - comment on the client's overall language skills
  - describe the language problems as revealed by the tests
  - comment on the unique language difficulties the tests help assess (e.g., agrammatic speech; naming problems; fluent but meaningless speech; confused, distracted, or irrelevant responses; difficulties with abstract language; and so forth)

(continues)

Adult Assessment Report Outline (continued)

- ○ describe the pragmatic or conversational skills observed and those that are judged inappropriate or missing
- Summarize the results of your language sample analysis
  - ○ describe the observed semantic, morphologic, syntactic, and pragmatic language skills the client produced during the language sampling
  - ○ compare the results of language sample analysis with those of standardized tests
  - ○ comment on the client's language comprehension as noted throughout the assessment session
- Write a summative statement about the existing and missing language skills that integrates observations based on standardized tests, language sample, and any other procedures used.

Fluency

Results will have been recorded on protocols included in Chapter 16.

Note that this section will be detailed if the client has been assessed for a fluency disorder; if not, general comments about fluency may be made in the report.

- Summarize the results of the speech sample analysis; state the percent dysfluency rate.
- Describe the types of dysfluencies the client produced during assessment.
- Describe the speech situations, specific conversational partners, and words the client typically avoids.
- Describe the client's negative emotional reactions as assessed through interviews or standardized assessment batteries.
- Describe in general terms the motor behaviors (e.g., eye blinks, hand and feet movements, facial grimaces) that are associated with dysfluencies.

Voice

Results will have been recorded on protocols included in Chapter 18.

Note that this section will be detailed if the client has been assessed for a voice disorder; if not, general comments about the client's voice may be made in the report.

- Summarize the results of clinical observations and results of specific assessment tasks presented to the client.
- Summarize the results of instrumental assessment of vocal parameters.
- Describe the voice disorders that have been observed and measured during assessment.

- Describe the resonance disorders that have been observed and measured during assessment.

- Comment on potential and suspected laryngeal pathologies associated with the noted voice problems.

- Describe the vocally abusive behaviors, if relevant.

- Summarize the laryngologist's report, if one is available.

Associated Clinical Conditions

Information on any associated clinical conditions will be extracted from the case history, interview, and any report received from other professionals (e.g., psychologists, psychiatrists, physicians, and audiologists).

Note that this section may be omitted if associated clinical conditions are absent.

- Describe any associated clinical conditions and the observed behavioral characteristics, including:
  - hearing loss
  - intellectual disabilities
  - neurological disorders
  - laryngeal pathologies
  - psychiatric or behavioral problems, including depression, hallucination, and obsessive compulsive behaviors
  - any other clinical condition noted or reported
- Summarize the reports of relevant specialists, if available.

Diagnostic Summary and Prognosis

Write a section on diagnostic summary and prognosis in which you:

- Summarize your major findings.
- State your diagnosis, if appropriate.
- Estimate a level of severity.
- Discuss strengths and weaknesses of the client.
- Give a prognostic statement based on your observation, judged motivation, family support, general health of the client, and response to any previous treatment:
  - prognosis with treatment, if recommended
  - prognosis without treatment
  - conditions under which a good prognosis may be obtained (more or less intensive treatment, follow-up by caregivers, completion of assigned work at home)

(continues)

Adult Assessment Report Outline (continued)

Recommendations

Cover the following in making your recommendations:

- State whether you recommend speech, language, voice, or fluency therapy.
- Estimate the frequency and duration of treatment.
- Make needed referrals to other professionals, including a medical specialist, an audiologist, or other specialists.
- Discuss areas where additional data need to be collected (i.e., additional assessment, a home speech sample, or diagnostic therapy).
- Describe recommended treatment goals.

Reference

Hegde, M. N., & Pomaville, F. (2008). *Assessment of communication disorders in children.* San Diego, CA: Plural.

PART II

Assessment of Motor Speech Disorders in Adults

CHAPTER 3

Assessment of Apraxia of Speech (AOS): Resources

- Description of AOS
- Epidemiology and Etiology of AOS
- Overview of Assessment of AOS
- Screening for AOS
- Standardized Tests for AOS
- Analysis and Integration of Assessment Results
- Diagnostic Criteria and Differential Diagnosis
- Postassessment Counseling

Description of AOS

AOS is a motor speech disorder characterized by deficits in the planning and programming of speech movements. Although the movement disorder known as *apraxia* has been studied for more than 100 years (Liepmann, 1900), the term *apraxia of speech* was not introduced until the late 1960s. In his presentation to the American Speech and Hearing Association Annual Convention in 1969, Darley introduced many of the traditional characteristics of AOS when he described this disorder as, "an articulatory disorder resulting from impairment, as a result of brain damage, of the capacity to program the positioning of speech musculature and the sequencing of muscle movements for the volitional production of phonemes. No significant weakness, slowness, or incoordination in reflex and automatic acts. Prosodic alterations may be associated with the articulatory problem, perhaps in compensation for it." The key points of Darley's definition are that (a) AOS affects articulation, (b) AOS is a problem of positioning and sequencing the articulators, (c) AOS is not caused by weakness or related neuromuscular deficits, and (d) AOS affects prosody.

These characteristics have been expanded and refined by many researchers since Darley first presented them, perhaps most notably by Wertz, LaPointe, and Rosenbek (1984), who suggested that AOS was " . . . a neurogenic phonologic disorder resulting from sensorimotor impairment of the capacity to select, program, and/or execute in coordinated and normally timed sequences, the positioning of the speech musculature for the volitional production of speech sounds" (p. 4). This definition highlights several additional characteristics of AOS, such as (a) its effect on volitional speech (as opposed to automatic utterances), (b) its impairment of selecting and executing movement sequences, and (c) its basis as a phonologic disorder.

These two definitions hint at the difficulty researchers have experienced over the years in describing the characteristics of AOS. The large number of published AOS definitions since Darley's time clearly show the difficulty researchers have had in describing this disorder. Even today there is no universal agreement on the errors that are associated with AOS. For example, inconsistent articulation errors have been a hallmark of AOS for many years, but studies over the past decade have suggested that the articulation errors in this disorder actually are fairly consistent for location and type during repeated trials (McNeil, Doyle, & Wambaugh, 2000). Not all researchers fully embrace these new views (Strand, 2010), but it is striking to note that after so much investigation, we still are struggling with the basic characteristics of this complex disorder. These reconsiderations and discussions can be frustrating for clinicians seeking the best diagnostic and treatment procedures for their clients with AOS, but they are an inevitable and valuable part of the research process.

The importance of accurately defining a complex disorder like AOS should not be minimized. By determining the "defining characteristics" of AOS, researchers assist clinicians in distinguishing it from related disorders like dysarthria and aphasia. When clinicians know which characteristics are needed for the diagnosis (and those that are not), they are better able to make accurate determinations of whether or not AOS is present in a client's speech. Recognizing this need to form a comprehensive description of AOS, McNeil, Robin, and Schmidt (2009) offered the following detailed definition of this disorder:

Apraxia of Speech is a phonetic-motoric disorder of speech production. It is caused by inefficiencies in the translation of well-formed and filled phonologic frames into previously learned kinematic information used for carrying out intended movements. These inefficiencies result in intra- and interarticulator temporal and spatial segmental and prosodic distortions. It is characterized by distortions of segment and intersegment transitionalization and coarticulation resulting in extended durations of consonants; vowels; and time between sounds, syllables and words. These distortions are often perceived as sound substitutions and as the misassignment of stress and other phrasal and sentence-level prosodic abnormalities. Errors are relatively consistent in location within the utterance and invariable in type. It is not attributable to deficits of muscle tone or reflexes, nor to primary deficits in the processing of sensory (auditory, tactile, kinesthetic, proprioceptive), or language information. In its extremely infrequently occurring isolated form, it is not accompanied by the above listed deficits of basic motor physiology, perception, or language. (p. 264)

The key components of this definition are that AOS is primarily characterized by (a) an overall slowed rate of speech, (b) slow, distorted movements during the productions of phonemes, syllables, and words that listeners often perceive as phoneme substitutions, and (c) prosodic errors. An additional important element is the finding that isolated (pure) AOS is rare and that when a client does have it, there is no co-occurring muscle, sensory, or language disorders. Probably the most controversial aspect of this definition is the previously mentioned assertion that AOS errors are relatively consistent for location and type. Despite any controversy, this definition has been recognized by many AOS researchers. Wambaugh, Duffy, McNeil, Robin, and Rogers (2006 a, b) used it as the foundation of their landmark AOS treatment guidelines papers. They suggested that there is considerable research indicating that this definition of AOS is the most complete and accurate at the present time.

Epidemiology and Etiology of AOS

Definitive data on the epidemiology of AOS is not available. The most detailed information on the prevalence of this disorder was reported by Duffy (2005). Based on 10,444 cases with a diagnosis of an acquired neurologic communication disorder seen at the Mayo Clinic from 1987–1990 and 1993–2001, only 4% of the patients had AOS. This suggests that AOS is not particularly common in comparison to other motor speech disorders. Moreover, when AOS does appear, it nearly always is with a co-occurring disorder. To assess how frequently it occurs with another condition, McNeil, Doyle, and Wambaugh (2000) reviewed the published literature for reports of comorbidity. By averaging the results across studies, they found that AOS and dysarthria appeared together in 31% of the reported cases; AOS and aphasia co-occurred in 81% of the cases; AOS and nonverbal oral apraxia in 68%; AOS and limb apraxia in 67%; and AOS, limb apraxia, and nonverbal oral apraxia in 83%.

Duffy (2005) reported similar co-occurrence data: AOS and dysarthria were found together in 29% of 155 reviewed cases at the Mayo Clinic; AOS and aphasia were found together in 72% of 155 reviewed cases; AOS and nonverbal apraxia of speech were in 63% of 107 reviewed cases. Isolated AOS occurred in 8.3% of 155 reviewed cases. Duffy cautioned that the percentages for dysarthria and aphasia comorbidity probably are low because the reported cases did not include those where dysarthria or aphasia was the primary communicative disorder. Conversely, Duffy suggested that the percentages for isolated AOS probably were high because the reviewed cases only included those where AOS was the primary disorder. Duffy's finding that isolated AOS is rare has been confirmed by other studies (Dronkers, 1996; Square-Storer, Roy, & Hogg, 1990).

There is limited information on AOS etiology and site of lesion. The most detailed information on etiology comes from Duffy (2005). In a review of 155 quasirandomly selected cases at the Mayo Clinic, he reported the following causes of AOS:

- Single left hemisphere stroke—41%
- Multiple stroke that included the left hemisphere—8%
- Unspecific degenerative disease of the CNS—10%
- Primary progressive aphasia or apraxia, or both—7%
- Alzheimer's disease or dementia—3%
- Other degenerative diseases—7%
- Surgical trauma—14%
- Closed head injury—1%
- Tumor in the left hemisphere—4%
- Other—6%

These findings indicate that stroke is by far the most common cause of AOS, accounting for 49% of the total cases. Site of lesion data are less clear. Researchers tend to agree that AOS can occur when the language dominant hemisphere is damaged, but there are contradictory findings on which specific region is responsible for motor speech programming. Studies have suggested that AOS is the result of damage to the insula (Dronkers, 1996; Donnan, Darby, & Saling, 1997), Broca's area (Hillis, Work, Barker, Jacobs, Breese, & Maurer, 2004), or the facial portion of the post central gyrus (McNeil, Weismer, Adams, & Mulligan, 1990). Other studies have suggested that subcortical lesions can be associated with AOS (Peach & Tonkovich, 2004). A study of patients with progressive aphasia with AOS revealed involvement of the insula, Broca's area, and subcortical structures (Wildgruber, Ackermann, & Grodd, 2001). Overall, this research suggests that the inferior frontal and parietal lobes of the language dominant hemisphere are involved in motor speech programming, but more precise information on localization needs to wait for better imaging techniques and more specific diagnostic criteria.

Overview of Assessment of AOS

Assessment of AOS can be challenging because of the high probability of co-occurring conditions and conflicting definitions of AOS. Before beginning the specifics of an AOS assessment, the clinician needs to understand the client's (a) current and projected health condition, (b) current communication deficits and needs, (c) overall quality of life, (d) strengths and family and social support systems, (e) expectations on returning to the previous or a new employment setting, (f) expectations of treatment and rehabilitation, and (g) cultural and verbal background. Much information on these variables may be obtained from a detailed case history, reports from the medical and rehabilitation professionals, and a carefully conducted interview of the client and the caregivers. Specific assessment procedures, when completed, will help build a profile of the client and the family.

Assessment includes both standard and special procedures specific to AOS. To complete a thorough assessment, the clinician will:

- Have the client or the family fill out a case history form
- Hold an interview with the client and the caregiver
- Administer a hearing screening test
- Complete an orofacial examination and assess diadochokinetic rates
- Possibly administer a standardized test
- Assess speech production
- Assess narrative and conversational skills
- Assess functional communication skills
- Assess communication-related quality of life
- Analyze and integrate the assessment results
- Offer postassessment counseling

The clinician can use the standard case history form given in Chapter 2. During the interview, the clinician may ask specific questions about the onset of stroke or other events that caused the AOS, subsequent medical management, current health status of the client, cultural and verbal background of the client and the family, and so forth. The clinician may use additional protocols given in Chapter 2 to make an orofacial examination, assess the diadochokinetic rates, and screen the client's hearing. The clinician will then proceed to collect diagnostic data from a conversational speech and language sample and nonstandardized assessment procedures. To assess AOS, clinicians usually assess a variety of skills that are either impaired or preserved in clients. These include speech rate, repetition, conversational speech, speech sound production, serial (automatic) speech, and perhaps singing. The degree to which each of these and other skills are assessed will depend on the individual client and the apparent severity of symptoms. Not all skills necessarily need to be assessed in depth in all clients. At the end of the assessment, the clinician will counsel the client and the caregivers about the assessment results, discuss speech-language treatment options, suggest a prognosis, and answer any questions the client and the caregivers may ask.

Screening for AOS

Clinicians working in hospitals and other medical settings may need to screen specific patients for AOS. It is prudent to screen patients before embarking on a time-consuming diagnostic assessment. Clinicians may use their own established procedures or an informal screening test to determine if an individual should be assessed further.

Experienced clinicians may use quick procedures based on their own clinical expertise. Patients recently admitted to hospitals for a cerebrovascular accident or other neurological problems that may be associated with AOS are candidates for a quick bedside screening. The clinician may screen patients by having them perform a few standard tasks. For instance, the clinician may not only engage the patient in conversation for a few minutes, but also ask the client to describe objects or pictures; count numbers, recite the names of months and days of the week; repeat a few words, phrases, and sentences; and answer questions about orientation to time, space, and person. The patient's responses may be sufficient to determine whether more in-depth assessment is necessary.

Standardized Tests for AOS

The only standardized, norm-referenced assessment of AOS is the *Apraxia Battery for Adults-Second Edition* (ABA-2) (Dabul, 2000). It is designed to diagnose AOS in adolescents and adults, as well as measure severity. Compared to the first edition, the ABA-2 includes more difficult items for detecting mild AOS and has updated norm data (49 normal individuals and 40 with apraxia). It also includes suggestions for treatment planning, recognizing atypical profiles, and tracking changes in speech production over time. The administration time is short, only about 20 minutes. The test manual includes psychometric data for reliability, content validity, criterion-related validity, and construct validity. No data are reported for intrajudge reliability, interjudge reliability, or test-retest reliability. The ABA-2 contains six subtests:

- Diadochokinetic Rate—the client is asked to say the syllable combinations "puh-tuh," "tuh-kuh," and "puh-tuh-kuh" for 3 seconds over three trials. The clinician records how many repetitions are produced on each trial, with the highest number recorded as a "Best Trial."

- Increasing Word Length—the client is asked to repeat three words of increasing length (e.g., thick-thicker-thickening). The clinician scores the productions on a scale of 0 to 2.

- Limb Apraxia and Oral Apraxia—the client is asked to perform hand and arm movements (e.g., "Show me how you make a fist.") and nonverbal oral movements (e.g., "Stick out your tongue."). The client's responses are scored on a scale of 0 to 5.

- Latency Time and Utterance Time for Polysyllabic Words—the client is asked to name pictures; the clinician records how long it takes from the initial presentation of the picture to the beginning of the utterance (latency time) and how long it takes to say the target word or words (utterance time).

- Repeated Trials Test—the client is asked to repeat target words three times. The clinician counts the number of errors in each production and then compares the number of errors in the first and third productions, scoring a minus if there are fewer errors in the first attempt compared to the third; scoring a plus if there are more in the first compared to the third; and scoring a zero if there is no difference.

- Inventory of Articulation Characteristics of Apraxia—the clinician obtains and analyzes speech samples from the client (see the following paragraph).

The final subtest of the ABA-2 (Inventory of Articulatory Characteristics of Apraxia) asks the clinician to obtain several speech samples by asking the client to describe a picture, read aloud, and to count to 30. Based on these three samples, the clinician determines the presence or absence of 15 speech behaviors. If 5 or more of them are present in the sample, the client may have a diagnosis of AOS:

1. Exhibits phonemic anticipatory errors
2. Exhibits phonemic perseverative errors
3. Exhibits phonemic transposition errors
4. Exhibits phonemic voicing errors
5. Exhibits phonemic vowel errors
6. Exhibits visible/audible searching
7. Exhibits numerous off-target attempts at the word
8. Errors are highly inconsistent
9. Errors increase as phonemic sequence increases
10. Exhibits fewer errors with automatic speech than volitional speech
11. Exhibits marked difficulty initiating speech
12. Intrudes schwa sound between syllables or in consonant clusters
13. Exhibits abnormal prosodic features
14. Exhibits awareness of errors and inability to correct them
15. Exhibits expressive-receptive gap

Although the behaviors on this list are reflective of the traditional characteristics of AOS, some researchers have questioned whether all the items have the ability to differentiate AOS from those found in other speech and language disorders, such as the literal paraphasias in fluent aphasia. For example, Pierce (1991) reported that only three of these (difficulty initiating speech, intrusion of the schwa, and abnormal prosody) are observed primarily in AOS; most of the others can be seen in clients with either AOS or fluent aphasia. McNeil, Robin, and Schmidt (2009) go even further and suggest that only the intrusion of the schwa and abnormal prosody are exclusively seen in individuals with AOS. All the remaining items are observed exclusively in cases of fluent aphasia (anticipatory, perseverative, and transposition errors; very inconsistent errors) or in either disorder (the remaining nine items). Until these questions are resolved with further research, clinicians using the ABA-2 may want to interpret the results with caution or confirm the test's findings with additional assessment.

Analysis and Integration of Assessment Results

An overall analysis and integration of assessment results is essential for making valid clinical decisions. Assessment of AOS can be more of an "ongoing" process than it is for other communication disorders, such as stuttering. For example, the client's health status might improve or deteriorate, depending on disease complications that are associated with AOS. With such changes, the severity of the AOS will also change for the better or for worse. The assessment of AOS will likely be complicated by the common co-occurrence of aphasia, dysarthria, or both. Sometimes the severity of the client's aphasia can prevent an accurate assessment of the accompanying AOS. To track these changes and situations, the clinician needs to make periodic, even if brief, assessments to ascertain the client's communication skills at different points during treatment and rehabilitation.

The clinician might take the following steps to analyze and integrate the assessment results before writing a diagnostic report:

- **The case history and interview information should be summarized.** The time and the conditions of the onset of AOS and the symptoms that preceded and followed the onset may be summarized as reported by the caregivers and the client. The client's family constellation and the ethnocultural (including verbal) background should be described. History of the client's health, education, occupation, hobbies, literacy skills, and interests should be summarized.

- **Medical assessment and treatment should be summarized.** The medical procedures (e.g., neurological examinations, imaging) done on the client, and specific neurological and medical diagnosis made on the client (e.g., stroke, tumor) should be summarized. The current medical treatment the client is undergoing should be noted. The current physical condition of the client (e.g., stable, deteriorating, improving) should be described. The recommendation of medical specialists for rehabilitation, including speech-language treatment, should be specified.

- **AOS assessment results should be described.** The clinician should analyze all the assessment procedures performed on the client, including the interview, observations, standardized test (if done), and any client-specific or criterion-referenced measures. This analysis will help identify the types of speech errors demonstrated by the client. This is probably the most important part of an AOS assessment. The diagnosis of AOS depends on the accurate identification and classification of speech errors, which are then compared to the known characteristics of AOS. Only by determining how many of the client's speech errors match those that are associated with AOS can the clinician make the diagnosis of this disorder.

- **Recommendations may be specified.** The analysis and integration of assessment data will result in the clinician's recommendations for the client, family members, and other caregivers. Treatment for clients with AOS is known to be effective, and typically is recommended (Ballard & Robin, 2002; Wambaugh, et al., (2006 a, b).

Diagnostic Criteria and Differential Diagnosis

Making an accurate diagnosis of AOS sometimes can be challenging for a number of reasons: the complexity of the disorder, the common co-occurrence of other neurological disorders, and the paucity of standardized AOS tests. Clinicians must use clinical judgment and experience to determine if the speech errors demonstrated by their client match the diagnostic criteria of AOS. Fortunately, as the clinical characteristics of AOS become better understood, making the correct diagnosis is less and less problematic. In their review of practice guidelines for treatment, Wambaugh, Duffy, McNeil, Robin, and Rogers (2006a) provided a useful list of diagnostic criteria for this disorder. They divided their diagnostic descriptors into three categories: (a) those that are observed primarily in AOS and are especially helpful in making a diagnosis (*primary clinical characteristics*), (b) those that occur in AOS but also can be found in other disorders (*nondiscriminative clinical characteristics*), and (c) those that should not be used to diagnose AOS because they are most often found in other disorders. They also listed three speech characteristics that rule out the diagnosis of AOS.

Primary Clinical Characteristics of AOS

These are the clinical characteristics that are *most useful* for diagnosing AOS. As a group, they are observed nearly exclusively in clients with AOS (Wambaugh, Duffy, McNeil, Robin, and Rogers, 2006a):

- Slow speech rate due to lengthened productions of vowels or syllables, or both
- Slow speech rate due to lengthened durations between sounds, syllables, words, and phrases—sometimes filled with a schwa sound
- Sound distortions of consonants and vowels
- Distorted phoneme substitutions
- Fairly consistent errors during repeated attempts at producing a target word, both for type of error (distortion, substitution, omission) and location of error
- Abnormal prosody

Nondiscriminative Clinical Characteristics of AOS

These are the nondiscriminative clinical characteristics that are *suggestive* of AOS. These are likely to be present in AOS, but because they also can be found in other disorders, they alone should not be used to make the diagnosis:

- Groping for articulatory positions; this groping can be visibly or audibly evident, or both.
- Perseverative errors of movement
- Increased errors with increased word length
- Difficulties initiating utterances
- Clients are aware of their errors
- Clients' automatic speech is produced more accurately than their propositional speech
- There are moments of error-free speech

Clinical Characteristics Most Often Associated with Other Disorders

These are the clinical characteristics that *should not be used* to diagnose AOS because they are more characteristic of other disorders than they are of AOS:

- Anticipatory articulation errors
- Transpositions of sounds or syllables
- A differential between expressive-receptive speech and language abilities
- The presence of limb apraxia or nonverbal oral apraxia

Characteristics Contraindicating AOS

Three items were found to be *exclusionary characteristics* for AOS, meaning that their presence in a client's speech rules out the diagnosis of AOS:

- A fast rate of speech
- A normal rate of speech
- Normal prosody

After completing the AOS assessment tasks in Chapter 4, clinicians should analyze their findings to determine how many of their client's speech errors fall into these categories. Here is a rough guideline for making a diagnosis based on these criteria:

- If your client demonstrates all six primary characteristics, there is a **high probability** that AOS is the diagnosis.
- If your client predominately demonstrates nondiscriminative characteristics along with most of the primary characteristics, there is a **moderate probability** that AOS is the diagnosis.
- If your client predominately demonstrates the four "should not use" characteristics, there is a **low probability** that AOS is the diagnosis.
- If your client demonstrates any of the exclusionary characteristics, he or she **does not have AOS.**

Distinguishing AOS From Aphasia

One of the more demanding assessment tasks for many clinicians is distinguishing between the errors in AOS and those in aphasia. Determining whether a client's errors are the result of AOS, fluent aphasia, or nonfluent aphasia sometimes can be particularly difficult for beginning clinicians. Fortunately, one of the easier diagnostic tasks is differentiating pure AOS and aphasia.

Pure AOS and Aphasia—As mentioned by McNeil, Robin, and Schmidt (2009), clinicians may only see one or two individuals with pure AOS in their entire careers, and although this is probably true, clinicians working in large clinics and busy medical centers may come upon it somewhat more often. When they do encounter it, they may be challenged by the diagnostic task because the errors of both conditions can appear to be similar, at least initially. For example, both include sound substitutions and distortions in their list of symptoms. However, careful analysis of a client's speech and language abilities will show one definite difference between pure AOS and aphasia:

- Pure AOS only affects the client's verbal output: Auditory comprehension, reading, and writing abilities are within normal limits. In aphasia, all four language modalities (verbal expression, auditory comprehension, reading, and writing) are affected to one degree or another.

AOS and Literal Paraphasias—Distinguishing between clients with AOS and those with fluent aphasia also can be a challenge because the literal paraphasic errors in fluent aphasia can superficially resemble those in AOS. Literal paraphasias are common in many cases of fluent aphasia. They include such errors as phonemes and syllable substitutions, sound transpositions, and added phonemes. The beginning clinician can be confused by these errors, but a careful examination of clients with AOS and fluent aphasia can reveal differences. Kent (1976) provided several concise suggestions to help clinicians tell the two apart:

- The substitutions in AOS tend to be close to the target phoneme, such as a /p/ substituted for a /b/. Literal paraphasias can produce substitutions that are quite different from the target sound, such as a stop consonant substituting for a fricative or even a vowel for a consonant.

- There often are delays at the beginning of an utterance in AOS while the client attempts to find the correct articulatory position. Such delays in the initiation of utterances are rare in fluent aphasia.

- The slow, halting speech production of AOS results in disturbed prosody. In fluent aphasia, prosody has a flow and rhythm that sounds much more normal.

- AOS commonly co-occurs with Broca's aphasia. Literal paraphasias usually are associated with Wernicke's or conduction aphasia.

- AOS usually occurs after anterior brain damage and can co-occur with right-hemiparesis. Literal paraphasias are most common after posterior brain damage and usually do not co-occur with hemiparesis.

McNeil, Robin, and Schmidt (2009) suggested additional characteristics that can help clinicians tell the difference between AOS and literal paraphasias:

- Clients with AOS demonstrate a slow rate of speech on phrases and sentences, even in utterances that are free of errors. Clients with literal paraphasias often demonstrate a nearly normal rate of speech in error-free utterances.

- Clients with AOS cannot increase their rate of speech and maintain accurate phoneme production. Clients with literal paraphasias sometimes can increase their rate of speech and maintain accurate phoneme production.

- Clients with AOS often demonstrate prolonged phoneme-to-phoneme movement transitions, prolonged intervals between words (even on phonemically correct utterances), and prolonged vowels in multisyllabic words or in sentences. Clients with literal paraphasias tend to demonstrate much more normal time intervals on these three features.

- In clients with AOS, self-initiated attempts to repair errors do not result in more accurate productions. In clients with literal paraphasias, such attempts tend to result in more accurate productions.

- Clients with AOS demonstrate phoneme distortions. Those with literal paraphasias do not.

Distinguishing AOS From Dysarthria

Another challenging differential diagnosis is between AOS and dysarthria. However, as with distinguishing between AOS and aphasia, the task is not too difficult when the characteristics of both conditions are examined carefully:

- Automatic and reactive (emotional) speech is often produced normally in AOS. For example, most clients with AOS can verbally count 1–10 with a majority of the words being said correctly. In dysarthria, speech errors tend to be fairly consistent during these overlearned types of verbal tasks.

- The strength, coordination, muscle tone, and range of motion of speech muscles are normal in AOS. In dysarthria, one or more of these motor elements probably will be impaired.

- AOS usually is associated with left-hemisphere, lower-frontal, or parietal lobe damage. Depending on the type, dysarthria can be associated with damage to many parts of the central and peripheral nervous system, including upper and lower motor neurons and the cerebellum.

- In AOS, speech errors tend to increase with increasing word length and complexity. In dysarthria, speech errors tend to be constant across both short and long words.

- Effortful groping for articulatory positions can be evident in AOS, especially on initial phonemes. Such groping is less common in dysarthria.

- AOS is primarily a disorder of articulation and prosody. Dysarthria often involves disorders of respiration, phonation, and resonation, in addition to problems with articulation and prosody.

- AOS occurs much more frequently with aphasia than dysarthria does.

Postassessment Counseling

Conclude the AOS assessment with postassessment counseling of the client and family. During this session, the clinician shares the assessment information with the client, accompanying family members, and other caregivers. Subsequent to the postassessment counseling, the clinician makes an analysis of information obtained from the case history and interview, reports from other specialists, clinical assessment results, instrumental evaluations, and results of questionnaires or other tests. Integrating the information collected from all sources and means, the clinician writes a diagnostic report. See Chapter 1 for details on the analysis and integration of assessment data and clinical report writing.

During the postassessment counseling session, the clinician makes a diagnosis, offers recommendations, and suggests a prognosis. The clinician also answers questions from the client and the family members about the disorder and the planned clinical services.

Make a Tentative Diagnosis

Although a final analysis of assessment results may not be completed yet, the clinician nonetheless will have come to tentative but generally valid clinical conclusions at the end of the assessment session. The clinician can make statements about the nature of the speech disorder, its prognosis, and treatment options. The clinician might describe the client's speech characteristics (e.g., substituting phonemes, difficulty finding the correct articulatory positions) that justify the diagnosis. The clinician also might point out disorders that are *not* indicated by the assessment. For example, a client may worry that changes in speech are early signs of a degenerative condition such as Parkinson's disease. If the medical reports and motor speech evaluation rule out this type of disorder, the clinician should share this important information with the client.

Make Recommendations

The clinician may recommend treatment for the AOS, depending on the type and severity of the disorder. Whether the client has had a medical evaluation for the speech problem or the SLP is the first professional to be consulted will determine the immediate course of action, however. A client with possible neurological involvement should be referred first to a neurologist if this has not already been done.

Suggest a Prognosis

It usually is difficult to make a firm prognosis for improved speech production in clients with AOS because of the numerous variables that are involved. A few of these variables include the severity of the AOS and the motivation of the client. Co-occurring conditions such as aphasia or dysarthria also make it difficult to offer an accurate prognosis. In general, individuals with a mild or moderate AOS can expect to show some improved speech production with treatment. The extent of the improvement will not be known during the postassessment counseling session, so it often is wise to avoid specific predictions when discussing the prognosis with the client and family. Some individuals with severe AOS also can show improved speech production with treatment, but the gains typically take longer and are less pronounced than for individuals with milder AOS. Other individuals with severe AOS (or those with AOS due to a degenerative disease) will not show improved speech production, and the treatment options for them might involve alternative and augmentative communication procedures.

Answer the Client's Questions

The client and family members will have questions about AOS and its treatment during the postassessment counseling session. They deserve honest and scientifically justified answers. Some commonly encountered questions and their answers are described here, but the clinician should be ready for other questions. Clients with complicated medical conditions will have additional questions specific to those conditions. The clinician also needs to modify the terms to suit the educational level of the client and the accompanying family members.

What causes AOS? AOS can be caused by any condition that damages a part of the brain called the *motor speech programmer*. In most individuals, this damage is caused by a stroke, but physical trauma, degenerative diseases, infections, and a number of other conditions also have been linked to AOS. [*The clinician provides an explanation of AOS, give examples.*] For example, a head wound that primarily affects the anterior, left side of the brain can damage the motor speech programmer. In a few individuals, AOS can be the result of a degenerative disease that causes the loss of neurons in the motor speech programmer. Treatment in such cases is initially medical, followed by speech therapy after the condition is stabilized. [*The clinician addresses the client's specific cause of AOS and gives more details.*]

How long does it take to treat AOS effectively? It depends on the severity of the AOS and if there are co-occurring conditions like aphasia and dysarthria. In some individuals with severe AOS, there really is little that can be done to improve the client's speech, and the use of alternative communication systems is recommended. Sometimes individuals need significant amounts of medical attention before or during speech therapy; this tends to extend the treatment time. Usually, the progress will be faster if we start the treatment soon, and if we are consistent rather than if we delayed it or have frequent interruptions. We offer treatment twice a week. [*If not, the clinician gives the actual schedule.*] If you work at home on our assignments and family members offer support, the progress might be even better. As you can guess, severe problems and problems with additional medical complications take more time to treat. [*The clinician expands the answer to give additional information relevant to the client's AOS.*]

What are some of the treatment options? There are several treatment options for AOS. The type of recommended treatment depends on the severity of the AOS and which type of treatment best addresses an individual's problem. A number of treatment procedures use a verbal and visual model from the clinician to get the client to say a word correctly, and the client then repeats the word many times. Another type of AOS treatment concentrates on the melody and rhythm of saying words during the beginning sessions and then fades the melody as the client becomes more independent in saying the words. A third type of AOS treatment uses a "hands on" approach, where the clinician uses his or her hands to help move a client's articulators into the correct positions to say various syllables, words, and phrases. Clients respond differently to these techniques, with one procedure often working better for a given individual than the others. Overall, the clinician and client work together to minimize the effects of AOS on speaking and to enhance the client's ability to produce the most natural sounding speech possible. [*The clinician expands the answer to give more treatment information relevant to the client's AOS.*]

When do we start treatment? It usually is better to start treatment as soon as possible. The sooner we start, the better might be the outcome. [*The clinician gives additional information, depending on whether the client needs to be referred to other specialists before starting treatment; also, depending on the service setting, the clinician tells when and how the treatment might begin.*]

References

Ballard, K. J., & Robin, D. A. (2002). Assessment of AOS for treatment planning. *Seminars in speech and language: Apraxia of speech: From concept to clinic, 4,* 23, 281–291.

Dabul, B. (2000). *Apraxia battery for adults* (2nd ed.). Austin, TX: Pro-Ed.

Darley, F. L. (1969, November). *Aphasia: Input and output disturbances in speech and language processing.* Paper presented to the annual meeting of the American Speech-Language-Hearing Association, Chicago, IL.

Donnan, G. A., Darby, D. G., & Saling, M. M. (1997). Identification of brain region for coordinating speech articulation. *The Lancet,* 221–222.

Dronkers, N. F. (1996). A new brain region for coordinating speech articulation. *Nature, 384,* 159–161.

Duffy, J. R. (2005). *Motor speech disorders: Substrates, differential diagnosis, and management* (2nd ed.). St. Louis, MO: Elsevier Mosby.

Hillis, A. E., Work, M., Barker, P. B., Jacobs, M. A., Breese, E. L., & Maurer, K. (2004). Reexamining the brain regions crucial for orchestrating speech articulation. *Brain, 127,* 1479–1487.

Kent, R. (1976). *Study of vocal tract characteristics in the dysarthrias.* Presented to the Veterans Administration Workshop on Motor Speech Disorders, Madison, WI.

Liepmann, H. (1900). Das Krankheitsbild der apraxia (motorischen asymboli) auf Grund eines Fallesvon einseitiger apraxie. *Monatschrift fur Psychiatrie and Neurologie, 9,* 15–40.

McNeil, M. R., Doyle, P. J., & Wambaugh, J. (2000). Apraxia of speech: A treatable disorder of motor planning & programming. In S. E. Nadeau, L. J. Gonzales Rothi, & B. Crosson (Eds.), *Aphasia and language: Theory to practice* (pp. 221–266). New York, NY: Guilford.

McNeil, M. R., Robin, D. A., & Schmidt, R. A. (2009). Apraxia of speech: Theory and differential diagnosis. In: McNeil M. R. *Clinical Management of Sensorimotor Speech Disorders* (2nd ed.). New York, NY: Thieme Medical.

McNeil, M. R., Weismer, G., Adams, S., & Mulligan, M. (1990). Oral structure nonspeech motor control in normal, dysarthric, aphasic, and apraxic speakers: Isometric force and static position control. *Journal of Speech and Hearing Research, 33,* 355–368.

Peach, R., & Tonkovich, J. (2004). Phonemic characteristics of apraxia of speech resulting from subcortical hemorrhage. *Journal of Communication Disorders, 37*(1), 77–90.

Pierce, R. S. (1991). Apraxia of speech versus phonemic paraphasia: Theoretical, diagnostic, and treatment considerations. In D. Vogel & M. P. Cannito (Eds.), *Treating disorders speech motor control: For clinicians by clinicians* (pp. 185–216). Austin, TX: Pro-Ed.

Square-Storer, P. A., Roy, E. A., & Hogg, S. C. (1990). The dissociation of aphasia from apraxia of speech, ideomotor limb, and buccofacial apraxia. In G. E. Hammond (Ed.), *Cerebral control of speech and limb movements* (pp. 451–476), Amsterdam, North Holland: Elsevier Science.

Strand, E. A. (2010, November). *Differential diagnosis of acute and progressive apraxia of speech in adults.* Paper presented to the annual meeting of the Academy of Neurologic Communication Disorders and Sciences, Philadelphia, PA.

Wambaugh, J., Duffy, J., McNeil, M., Robin, D., & Rogers, M. (2006a). Treatment guidelines for acquired apraxia of speech: A synthesis and evaluation of the evidence. *Journal of Medical Speech-Language Pathology, 14*(2), xv–xxxiii.

Wambaugh, J., Duffy, J., McNeil, M., Robin, D., & Rogers, M. (2006b). Treatment guidelines for acquired apraxia of speech: Treatment descriptions and recommendations. *Journal of Medical Speech-Language Pathology, 14*(2), xxxv–lxvii.

Wertz, R. T., LaPointe, L. L., & Rosenbek, J. C. (1984). *Apraxia of speech in adults: The disorders and its management.* Orlando, FL: Grune and Stratton.

Wildgruber, D., Ackermann, H., & Grodd, W. (2001). Differential contributions of motor cortex, basal ganglia, and cerebellum to speech motor control: Effects of syllable repetition rate evaluated by fMRI. *NeuroImage, 13*, 101–109.

CHAPTER 4

Assessment of Apraxia of Speech (AOS): Protocols

- Overview of AOS Protocols
- Assessment of AOS: Interview Protocol
- AOS Assessment Protocol 1: Oral Apraxia
- AOS Assessment Protocol 2: Speech Production in AOS
- AOS Assessment Protocol 3: Comparing Alternate Motion Rates (AMRs) and Sequential Motion Rates (SMRs)
- AOS Assessment Protocol 4: Connected Speech

Overview of AOS Protocols

Assessment protocols provided in this chapter help assess AOS in adults in an efficient manner. The protocols offer ready-made formats that clinicians can use in structuring their client and family interviews and assessing various parameters of AOS.

The protocols offered in this chapter also are available on the accompanying CD. The clinician may print the needed protocols in evaluating his or her clients. The clinician may combine these protocols in suitable ways to facilitate the evaluation of an adult's AOS disorders.

In assessing adults with multiple disorders, the clinician may combine these protocols with protocols from other chapters. For example, the clinician may combine these AOS assessment protocols with dysarthria assessment protocols (Chapter 6) or aphasia assessment protocols (Chapter 5).

The protocols given in this chapter are specific to AOS in adults. To complete the assessment on a given client, the clinician should combine these disorder-specific protocols with the common assessment protocols given in Chapter 2:

- The Adult Case History
- Orofacial Examination and Hearing Screening Protocol
- Diadochokinetic Assessment Protocol for Adults
- Adult Assessment Report Outline

Assessment of AOS: Interview Protocol

Name _____ DOB _____ Date _____ Clinician _____

Individualize this protocol on the CD and print it for your use. 💿

Preparation

- Review the guidelines given under *The Initial Clinical Interview* in Chapter 1.
- Arrange for comfortable seating and lighting.
- Record the interview on audio or video.
- Initially interview the client alone and then have the accompanying person join the interview.
- Review the case history ahead of time and take note of areas you want to explore during the interview.

Introduction

Introduce yourself. Describe the assessment plan and tell the client the time it will take.

Example: "Hello Mr./Mrs. [*client's name*]. My name is [*your name*] I am the speech-language pathologist who will be assessing you today. I would like to start by reviewing the case history and asking you a few questions. After we finish talking, I will work with you. Today's assessment should take about [*estimate the amount of time you plan to spend*]."

Interview Questions

The questions are generally directed toward the adult client with suspected AOS. When interviewing the client and the accompanying person together, it is essential to pose the same, but reworded, question to the accompanying person. A few examples are shown within the brackets; the clinician may use this strategy whenever necessary.

- What is your main concern regarding your speech? [What do you think is his (her) main problem?]
- How would you describe your speech problem? [How would you describe her (his) speech problem?]
- When did you first notice that your speech was different? [When did you notice that his (her) speech was different?]
- Has your speech changed over time? If so, how?
- Have you seen your family doctor about your speech?
- Did your family doctor refer you to a specialist?
- What did the doctor(s) tell you?

(continues)

Assessment of AOS: Interview Protocol (continued)

- Besides a speech problem, are you concerned with any aspects of your talking?

- How would you describe these other talking problems? [How would you describe his (her) overall speech?]

- Are there times when your speech is better or worse? For example, is it better in the morning than in the evening? [Do you also think her (his) speech varies throughout the day?]

- Do you believe that your speech problem is affecting your social interactions? Would you describe how?

- Do you think that your speech problem is affecting your job performance? How is it affected?

- Has anyone else in your family ever experienced speech problems?

- Do you have any other chronic health conditions or concerns?

- Are you currently on any medications?

- It looks like I have most of the information I wanted from you. Do you have any questions for me at this point?

- Thank you for your information. It will be helpful in my assessment. I will now work with you to better understand your speech problem. When we are done, we will discuss our findings.

Review the case history again and ask additional questions if needed.

AOS Assessment Protocol 1: Oral Apraxia

Name _____ DOB _____ Date _____ Clinician _____

Individualize this protocol on the CD and print it for your use. 💿

Instructions: Answer the following questions about the client's nonspeech muscle movements. The clinician also may make an estimate of severity (0 = *No deficit*, 1 = *Mild*, 2 = *Moderate*, 3 = *Severe*).

Assessment of Oral Apraxia	Yes	No	Severity
Can the client pucker the lips?			
Can the client pucker and smile alternately?			
Can the client quickly move the tongue from side to side?			
Can the client puff out the cheeks?			
Can the client produce a voluntary cough on command?			
Can the client touch the tongue to the upper lip?			
Can the client chatter the teeth as if cold?			
Can the client click the tongue?			
Can the client smile on command?			
Can the client protrude and retract the tongue quickly?			
Can the client open the mouth completely, as if yawning?			
Can the client clear the throat on command?			
Can the client lick the lips?			
Can the client whistle?			
Can the client bite the lower lip?			
Can the client touch the tongue to the chin?			
Can the client round the lips?			
Can the client show the teeth on command?			
Can the client show how to blow out a candle?			
Can the client use the tongue tip to protrude the cheek?			
Clinician's summative statement:			

AOS Assessment Protocol 2: Speech Production in AOS

Name _____ DOB _____ Date _____ Clinician _____

Individualize this protocol on the CD and print it for your use. 💿

Instructions: Ask the client to produce the following words, phrases, and sentences, indicating whether the responses were correct or incorrect. The clinician also may make an estimate of severity (0 = *No deficit*, 1 = *Mild*, 2 = *Moderate*, 3 = *Severe*).

Assessment of Speech Production	Correct	Incorrect	Severity
Multisyllabic words			
1. Shadow			
2. Discharge			
3. Fullness			
4. Vegetarian			
5. Provision			
6. Mechanical			
7. Insensitive			
8. Embarrassing			
9. Refrigerator			
10. Inflammable			
Phrases			
1. National forest			
2. Fascinating storyteller			
3. Computer specialist			
4. Beautiful monument			
5. Glimmering brightly			
6. Constitutional amendment			
7. Vice chancellor			
8. Misrepresented information			
9. Complex organization			
10. Congressional appointment			

Assessment of Speech Production	Correct	Incorrect	Severity
Sentences			
1. He followed each line.			
2. It was a big quarrel.			
3. Marsha's specialty is international law.			
4. The rarest parrot is the Norwegian Blue.			
5. His accomplishments are many.			
6. It is a handy reference book.			
7. Roberta is learning a musical instrument.			
8. Jerry's imagination is bottomless.			
9. It is an expression of affection.			
10. Oceanographers must not get seasick.			
Sequences			
1. Have the client say the days of the week.			
2. Have the client say the alphabet.			
3. Have the client count from 1 to 20.			
4. Have the client count from 20 back to 1.			
Increasing Word Length			
1. Hap-happen-happening			
2. Guard-guarding-guardian			
3. Tic-tickle-tickling			
4. Sin-sincere-sincerely			
5. Note-noting-notable			
6. Pro-provide-providing			
7. Lit-litter-littering			
8. Cow-coward-cowardly			
9. Ad-advance-advancement			
10. In-indent-indentation			

(continues)

AOS Assessment Protocol 2: Speech Production in AOS (continued)

Assessment of Speech Production	Correct	Incorrect	Severity
Repeated Trials (Have the client say each word three times)			
1. Underscore			
2. Thoughtful			
3. Judgment			
4. Goodness			
5. Grumble			
6. Entertainment			
7. Voluntary			
8. Favorable			
9. Enchanted			
10. Quibble			
Clinician's summative statement:			

AOS Assessment Protocol 3: Comparing Alternate Motion Rates (AMRs) and Sequential Motion Rates (SMRs)

Name _____ DOB _____ Date _____ Clinician _____

Individualize this protocol on the CD and print it for your use. ◉

Instructions: Compare the client's ability to produce AMRs and SMRs. Typically, a client with AOS can successfully produce the AMR phonemes but will demonstrate significant difficulty producing the three phonemes in the SMR task. The clinician also may make an estimate of severity (0 = *No deficit*, 1 = *Mild*, 2 = *Moderate*, 3 = *Severe*). Normal rates for AMRs are approximately 6 productions per second, although "kuh" productions may be slightly slower (Kent, Kent, & Rosenbek, 1987).

Assessment of Alternate Motion Rates (AMRs)	Yes	No	Severity
1. Have the client take a single, deep breath and say "puh-puh-puh" as rapidly and evenly as possible. Demonstrate.			
Duration and quality of trial one:			
2. Now have the client say "tuh-tuh-tuh" as rapidly and evenly as possible. Demonstrate.			
Duration and quality of trial one:			
3. Now have the client say "kuh-kuh-kuh" as rapidly and evenly as possible. Demonstrate			
Duration and quality of trial one:			
4. Judge the quality of the client's AMRs			
Are the AMRs produced evenly (i.e., rhythmically)?			
Is the client's pitch normal during productions?			
Is the client's loudness within normal limits?			
Is the articulation clear and precise?			
Is articulatory groping present?			
Is an obvious delay evident before the productions?			
Assessment of Sequential Motion Rate (SMR)	Yes	No	Severity
1. Have the client take a single, deep breath and say "puh-tuh-kuh" as rapidly and evenly as possible. Demonstrate.			
Duration of trial one:			
Duration of trial two:			
Duration of trial three:			

(continues)

AOS Assessment Protocol 3: Comparing AMRs and SMRs (continued)

Assessment of Sequential Motion Rate (SMR)	Yes	No	Severity
2. Judge the quality of the client's SMR.			
Are the productions of each syllable smooth?			
Are there hesitations, substitutions, or omissions of phonemes?			
Are there transpositions of phonemes?			
Are there anticipatory errors in the speech?			
Does the client show awareness of speech errors?			
Clinician's summative statement			

AOS Assessment Protocol 4: Connected Speech

Name _____ DOB _____ Date _____ Clinician _____

Individualize this protocol on the CD and print it for your use. 💿

Instructions: Have the client read aloud the following paragraph or a standard reading passage such as "My Grandfather." Judge the client's speech by answering the following questions.

> One summer night a man stood on a low hill overlooking a wide expanse of forest and field. A light mist lay along the earth, partly veiling the lower features of the landscape, but above it the taller trees showed in well-defined masses against a clear sky. Two or three farmhouses were visible through the haze, but in none of them, naturally, was a light.
>
> (From Ambrose Bierce's "A Resumed Identity")

Assessment of Connected Speech	Yes	No	Severity
1. Does the client produce phonemes clearly?			
2. Is the speech rate too slow?			
3. Are there inappropriate silent pauses between words?			
4. Is loudness adjusted appropriately while reading?			
5. Is monoloudness present?			
6. Is monopitch present?			
7. Does the client frequently revise productions of words?			
8. Does the client show articulatory groping while reading?			
9. Are multisyllabic words more difficult for the client to produce than single-syllable words?			
10. Are there periods of error-free speech production?			
11. Are there any perseverative errors?			
12. Is overall prosody abnormal?			
Clinician's summative statement			

Reference

Kent, R. D., Kent, J. F., & Rosenbek, J. C. (1987). Maximum performance test of speech production. *Journal of Speech and Hearing Disorders, 52,* 367–387.

CHAPTER 5

Assessment of Dysarthria: Resources

- Types of Dysarthria
- Epidemiology of Dysarthria
- Etiology of Dysarthria
- Overview of Dysarthric Speech
- Overview of Assessment of Dysarthria
- Standardized Tests for Dysarthria
- Diagnostic Criteria and Differential Diagnosis
- Postassessment Counseling

Types of Dysarthria

Dysarthria literally means a disorder of articulation (*dys* meaning disorder and *arthria* meaning to speak clearly). While this definition is concise, it is incomplete. Dysarthria is more than just an articulation deficit. It actually is a speech production disorder caused by neuromotor damage to the central or peripheral nervous system, and it can involve deficits of respiration, phonation, resonation, prosody, and articulation. Dysarthria and apraxia of speech often are described as *motor speech disorders* because they both affect the normal neuromotor execution of speech. Furthermore, dysarthria is not a single disorder. The word *dysarthria* actually is an umbrella term that covers a collection of seven separate subcategories of dysarthria, each with its own etiology and characteristics. Six of the dysarthrias are pure (flaccid, spastic, unilateral upper motor neuron dysarthria, ataxic, hypokinetic, and hyperkinetic), meaning they are the result of damage to only one part of the motor system. The seventh subcategory, mixed dysarthria, can occur when damage extends to more than one part of the motor system, such as when a brainstem stroke damages upper and lower motor neurons and results in a flaccid-spastic mixed dysarthria. The following paragraphs examine each of the seven dysarthrias, describing the qualities that make them unique and reviewing their neurological bases.

Overview of Flaccid Dysarthria

Flaccid dysarthria is caused by any condition that damages the cranial or spinal nerves used in speech production. The damage can occur anywhere along the length of the nerve, from its origins in the brainstem (or spinal cord) to its ending at the neuromuscular junction, where it makes synaptic contact with muscles cells. Flaccid dysarthria is primarily associated with muscle weakness or paralysis caused by reduced or absent motor impulses secondary to nerve damage. The specific characteristics of flaccid dysarthria depend on which cranial or spinal nerve is damaged. If, for example, only the left branch of the facial nerve (VII) is damaged, the resulting speech problem would be a mild articulation deficit for bilabial or labiodental phonemes. But if all the speech production cranial nerves were significantly damaged, the resulting flaccid dysarthria could be severe, seriously affecting phonation, resonation, articulation, and prosody. Of the 12 cranial nerves, 6 are used in speech production. Each plays a specific role in allowing us to produce intelligible speech:

- Trigeminal (V)—Although this cranial nerve mostly contains sensory neurons, its lower motor neurons innervate the jaw and the tensor veli palatini muscle. Damage to just the left or right branch of this cranial nerve usually has little effect on speech production because the undamaged, opposite branch will fully innervate the jaw muscles on that other side of the face, allowing the jaw to close more or less normally. However, when both the left and right branches of the trigeminal nerve are damaged, the jaw can hang loosely and be unable to close far enough to allow labial and lingual articulation of speech sounds.

- Facial (VII)—As its name implies, the facial nerve innervates the muscles of the face. The cervicofacial branch of the facial nerve innervates the muscles of the lower face, and when it is damaged, it can cause upper and lower lip weakness, resulting in imprecise bilabial or labiodental consonants.

- Glossopharyngeal (IX)—Like the trigeminal nerve, the glossopharyngeal nerve primarily contains sensory neurons; however, its motor neurons do have a role in speech production. The motor neurons in this cranial nerve innervate the stylopharyngeus and superior pharyngeal muscles, both of which are used to shape the pharynx during speech. Damage to this cranial nerve may cause distorted vowels.

- Vagus (X)—The vagus is a critically important cranial nerve for speech production. Three of its branches innervate key muscles in the speech mechanism. The *pharyngeal branch of the vagus nerve* innervates the levator veli palatini muscle, which is essential for elevating the velum and closing the velopharyngeal port. Damage to this branch can result in hypernasal speech. The pharyngeal branch also innervates the superior and middle pharyngeal constrictor muscles, which are used in shaping the pharynx for vowel production. The *external superior laryngeal nerve branch of the vagus nerve* innervates the cricothyroid muscle, which helps stretch and tense the vocal folds. Damage to this nerve branch can reduce pitch changes during speech, as well as cause decreased loudness and increased breathiness during phonation. The *recurrent nerve branch of the vagus nerve* innervates all the intrinsic muscles of the larynx, except for the previously mentioned cricothyroid muscle. This means that nearly all the adductor, abductor, and tensor muscles of the larynx are innervated by this one nerve branch. Damage to the recurrent nerve may result in breathy or hoarse phonation (i.e., phonatory incompetence), as well as inhalatory stridor.

- Accessory (XI)—The cranial root of the accessory nerve merges with the vagus nerve shortly after leaving the brainstem. Its motor neurons work together with those of the vagus nerve to innervate the velum, pharynx, and larynx. Damage to the accessory nerve can cause many of the same speech errors previously described for the vagus nerve.

- Hypoglossal (XII)—This cranial nerve innervates all the intrinsic and most of the extrinsic tongue muscles. Damage to this nerve will cause weak and imprecise tongue movements, resulting in distorted lingual phonemes.

- Spinal nerves—Spinal nerves also are involved in speech production. Many of those that branch from the cervical and thoracic sections of the spinal cord innervate the respiratory muscles (i.e., intercostal muscles and diaphragm). When spinal nerve damage is widespread, it can affect respiration for speech production, resulting in decreased speech loudness, shortened utterances, impaired prosody, and strained vocal quality.

Overview of Spastic Dysarthria

Spastic dysarthria is caused by bilateral damage to upper motor neurons. Upper motor neurons are neural tracts in the central nervous system that make synaptic contact with the lower motor neurons in the cranial and spinal nerves. A simplified way to understand the role of upper motor neurons is this: Upper motor neurons take the motor impulses created in the brain and transmit them to lower motor neurons in the cranial and spinal nerves (which then send the impulses to the muscles). There are two broad collections of upper motor neurons. One is the **pyramidal system**, which transmits skilled voluntary movements (such as speech movements) from the cortex down to the cranial and spinal nerves. The other is the **extrapyramidal system** (i.e., the upper motor neuron tracts that are extra or in addition to the pyramidal system). The extrapyramidal tracts transmit motor impulses from the brain that regulate posture, muscle tone, and reflexes. When an individual has bilateral damage (left and right side damage) to the pyramidal and extrapyramidal tracts, the result can be spastic dysarthria.

Because spastic dysarthria is caused by combined damage to both of these upper motor neuron tracts, the characteristics of this dysarthria are a combination of what we would expect if just one of these tracts was damaged individually. Individuals with spastic dysarthria demonstrate speech movements that have *weakness*, *slowness*, *spasticity* (too much muscle tone), and, in some cases, *abnormal reflexes*. When listening to someone with spastic dysarthria, the weakness and slowness may be most *perceptually* evident in the tongue and lip movements, causing distorted consonants. The spasticity may be most *perceptually* evident in the larynx, where the tight, hyperadduction of the vocal folds can give the individual's phonation a harsh or strained-strangled quality.

Overview of Unilateral Upper Motor Neuron Dysarthria

As its name implies, this type of dysarthria is caused by upper motor neuron damage that is restricted to one side of the central nervous system. For the speech musculature, this upper motor neuron damage usually only affects the half of the lower face and tongue that is opposite to the damage. For instance, if upper motor neuron damage is in the left hemisphere, the right side of a client's lower face and tongue will demonstrate weak and slow movements. Unilateral upper motor neuron dysarthria usually results in a relatively mild or moderate articulation disorder because only the tongue and lips on one side of the face are affected by the lesion. Consequently, imprecise consonants and slow alternate motion rates are the two most common speech characteristics of unilateral upper motor neuron dysarthria (Duffy, 2005).

Overview of Ataxic Dysarthria

Ataxic dysarthria is associated with damage to either the cerebellum or the neural tracts leading to and from the cerebellum. The cerebellum is an important component of the motor system. At any given moment, the cerebellum has access to nearly all the body's sensory information, and it uses this information to refine and coordinate planned voluntary movements before they are actually performed. The cerebellum coordinates planned movements with the body's immediate circumstances so that the timing, force, speed, and direction of actions are accomplished smoothly and accurately. In addition to refining planned movements, the cerebellum also has connections to the extrapyramidal system that allow it to rapidly adjust an individual's posture during an ongoing movement, such as stumbling on a cracked sidewalk while walking. The cerebellum can "sense" the loss of balance and make quick postural adjustments to ensure that the person does not fall.

When the cerebellum or its neural tracts are damaged, movements can become uncoordinated and impaired. When speech production is affected by cerebellar damage, the result is ataxic dysarthria. This dysarthria is characterized primarily by articulation and prosody disorders. Imprecise consonants, distorted vowels, and irregular articulatory breakdowns are common articulation errors in ataxic dysarthria. Excess and equal stress, prolonged phonemes, and prolonged intervals between phonemes are common prosodic errors. Many individuals with ataxic dysarthria describe their speech as having a drunken quality. Others have described the speech of someone with ataxic dysarthria as being blurred or sounding like it is dragging.

Overview of Hypokinetic Dysarthria

Hypokinetic dysarthria is almost exclusively associated with idiopathic Parkinson's disease. The term *hypokinetic* means too little movement, and this is a particularly good description of this disease because voluntary movements can be significantly attenuated or "compressed," especially in the later stages of the condition. Parkinson's disease is the result of an imbalance between two neurotransmitters in the basal ganglia—dopamine (inhibitory) and acetylcholine (excitatory). In the normally functioning basal ganglia, the actions of these two neurotransmitters are properly balanced, allowing the basal ganglia to accurately refine voluntary movements. In cases of Parkinson's disease, however, the neurons that produce dopamine gradually die, which leaves the basal ganglia overexcited with too much acetylcholine. As the basal ganglia slowly become more and more overexcited, the typical characteristics of parkinsonism begin to appear:

- **Tremor** is one of the most common symptoms of Parkinson's disease, and it often is the first one noticed by patients with this condition. It is a resting tremor, meaning it is most evident while the body is at rest. When the body is in motion, the tremor tends to be greatly reduced, or it will disappear completely.

- **Bradykinesia** is the slowed and reduced range of movement seen in this disease. Voluntary movements are labored, slow, and limited, such as seen in the shuffling walk demonstrated by clients with Parkinson's disease. It is important to note that bradykinesia is caused by the neurochemical imbalance in the basal ganglia, not by muscle weakness, as might be assumed by watching someone with this condition struggle to complete simple tasks.

- **Muscle rigidity** is frequently seen in Parkinson's disease. It is due to increased muscle tone, especially in the neck, torso, and limbs. When pulling an affected limb to full extension, constant resistance to the movement will be noted.

- **Akinesia** causes a delay in the initiation of a voluntary movement. Usually, the delay is only for a few seconds, but it may be significantly longer with some clients. In the most serious cases of akinesia, clients can become "frozen" in position and will be unable to move voluntarily.

- **Disturbed postural reflexes** are most evident when the affected individual is attempting to perform normal movements, such as walking, getting up from a chair, or standing still. For example, if lightly pushed while standing, the client may fall because of an inability to rapidly shift his or her center of balance.

The speech characteristics of hypokinetic dysarthria include deficits of prosody, articulation, phonation, and respiration. The prosodic errors include monopitch, monoloudness, and reduced stress. Inappropriate silences and short rushes of speech also may be evident. About 20% of individuals with hypokinetic dysarthria have an increased rate of speech, often resulting in blurred articulation that severely affects intelligibility. The most common articulation error is imprecise consonants. Phonation errors include a harsh or breathy voice quality, and a few individuals may have low pitch. Respiration can be affected by reduced range of movement in the respiratory muscles, resulting in shallow breathing, poor control of exhalations, and short breathing cycles. Interestingly, resonance is rarely affected in this type of dysarthria.

Overview of Hyperkinetic Dysarthria

Hyperkinetic dysarthria is caused by involuntary movements (hyperkinesia) that interfere with speech production. There are a number of disorders that have hyperkinesia as one of their symptoms, and the variety of these involuntary movements can be striking. In some disorders, the movements only may be subtle contractions of the pharyngeal muscles, but in others they involve the whole body, making such tasks as walking and speech nearly impossible. Basal ganglia dysfunction is the suspected cause of most hyperkinetic disorders, but a number of them have unknown etiologies. Hyperkinetic dysarthria has been associated with the following disorders:

- *Chorea*—This is a hyperkinetic movement disorder with involuntary movements that tend to change quickly and sometimes appear to be purposeful. When chorea affects the limbs and torso, the resulting movements have been described as being "dance like" because of their flowing nature. Huntington's disease is the most well-known disorder that has chorea as a prominent symptom. It is an inherited disease that causes the progressive degeneration of neurons in the cerebral cortex and the basal ganglia. The first symptom of Huntington's is often a nearly imperceptible decline in cognitive abilities, usually only detectable by specialized testing. But as the disease progresses, these cognitive disorders become more evident. Personality changes, and word-finding difficulties and depression are common. As the cognitive disorders become more obvious, chorea also gradually appears in affected individuals. In Huntington's disease, choreic movements may first appear to be only a generalized restlessness, but over time they increase in severity to the point where the involuntary movements affect the entire body, thus causing hyperkinetic dysarthria. The random, quickly changing nature of choreic movements results in a large number of potential speech errors, including imprecise consonants, variable pitch, monopitch, and prolonged interval between phonemes or words.

Tardive dyskinesia also is associated with chorea and is characterized by involuntary movements of the face, mouth, and neck. This condition is caused by the use of antipsychotic drugs for long periods. The involuntary mouth movements in this disorder often involve repetitive "lip smacking," which affects speech production.

- Myoclonus—This condition results in brief, involuntary contractions of single muscles or of whole muscle groups. Depending on the type of myoclonus, the contractions can occur (a) only once, (b) in a nonrhythmic repetition, (c) or in a regular pattern. Palatopharyngolaryngeal myoclonus is a good example of myoclonic contractions causing hyperkinetic dysarthria. In this disorder, the muscles of the velum, pharynx, and larynx involuntarily contract rhythmically, about one to three times a second. The effects of these contractions sometimes are evident in connected speech, but frequently they are only noted during a prolonged vowel.

- Tic Disorders—Tics are involuntary movements that can be voluntarily suppressed for a short time. The affected body parts vary depending on the type of tic. Motor tics include repetitive eye blinking, grimaces, kicking, and hopping. Vocal tics can appear as throat clearing, growling sounds, shouting, and barking. In rare cases, vocal tics include coprolalia, the involuntary production of obscene words. When tics interfere with speech production, they can cause hypokinetic dysarthria. The most well-known tic disorder is Gilles de la Tourette syndrome, a condition where multiple motor and vocal tics change and evolve over time.

- Essential Tremor—Sometimes called *organic tremor*, this is a benign hyperkinetic disorder of unknown origin. It is the most common type of hyperkinesia seen by neurologists. It causes rhythmic action tremors in affected body parts, which can include the hands, arms, neck, and head. When these tremors affect the larynx, the result is *essential voice tremor*. Individuals with essential voice tremor demonstrate tremulous, "shaky" phonations because of the involuntary contractions of their vocal cords.

- Dystonia—This condition results in involuntary muscle contractions that typically have more of a sustained or prolonged quality than those seen in chorea. Dystonic muscle contractions often have a "waxing and waning" characteristic, meaning that they gradually come and go over a period of seconds or minutes. However, they also can be constant, causing fixed contractions of the affected body part. Dystonia is categorized into four types: focal (contractions of only one body part), segmental (contractions of two or more body parts), generalized (contractions affecting all limbs and the torso), or hemidystonia (contractions on one side of the body, affecting two or more body parts). Any of these dystonias can cause hyperkinetic dysarthria if they affect the speech muscles. For example, a focal dystonia may cause a prolonged protrusion of the tongue, making articulation difficult or impossible. A generalized dystonia could affect nearly all components of the speech mechanism, causing difficulties with respiration, articulation, resonance, phonation, and prosody.

Overview of Mixed Dysarthria

Mixed dysarthria is the most common type of dysarthria (Duffy, 2005). It occurs when there is damage to two or more parts of the motor system. For instance, a condition that damages lower motor neurons in the cranial nerves and also damages upper motor neurons bilaterally can cause a flaccid-spastic mixed dysarthria. The speech characteristics of this type of mixed dysarthria are a combination of those seen in the individual dysarthrias. In this example, the affected client will demonstrate a dysarthria that has both flaccid and spastic qualities. The relative severity of the flaccid and spastic characteristics would depend on which areas of the motor system were most impaired. If both lower and upper motor neurons were more or less equally impaired, then both the flaccid and spastic aspects of the dysarthria would be approximately the same. If, however, there was more damage to upper motor neurons than lower motor neurons, the spastic qualities would be more evident. Nearly any combination of the individual dysarthrias is possible, with the exception of a spastic-unilateral upper motor neuron mixed dysarthria (the bilateral damage that causes the spastic dysarthria would "cancel out" the unilateral damage).

Epidemiology of Dysarthria

The incidence and prevalence of dysarthria is not known, but it is not a rare condition. Dysarthria is closely associated with a number of well-known disorders such as stroke, Parkinson's disease, multiple sclerosis, amyotrophic lateral sclerosis, and Huntington's disease. For example, Ramig, Fox, and Sapir (2004) reported that a high percentage of individuals with Parkinson's disease either have dysarthria, a voice disorder, or both. Similarly, Yorkston, Beukelman, Strand, and Bell (1999) suggested that 60% of individuals with traumatic brain injury have dysarthria during the acute stages of their recovery, and 10% have it long term. To date, the most informative data on the distribution of dysarthria comes from Duffy (2005). Of the 10,444 individuals seen for an acquired neurologic communication disorder at the Mayo Clinic from 1987–1990 and 1993–2001, 54% of them had dysarthria. The next most common disorder (16%) was "other cognitive-language disorders," which included dementia, traumatic head injury, confusion, and related conditions.

Duffy (2005) also reported the distribution of specific dysarthria types during the same period, based on 6101 patients with neurologic motor speech disorders:

- Mixed dysarthria—27%
- Hyperkinetic dysarthria—18%
- Ataxic dysarthria—10%
- Unilateral upper motor neuron dysarthria—8%
- Flaccid dysarthria—8%
- Spastic dysarthria—8%
- Hypokinetic dysarthria—8%
- Undetermined dysarthria—3%

Duffy noted that while the precise number of individuals with dysarthria is unclear, current evidence indicates that (a) it is seen frequently in medical settings, (b) it is associated with numerous medical disorders, and (c) it makes up a significant portion of the caseload in speech-language pathology clinics.

Etiology of Dysarthria

Dysarthria is caused by neurologic damage to the motor system. This damage can occur in most any area of the motor system used for speech production, including the cerebral cortex, subcortical structures, cerebellum, and cranial nerves. Damage or dysfunction in any of these areas can cause dysarthria. Moreover, the range of conditions that can impair the motor system is broad, including physical trauma, infections, degenerative diseases, strokes, and numerous other disorders. The causes of dysarthria vary, depending on which areas of the motor system are impaired. Even within each type of dysarthria, there are multiple conditions that can cause speech disorders.

Flaccid dysarthria is caused by damage to lower motor neurons inside the nerves that innervate the muscles of speech production. This damage may occur anywhere along the length of the nerve, from its origins in the brainstem or spinal cord to the end of its axon at the neuromuscular junction. The most common causes of flaccid dysarthria include the following conditions:

- Physical trauma to lower motor neurons—This damage may be the result of blows to the head and neck, falls, broken bones that cut or compress neurons, and rotational force that twists or stretch neurons, and even surgical mistakes that accidently nick or cut a nerve.

- Brainstem stroke—Because the cranial nerves originate in the inside of the brainstem (at points called the *cranial nerve nuclei*), a hemorrhagic or ischemic brainstem stroke can interrupt blood flow to the lower motor neuron cell bodies, which will kill the affected neurons. With the loss of these neurons, movement impulses will not be passed on to the speech muscles, resulting in weak or absent movements in the speech mechanism.

- Myasthenia gravis—This is an autoimmune disorder that affects the neuromuscular junction. In this disorder, immune system antibodies attach themselves to the neurotransmitter receptor sites in muscle tissue, blocking the reception of the chemical (acetylcholine) that signals a muscle to contract. Because of the blockage, only reduced amounts of acetylcholine are available to the muscles, resulting in their rapid fatigue during sustained contractions. Flaccid dysarthria can occur when the antibodies block muscle receptors in the speech muscles. During prolonged speech tasks, such as counting to 100, a client with myasthenia gravis can demonstrate the rapid appearance of imprecise consonants, hypernasality, slowed rate of speech, and breathy phonation.

- Guillain-Barre syndrome—This is an autoimmune disorder of unknown origin, although is often appears after an individual has had certain infections or immunizations. It causes the demyelination of neurons, primarily affecting lower motor neurons in cranial and spinal nerves. As the myelin degenerates, motor impulses traveling to the muscles are degraded, resulting in progressively weaker muscle contractions. The progression of the condition can be rapid, sometimes changing significantly in just a day. Flaccid dysarthria will result when the demyelination occurs in the nerves that innervate the speech muscles. Most individuals with Guillain-Barre syndrome recover fully. However, it is fatal in about 3% of cases, and others will always have some residual weakness.

- Tumors—Tumors growing in the brainstem, neck, or orofacial structures can affect a cranial nerve's ability to properly transmit neural impulses to the muscles, thereby causing flaccid dysarthria.

Spastic dysarthria is caused by bilateral damage to upper motor neurons in the pyramidal and extrapyramidal tracts. The pyramidal tracts transmit skilled voluntary movements from the cortex to the lower motor neurons in the cranial and spinal nerves. The extrapyramidal tracts transmit motor impulses that regulate posture, muscle tone, and posture. The motor impulses traveling through both of these tracts work together to allow us to carry out movements as intended. For example, when typing on a keyboard, the motor impulses traveling through the pyramidal tracts tell which finger to hit which key—that is, they transmit the skilled voluntary movements in this task. The motor impulses in the extrapyramidal tracts keep our hands, arms, back, and head in just the right position to allow our fingers to hit the correct keys—that is, they transmit the postural support needed for typing. When the upper motor neurons that innervate the cranial nerves of speech production are damaged bilaterally, speech movements will be slow and weak (because of the pyramidal tract damage) and also have spasticity and additional weakness (because of the extrapyramidal tract damage). Here is a listing of the conditions that can cause spastic dysarthria:

- Stroke—A stroke that is able to bilaterally damage the pyramidal and extrapyramidal tracts can cause spastic dysarthria. Usually, it is a brainstem stroke that can cause this damage because both the left and right axons of these tracts are very close together in the brainstem, enabling a single stroke to affect them all. Two separate strokes in each hemisphere also are able to cause this bilateral upper motor neuron damage.

- Traumatic head injury—Many head injuries result in widespread damage to both hemispheres of the brain. The shifting and twisting of the brain can stretch and tear axons in multiple locations, including those of the pyramidal and extrapyramidal tracts, consequently causing spastic dysarthria.

- Brainstem tumor—A single brainstem tumor can compress or destroy upper motor neurons bilaterally as it grows because those neural tracts are so close to each other in the brainstem.

- Cerebral anoxia—This is the loss of oxygen to brain cells. It can be caused by heart attack, drug overdose, electrocution, or any other condition that results in cardiovascular or respiratory failure. If the brain is deprived of oxygen for as little as 2–5 minutes, lasting brain damage can be the result. Cerebral anoxia can cause spastic dysarthria because it is able to produce bilateral damage to upper motor neurons.

- Cerebral infections—Viral and bacterial infections also have the ability to cause spastic dysarthria when they involve either the brainstem or both cerebral hemispheres.

Unilateral upper motor neuron dysarthria is caused by upper motor neuron damage that is restricted to only one side of the brain. It does not matter which hemisphere is affected. When the damage is in the left hemisphere, this type of dysarthria will often co-occur with aphasia, apraxia of speech, or with both. When the damage is in the right hemisphere, it will often co-occur with the perceptual and cognitive deficits associated with right-hemisphere syndrome. Unilateral upper motor neuron dysarthria usually is caused by conditions that result in focal lesions:

- Stroke—The most common cause of this dysarthria is a single stroke affecting one hemisphere. Duffy and Folger (1986) found that 91% of the cases they reviewed were caused by stroke. The location of the stroke can be varied (cortical or subcortical), as long as it affects upper motor neurons.

- Tumors—Although not a common cause of this dysarthria, tumors are able to compress upper motor neurons in one hemisphere as they grow, which can affect a neuron's ability to transmit information. Tumors also may compress arteries or veins and interrupt the normal flow of blood needed by upper motor neurons to function properly.

- Traumatic head injury—Because most head injuries result in diffuse brain damage, they are not common causes of unilateral upper motor neuron dysarthria. However, the effects of some head injuries can be restricted to one hemisphere, such as in cases of penetrating head wounds.

Ataxic dysarthria is caused by damage to the cerebellum or to the neural tracts leading in and out of the cerebellum. Cerebellar damage disrupts our ability to coordinate movements—the timing, force, speed, and direction of movement are impaired. Ataxic dysarthria frequently results in speech that has a clumsy, blurred quality, often described as sounding "drunken." A number of conditions can damage the cerebellum:

- Degenerative diseases—Autosomal dominant cerebellar ataxia of late onset is a degenerative disease that affects the cerebellum. It is an inherited disorder that causes ataxia, visual and hearing deficits, balance problems, and dementia. Its course is fairly quick, with affected individuals dying within several years of the first appearance of the symptoms. Other degenerative disorders that can cause ataxia are idiopathic sporadic late-onset cerebellar ataxia, Friedreich's ataxia, and olivopontocerebellar degeneration.

- Stroke—A number of large arteries supply blood to the cerebellum, and when the blood flow through them is interrupted by a stroke, ataxic dysarthria can be one of the results. One estimate is that 10% of intracerebral hemorrhages primarily affect the cerebellum (Heilman, Watson, & Greer, 1977).

- Toxicity and metabolic disorders—The function of the cerebellum can be affected by overexposure to a number of chemicals, such as lead, mercury, acrylamide, and cyanide. Chronic alcohol abuse can permanently damage the cerebellum, as can prolonged use of certain medications, such as the antiseizure drug Dilantin.

- Traumatic head injury—Rotational force head injuries may especially affect the neural tracts leading in an out of the cerebellum. The rapid twisting of the brain during this type of injury may stretch or break those axons, thereby impairing cerebellar function.

- Tumors—A tumor can develop either within the cerebellum or nearby, and as it grows, it can compress cerebellar neurons and impair their function. A tumor also can grow near the tracts leading in and out of the cerebellum and affect their ability to transmit information to the rest of the motor system.

- Infections—While not common causes of ataxic dysarthria, infections can selectively affect cerebellar tissue.

Hypokinetic dysarthria is caused by basal ganglia dysfunction. By far, the most common cause of this type of dysarthria is idiopathic Parkinson's disease.

- Parkinson's disease—This is a slowly progressive disorder primarily associated with the degeneration of neurons in the substantia nigra, which is a small collection of neuron cell bodies near the basal ganglia. In a normally functioning brain, neurons in substantia nigra neurons provide dopamine to large portions of the basal ganglia, a key part of the motor system for refining voluntary movements. Normal basal ganglia function is dependent on balanced amounts of an excitatory neurotransmitter (acetylcholine) and an inhibitory neurotransmitter (dopamine). In patients with Parkinson's disease, the neurons in the substantia nigra degenerate, causing dopamine levels in the basal ganglia to decline. This disrupts the balance of acetycholine and dopamine, leaving the basal ganglia in an overly excited state, which leads to the previously mentioned characteristics of parkinsonism: tremor, bradykinesia, muscular rigidity, akinesia, and impaired postural reflexes.

- Neuroleptic-induced parkinsonism—High dosages of certain antipsychotic drugs can affect the balance of acetylcholine and dopamine in the brain. If these medications are taken for several weeks, it is possible for the patient to begin showing signs of parkinsonism, such as tremor, rigidity, and bradykinesia. These negative side effects will disappear if the dosage is reduced.

- Postencephalitic parkinsonism—Viral encephalitis can damage the substantia nigra, causing a reduction of dopamine to the basal ganglia. The symptoms of postencephalitic parkinsonism are similar to those of idiopathic Parkinson's disease. It usually is treated with dopamine replacement medications.

Hyperkinetic dysarthria has a variety of etiologies, depending on what is causing the underlying hyperkinesia. In general, most cases of this dysarthria are associated with different types of basal ganglia dysfunction:

- Huntington's chorea—Although the precise cause of Huntington's chorea is known, a number of complex theories have been suggested, most of them concentrating on why basal ganglia neurons degenerate. One proposal is that the mutated Huntingtin protein makes key basal ganglia neurons fatally receptive to the neurotransmitter glutamine, a process known as excitotoxicity. When excitotoxicity is present, even normal amounts of glutamine will kill affected neurons.

- Myoclonus—This hyperkinetic condition has been associated with infections, strokes, kidney failure, drug overdose, tumors, and certain medications. Palatopharyngolaryngeal myoclonus is frequently linked to brainstem lesions.

- Tic disorders—The neurological cause of tic disorders is unknown, but dysfunction of the frontal lobe and basal ganglia are suspected. Tourette's syndrome appears to be an inherited condition, but environmental influences also are thought to influence its severity.

- Essential tremor—This hyperkinetic disorder has a genetic link in approximately 50% of cases, although the neurological basis of the tremor is not known.

- Dystonia—The cause of primary dystonias is unknown, but basal ganglia dysfunction and neurotransmitter imbalance are suspected. Environmental influences also may contribute to the appearance of this hyperkinesia.

Mixed dysarthria is caused by conditions that damage more than one area of the motor system, such as a brainstem stroke that affects the function of both upper and lower motor neurons, resulting in a flaccid-spastic mixed dysarthria. The list of conditions that can result in mixed dysarthria is long. Here are short descriptions of six disorders that can have mixed dysarthria as a common characteristic:

- Multiple sclerosis—This is a progressive disease that causes the degeneration of the myelin sheath around axons. It can affect myelin anywhere in the central nervous system: the spinal cord, cerebellum, cerebrum, and brainstem. The degeneration usually begins as an inflammation of the myelin, which can progress in intensity until the myelin and the cells that produce it are destroyed. The effects of multiple sclerosis can be focal or diffuse. In some individuals only one area will be affected, such as the cerebellum. Other individuals will develop lesions in many parts of the central nervous system. The cause of multiple sclerosis is not known, but it probably has genetic, infectious, and environmental factors that contribute to its development. The types of dysarthria most commonly associated with multiple sclerosis are difficult to identify because so much of the motor system can be affected by this disorder. Duffy (2005) stated that spastic and ataxic dysarthria, along with ataxic-spastic mixed dysarthria, probably are the most common in multiple sclerosis.

- Shy-Drager syndrome—This is a degenerative disorder of unknown origin that affects neurons in the autonomic nervous system, basal ganglia, cerebellum, and brainstem. Parkinson-like symptoms are common—bradykinesia, muscle rigidity, and akinesia all can be present. Spasticity also may develop in the neck, face, and limbs as upper motor neurons become affected. The effects of this disorder on the autonomic nervous system cause problems with bowel and bladder control, poor regulation of blood pressure, and impaired pupillary reactions to light. Linebaugh (1979) found spastic-ataxic-hypokinetic, ataxic-spastic, and hypokinetic-ataxic mixed dysarthria to be associated with Shy-Drager syndrome.

- Progressive supranuclear palsy—This also is a progressive degenerative disorder of unknown origin. It causes the degeneration of neurons in cerebellum, brainstem, and basal ganglia. One of the more unique characteristics of this condition is the gradual reduction of voluntary eye movements, which makes tasks such as reading and walking down stairs difficult. Parkinsonian symptoms include muscle rigidity. Other characteristics include spasticity in the arms, legs, neck, or face; dementia; dysphagia; and mixed dysarthria. Duffy (2005) found that hypokinetic, spastic, or ataxic dysarthria can be found in different mixed combinations in this disorder.

- Olivopontocerebellar atrophy—As its name indicates, this disease results in the degeneration of neurons in the brainstem's olivary nucleus, the pons, and the cerebellum. The cause of this rare condition is not known, although a genetic link has been established in some cases. The symptoms are diverse: tremor, balance difficulties, numbness in the hands and feet, and uncoordinated movements of the limbs. The types of dysarthria associated with olivopontocerebellar atrophy also are varied. A mixed dysarthria with combinations of ataxic, spastic, flaccid, and hypokinetic qualities is possible (Duffy, 2005).

- Amyotrophic lateral sclerosis—This progressive neurologic disease causes the deterioration of motor neurons. Although all upper and lower motor neurons ultimately degenerate as the disease progresses, in some clients it is the lower motor neurons that are first affected. In other clients, it is the upper motor neurons that show the first signs of degeneration. In yet another group of clients, upper and lower motor neurons degenerate at approximately the same rate. Almost all cases of amyotrophic lateral sclerosis are persistently progressive, with weakness and muscle atrophy preventing nearly all voluntary movements in the later stages. Dementia is not associated with this disorder, but some cognitive decline can be noted. Eye movements, body sensation, and bladder control typically remain intact. The dysarthria associated with this condition varies according to which motor neurons degenerate first. Those clients with initial lower motor neuron involvement will first show a flaccid dysarthria (which evolves into a flaccid-spastic mixed dysarthria as upper motor neurons are affected). Those with initial upper motor neuron involvement will first show a spastic dysarthria (which then evolves into mixed dysarthria as the lower motor neurons are affected.) Those with both sets of motor neurons degenerating at about the same rate will demonstrate a flaccid-spastic mixed dysarthria throughout the course of the disease. In the final stages of this disorder, intelligible speech is not possible.

- Wilson's disease—Another progressive neurologic disorder, Wilson's disease is an inherited condition where the affected individual cannot metabolize the small amounts of dietary copper found in food. Rather than being excreted, the copper is deposited in the brain, liver, kidney, and corneas of the eyes. Over time, the buildup of this metal can reach toxic levels and affect the functioning of the central nervous system. The symptoms of Wilson's disease are extensive, including dementia, tremor, bradykinesia, muscle rigidity, limb ataxia, and dysphagia. There also are psychiatric symptoms, such as depression, mania, and schizophrenic-like behaviors. Effective treatments are available, but permanent damage or death may occur if the intervention is not started soon enough in its progression. The dysarthria most associated with Wilson's disease is of the ataxic-spastic-hypokinetic mixed type.

- Friedreich's ataxia—This condition causes a progressive degeneration of neurons in the spinal cord, brainstem, and cerebellum. It is a rare, inherited disorder that is untreatable. It is fatal for most individuals about 10–15 years after the first appearance of symptoms, which usually include ataxic movements of the arms and legs. Limb muscle atrophy and weakness, visual impairment, and hearing loss may be evident in the later stages. Dementia sometimes occurs in individuals with this condition. Spastic dysarthria, ataxic dysarthria, and ataxic-spastic mixed dysarthria can be found in the speech of individuals with Friedreich's ataxia.

There are numerous other conditions that can cause mixed dysarthria, with widely varied etiologies. For instance, Duffy (2005) reported the following causes of mixed dysarthria at the Mayo Clinic from 1969–1990 and 1999–2001:

- Degenerative disorders (66%), including amyotrophic lateral sclerosis, Parkinson's disease, nonspecific CNS degenerative disease, and others.

- Vascular disorders (11%), including multiple or single strokes, and vascular malformations.

- Traumatic (5%), including closed head injury and surgical trauma.

- Multiple causes (5%), including varied strokes, cerebellar degeneration, encephalopathy, and others.

- Demyelinating disorders (4%), including multiple sclerosis and others.

- Tumor (4%), including mass and paraneoplastic.

- Undetermined (3%)

- Toxic or metabolic (1%), including hypothyroidism, central pontine myelinolysis, neuroleptic toxicity, and others.

- Inflammatory (1%), including postviral encephalopathy, progressive encephalopathy, and spongioform encephalopathy.

Overview of Dysarthric Speech

Many disorders that cause dysarthria have the potential to affect all components of speech production: respiration, phonation, resonation, articulation, and prosody. Depending on the type of dysarthria, deficits in some of these components will be more evident than in others. For example, disorders of phonation, resonation, articulation, and prosody are common in spastic dysarthria, but problems with respiration are rare. In other conditions, such as middle stage Huntington's disease, problems with all five components can be equally observable. The determining factor is the part of the motor system affected by the disorder that causes the dysarthria.

Speech Characteristics of Flaccid Dysarthria

Flaccid dysarthria is caused by lower motor neuron damage to the cranial and spinal nerves. Because these nerves are involved in all aspects of speech production, flaccid dysarthria has the potential to affect respiration, phonation, resonation, articulation, and prosody.

- **Hypernasality**—Caused by damage to the pharyngeal branch of the vagus nerve (X). Nasal emission, weak pressure consonants, and shortened phrase length also can be evident when hypernasality is present.

- **Imprecise consonant productions**—Errors in bilabial and labiodental phonemes are caused by damage to the facial nerve (VII), and errors in lingual phonemes are caused by damage to the hypoglossal nerve (XII). Rare cases of bilateral trigeminal nerve (V) damage can result in jaw paralysis, which would affect nearly all consonant and vowel productions.

- **Phonatory incompetence**—Incomplete adduction of the vocal folds during phonation is caused by damage to the recurrent nerve branch of the vagus nerve (X).

- **Reduced loudness and shortened phrase length**—Spinal nerve damage can lead to reduced respiratory abilities, resulting in decreased vital capacity and an impaired ability to control exhalations.

- **Monopitch** and **monoloudness**—Weak laryngeal muscles are not able to tense and relax the laryngeal muscles with sufficient strength or speed to produce normal pitch and loudness changes.

Speech Characteristics of Spastic Dysarthria

Spastic dysarthria is the result of bilateral upper motor neuron damage to the pyramidal and extrapyramidal tracts. This type of dysarthria has the potential to affect phonation, resonation, articulation, and prosody. Respiration usually is not affected in cases of this dysarthria.

- **Imprecise consonants**—This deficit may be due to incomplete articulatory contacts and incomplete productions of consonant clusters. Disturbances in voice onset time also may contribute to the client's articulation problems. Vowel distortions are sometimes noted as well.

- **Harsh or strained-strangled vocal quality**—Harsh vocal quality is caused by small amounts of air leaking through a slightly open glottis during phonation. Strained-strangled vocal quality is the result of air being pushed through a tightly constricted glottis. Low pitch also can be evident in the phonation of clients with spastic dysarthria.

- **Hypernasality**—This resonance deficit is common in this dysarthria. It is most likely caused by spasticity and weakness in the velar muscles, which reduces range of motion and slows velar movement.

- **Monopitch** and **monoloudness**—Both of these prosodic errors are caused by spasticity in the laryngeal muscles, which reduces the speed and flexibility of their contractions. The quick variations in vocal fold tension needed to adjust pitch and loudness are thereby impaired. Shortened phrases and slow rate of speech also are associated with spastic dysarthria.

Speech Characteristics of Unilateral Upper Motor Neuron Dysarthria

Unilateral upper motor neuron dysarthria is the result of damage to the upper motor neurons in one hemisphere of the brain. It is mostly a mild or moderate deficit of articulation that affects muscles of the lower face and tongue on the side of the head opposite the lesion. The other parts of the speech mechanism (e.g., velum, larynx, jaw, and pharynx) are rarely affected by this type of damage; consequently, resonance, respiration, phonation, and prosody are usually within normal limits.

- **Imprecise consonants**—Weakness in the half of the tongue and lower face opposite the lesion cause these articulation errors, which are frequently heard in labial and lingual phonemes.

- **Harsh vocal quality**—Sometimes is noted in a small number of clients with this type of dysarthria, perhaps because of mild vocal fold weakness following the event that caused the unilateral upper motor neuron damage.

- **Hypernasality**—Also can be heard in a few clients with unilateral upper motor neuron dysarthria, possibly because of mild velar weakness.

Speech Characteristics of Ataxic Dysarthria

Ataxic dysarthria is the result of damage to the cerebellum or the neural tracts that connect the cerebellum to the rest of the central nervous system. Articulation and prosody deficits are the primary speech characteristics of this dysarthria, although other components of speech production can be affected as well. The speech errors in this dysarthria occur when the cerebellum's ability to control the speed, direction, force, and timing of movement is impaired.

- **Imprecise consonants**—These errors are the result of the uncoordinated movements that are characteristic of ataxia. Vowel distortions also may be present in the speech of some individuals with this dysarthria.

- **Irregular articulatory breakdowns**—This is another articulation disorder that can be present in ataxic dysarthria. These articulatory errors occur intermittently during connected speech, and they can affect both consonants and vowels. Perceptually, irregular articulatory breakdowns sound as if the phonemes in a syllable have been compressed together; these breakdowns tend to occur in sentences with multisyllabic words.

- **Equal and excess stress**—This prosodic error occurs when an individual with ataxic dysarthria puts equal stress on syllables and words that should have varying stress patterns. It gives the impression that each syllable or word is being produced independently of the surrounding words. It can sometimes give the speaker's prosody a "robotic" quality.

- **Prolonged phonemes** and **prolonged intervals between phonemes**—Cerebellar damage can result in the slowing of movement, which can affect the speech muscles. These two errors contribute to the slow rate of speech that can be observed in ataxic dysarthria.

- **Monopitch** and **monoloudness**—These two prosodic errors probably are caused by hypotonia (reduced muscle tone) in the larynx.

- **Harsh vocal quality**—Although there are not many phonatory deficits in ataxic dysarthria, harsh vocal quality may be observed in a few clients. It most likely is the result of hypotonia in the larynx.

- **Exaggerated** or **paradoxical respiratory movements**—These difficulties can be the result of poorly coordinated respiratory muscles. The exaggerated movements sometimes can cause excessive loudness variations during conversation. Paradoxical movements occur when the intercostal muscles and the diaphragm do not contract in a coordinated manner, often directly working against each other during inhalation or exhalation. The result is reduced vital capacity for speech production.

Speech Characteristics of Hypokinetic Dysarthria

Hypokinetic dysarthria is almost exclusively associated with idiopathic Parkinson's disease. Articulation and prosody errors are the most obvious impairments in this dysarthria, but phonatory and respiratory errors also can be observed. Resonation deficits are rare. In general, these speech production difficulties are primarily caused by slow speed of movement and reduced range of motion (bradykinesia), difficulty in starting movements (akinesia), and muscle rigidity.

- **Imprecise consonants**—Many of these articulation errors are caused by reduced range of motion in the articulators, making stop consonants sound like fricatives and distorting other consonants (Duffy, 2005).

- **Monopitch** and **monoloudness**—These errors may be the result of reduced range of motion in laryngeal muscles, as well as a general lack of stamina in the contractions of those muscles. Related to these errors of prosody is **reduced stress** on syllables and words.

- **Inappropriate silences**—Because of akinesia, individuals with this dysarthria sometimes have difficulty initiating voluntary movements. These moments of silence may last for only a few seconds and usually occur at the beginning of utterances.

- **Increased rate of speech**—Noted in about 20% of individuals with hypokinetic dysarthria, it can give their speech a blurred quality and contribute to the imprecise consonant errors mentioned previously. Hypokinetic dysarthria is the only dysarthria where increased rate of speech can be present.

- **Short rushes of speech**—These bursts of speed during connected speech are more common than constantly increased rates of speech. They sometimes are preceded by a short pause, which can give their prosody a stop-and-go quality.

- **Harsh** or **breathy vocal quality**—These phonatory errors are probably the result of vocal folds that do not fully adduct during speech, allowing small amounts of air to make turbulent, "friction of air" sounds while passing through the glottis. In the most severe cases, a client's phonation will be not much more than a whisper.

- **Reduced vital capacity for speech**—Several respiratory deficits have been noted in this dysarthria, including paradoxical movements of the intercostal muscles and the diaphragm, reduced range of movement for respiratory muscles, and shortened breathing cycles. Any of these can produce shallow breath support for speech production.

Speech Characteristics of Hyperkinetic Dysarthria

Hyperkinetic dysarthria is the result of involuntary movements that interfere with the voluntary movements needed for speech production. There are a number of conditions that can cause this dysarthria, all of them having hyperkinesia as a common symptom. The types of speech errors present in hyperkinetic dysarthria are dependent on (a) which speech muscles are affected and (b) the severity of the involuntary movements. Some disorders like myoclonus may have only minor effects on speech production. Palatopharyngolaryngeal myoclonus typically can only be heard during prolonged vowel productions but not in connected speech. Other disorders like a focal lingual dystonia can so severely affect the speech mechanism that intelligible speech is impossible. Here is a partial listing of the speech errors that can occur in hyperkinetic dysarthria:

- Imprecise consonants
- Prolonged intervals between syllables or words
- Variable rate of speech
- Monopitch
- Inappropriate silences
- Excessive loudness variations
- Rapid inhalations or exhalations
- Harsh or strained-strangled vocal quality
- Irregular articulatory breakdowns
- Monoloudness
- Voice stoppage
- Short phrases
- Prolonged phonemes
- Distorted vowels
- Hypernasality

Speech Characteristics of Mixed Dysarthria

Mixed dysarthria may occur whenever a disorder affects more than one portion of the motor system. As mentioned previously, nearly any combination of the six pure dysarthrias can combine to form a mixed dysarthria, depending on the cause. Only a combination of spastic and unilateral upper motor neuron dysarthria is impossible. The speech characteristics of mixed dysarthria depend on the severity and extent of the damage. Damage that extends more or less equally to two or more parts of the motor system can result in a mixed dysarthria whose speech characteristics are equally prominent.

It is difficult to provide a concise list of speech characteristics for mixed dysarthria because of the numerous disorders and variables that can be involved, but detailed information is available regarding speech production in three conditions: multiple sclerosis, amyotrophic lateral sclerosis, and Wilson's disease. Darley, Brown, and Goldstein (1972) found that most individuals with **multiple sclerosis** did not have dysarthria (59%) and that a significant number (28%) had only minimal problems with their speech. The remaining individuals with this disease demonstrated the following speech production errors:

- Impaired loudness control
- Harsh vocal quality
- Imprecise articulation
- Impaired emphasis (also known as scanning speech)
- Decreased vital capacity
- Hypernasality
- Inappropriate pitch level
- Breathiness
- Increased breath rate
- Sudden articulatory breakdowns

Duffy (2005) indicated that ataxic-spastic mixed dysarthria is common in multiple sclerosis and that pure ataxic or spastic dysarthria also may be present in this disease.

The lower and upper motor neuron degeneration in **amyotrophic lateral sclerosis** causes flaccid-spastic mixed dysarthria in all individuals, although some may demonstrate a pure flaccid or spastic dysarthria early in the disease. This condition's effect on speech can be profound, often resulting in complete unintelligibility in the end stages. Darley, Aronson, and Brown (1969a, 1969b) reported the following speech characteristics of 30 individuals with this disorder:

- Imprecise consonants
- Hypernasality
- Harsh vocal quality
- Slow rate of speech
- Monopitch
- Short phrases

- Distorted vowels
- Low pitch
- Monoloudness
- Excess and equal stress

Wilson's disease is associated with both pure and mixed dysarthria. Berry, Darley, Aronson, and Goldstein (1974) examined the speech of 20 individuals with this disorder and found that ataxic-spastic-hypokinetic mixed dysarthria was common, with any of these three components being more evident in speech than the others. These researchers also noted that instances of pure ataxic, spastic, and hypokinetic dysarthria were present in some of the individuals they examined. Here is a listing of the speech errors noted by Berry et al. (1974) for Wilson's disease:

- Reduced stress
- Monopitch
- Monoloudness
- Imprecise consonants
- Slow rate
- Excess and equal stress
- Irregular articulatory breakdowns
- Hypernasality
- Inappropriate silences

Overview of Assessment of Dysarthria

There are two approaches to assessing dysarthria in adults. The first involves instrumentation to precisely measure the components of the client's speech. Computerized spectrograms of speech waves, aerodynamic measures of phonation, and electromyographic analysis of the larynx are all examples of this type of assessment. The benefits of these procedures include the precision of the measures, the objectivity of the results, and the storage of hard data for future study. When instrumentation is used in treatment, it also can provide instant visual and auditory feedback to clients working to improve their speech productions.

The second category of dysarthria assessment is perceptual. This procedure primarily uses the examiner's ears (and eyes) to detect the presence of dysarthria. Because the ear is the "real life" judge of whether dysarthria is present, it can be considered to be the most important item in the clinician's toolbox. This chapter will concentrate on the perceptual assessment of dysarthria. There are several reasons for this. First, a majority of clinicians do not have access to the equipment needed to perform an instrumental assessment. They must rely on their ears out of necessity. Second, because of limited access to speech analysis equipment, many clinicians have not had the practice needed to competently perform an instrumental assessment of dysarthria. Third, there are many excellent resources already published on instrumental assessment; the reader is urged to seek out those textbooks for further information.

Standardized Tests for Dysarthria

Compared to other adult communication disorders (such as aphasia), there are relatively few published standardized tests for dysarthria. One potential reason for this is the wide availability of detailed, informal dysarthria assessment tools inside a number of textbooks. Duffy (2005), McNeil (1997), and Yorkston, Beukelman, Strand, and Hakel (2010) each include complete assessment tools for dysarthria in their chapters on assessment of motor speech disorders. Nevertheless, the stand-alone standardized tests that are available do provide a few special features that are not found in the textbook-based assessments:

- *Frenchay Dysarthria Assessment-2* (Enderby & Palmer, 2008)—First published in 1983, the *Frenchay Dysarthria Assessment-2* is unique in that it is the only published test that aids in the differential diagnosis of the various dysarthrias and provides information on intelligibility. Moreover, this test also suggests which elements of the client's speech most affect intelligibility, something that can assist in developing treatment goals. The client's performance on a variety of tasks (reflexes, respiration, lips and tongue at rest and during movement, velopharyngeal closure, laryngeal function, and intelligibility for words, sentences, and conversation) is rated on a 9-point scale. The administration time is reasonably short. The authors report good intra- and inter-rater reliability and validity. Normative data are provided for ages 12 to 97 and for clients with specific types of dysarthria.

- *Assessment of Intelligibility of Dysarthric Speech* (Yorkston & Beukelman, 1981)— This test is a widely used standardized assessment of intelligibility. It examines single-word and sentence intelligibility of speakers with dysarthria. It also provides data on speaking rate. For the single-word assessment task, clients are asked to randomly read 50 words while being audiotaped. Later, a naïve listener judges the client's productions for intelligibility by listening to the audio recording. By determining the total number of words spoken and the total number that were correctly understood by the listener, a percent of intelligible words is easily calculated. A similar procedure is used for assessing sentence intelligibility. The client randomly reads 22 sentences, ranging in length from 5 to 15 words, while again being audiotaped. The naïve listener then transcribes the words in the sentences while listening to the recording, and thereby provides a percentage of words that was understood correctly. The rate of speech is calculated by dividing the time it takes to read the sentences into the total number of words spoken. The *Assessment of Intelligibility of Dysarthric Speech* also is able to provide estimates of severity and communication efficiency (i.e., how close the client's speech is to normal speech).

- *The Speech Intelligibility Test for Windows* (Yorkston, Beukelman, Hakel, & Dorsey, 2007)—This test is an updated version of the *Computerized Assessment of Intelligibility of Dysarthric Speech* (Yorkston, Beukelman, & Traynor, 1984). Like the *Assessment of Intelligibility of Dysarthric Speech*, the *Speech Intelligibility Test for Windows* provides measures of single-word and sentence intelligibility, rate of speech, and communication efficiency. The calculation of scores is done automatically by the computer program, allowing for a quick determination of intelligibility percentages and rate of speech. In addition, the program is able to determine a percentage of correct vowels and consonants (including specific scores for stops, fricatives, affricates, semivowels, nasals and pressure consonants). Interjudge reliability of this test is good.

- *Dysarthria Examination Battery* (Drummond, 1993)—This test was developed at the Arkansas Medical Center for day-to-day clinical use. It contains 15 rating scale items and 21 quantitative tasks. Client performance on these tasks is compared to data in the manual for estimates of severity and treatment suggestions. The *Dysarthria Examination Battery* is organized by speech production subsystems:

  o Respiration—counting, reading the Grandfather passage, resting breathing, maximum phonation time, and related tasks.

  o Phonation—fundamental frequency, intensity range, loudness, and quality of phonation.

  o Resonation—velar elevation, nasal emission, nasal resonance, and related tasks.

  o Articulation—tongue and jaw range of movement, tongue strength, and vowel and consonant productions.

  o Prosody—listener judgments of spontaneous speech and reading aloud, length of sentences, and range of fundamental frequency during sentence productions.

  o Intelligibility—listener judgments of single-word and sentence productions.

  The author does report validity and reliability data, but they tend to be less detailed than those in the previously described dysarthria assessment tools. Clinicians should be aware that the *Dysarthria Examination Battery* requires equipment that may not be available in all work settings. For example, a dry spirometer is needed to determine vital capacity, and speech analysis instrumentation is needed to find a client's fundamental frequency.

Diagnostic Criteria and Differential Diagnosis

Although diagnosing dysarthria can be difficult, especially for the beginning clinician, there are key characteristics or combinations of characteristics that are associated frequently with just one type of dysarthria. For example, phonatory incompetence and hypernasality are found only in flaccid dysarthria. By carefully analyzing a client's oral motor abilities and speech characteristics, even the inexperienced clinician can accurately diagnose dysarthria. The assessment of dysarthria usually begins with an examination of the client's medical records. Here the clinician can find information about a client's awareness and reaction to the problem, relevant medical history, educational and family background, and medical doctors' reports on their examinations. Of all the material that may be available in the medical chart, site of lesion information often is the most useful in determining the type of dysarthria that may be present.

Site of Lesion Information

Site of lesion information can be an invaluable aid in determining the correct dysarthria diagnosis because damage in specific portions of the central and peripheral nervous system are associated with specific types of dysarthria:

- Flaccid dysarthria—caused by *damage to lower motor neurons* in the cranial and spinal nerves in the peripheral nervous system.

- Spastic dysarthria—caused *by bilateral damage to upper motor neurons* in central nervous system.

- Unilateral upper motor neuron dysarthria—caused by *unilateral damage to upper motor neurons* in the central nervous system.

- Ataxic dysarthria—caused by *damage to the cerebellum* or to the neural tracts that connect the cerebellum to the rest of the central nervous system.

- Hypokinetic dysarthria—caused almost exclusively by *degeneration of neurons in the substantia nigra.*

- Hyperkinetic dysarthria—caused in most instances by *suspected dysfunction in the basal ganglia.*

- Mixed dysarthria—caused by *damage to more than one specific portion of the motor system.*

Although site of lesion information is not always available, it should be one of the first pieces of information the clinician looks for when reviewing the client's medical record.

Assessing the Client

After examining the medical record, the clinician should begin the dysarthria-specific protocols in Chapter 6. When assessing dysarthria, it may be best to concentrate on the oral motor and speech tasks in Chapter 6, rather than use the similar items in Chapter 2. The tasks in Chapter 6 are specifically designed to evoke behaviors that help in the differential diagnosis of dysarthria. The oral motor tasks in Chapter 2 are more general in nature and are appropriate for assessing the other adult communication disorders. Because there are certain assessment items that are particularly effective in evoking the speech production errors associated with specific types of dysarthria, the clinician should pay special attention to the client's performance on the tasks described in the following paragraphs.

Diagnosing Flaccid Dysarthria

The assessment tasks in Chapter 6 that may be particularly useful in detecting key characteristics of flaccid dysarthria include the following:

- *Vowel prolongation* can produce the breathy voice quality that is typical of phonatory incompetence as well as the respiratory weakness that can shorten the length of the client's production of the vowel.

- *Alternate motion rates* can evoke the slow production of phonemes that is common in this dysarthria.

- *Connected speech* during conversation or while reading aloud can evoke a client's monopitch and monoloud prosody, shortened phrases, articulation distortions, and hypernasality.

There are a number of physical symptoms and speech errors that are more characteristic of flaccid dysarthria than of the other dysarthrias. When any of the following are noted during the motor speech assessment in Chapter 6, the client may have flaccid dysarthria:

- Diminished or absent oral reflexes (e.g., gag reflex)—this contrasts with the hyperreflexes that can be present in spastic dysarthria.

- Muscle atrophy in the muscles of the speech mechanism—atrophy is the result of lower motor damage (which also is the cause of flaccid dysarthria).

- The combination of hypernasality and phonatory incompetence is a strong indicator of flaccid dysarthria.

- Inhalatory stridor (audible phonation during inhalation) suggests laryngeal weakness that often is associated with flaccid dysarthria.

- Diplophonia is more often associated with flaccid dysarthria than any other dysarthria.

Diagnosing Spastic Dysarthria

The assessment tasks in Chapter 6 that may be particularly useful in detecting key characteristics of spastic dysarthria include the following:

- *Vowel prolongation* can reveal the low pitch and harsh or strain-strangled vocal quality associated with this dysarthria.

- *Alternate motion rates* will highlight the slowed phoneme production often found in spastic dysarthria.

- *Connected speech* during conversation or reading aloud can reveal the client's monopitch and monoloud prosody, shortened phrases, articulation distortions, and hypernasality.

There are a number of the physical symptoms and speech errors more characteristic of spastic dysarthria than of the other dysarthrias. When any of the following are noted during the motor speech assessment in Chapter 6, the client may have spastic dysarthria:

- Hyperactive oral reflexes (such as an excessively sensitive gag reflex) contrast with the reduced or diminished reflexes that can be present in flaccid dysarthria.

- Pseudobulbar affect and drooling are more common in this dysarthria than the others.

- The combination of slow speech rate and harsh or strained-strangled vocal quality is unique to spastic dysarthria.

Diagnosing Unilateral Upper Motor Neuron Dysarthria

The assessment tasks in Chapter 6 that may be particularly useful in detecting key characteristics of unilateral upper motor neuron dysarthria include the following:

- The motor speech examination will reveal weakness on one side of the *lower face and tongue*. Weakness will not be evident in the upper face muscles.
- *Vowel prolongation* may reveal the harsh vocal quality that is present in a few individuals with this dysarthria.
- *Alternate motion rate* may reveal slightly slowed phoneme production.
- *Connected speech* during conversation or reading aloud can reveal the imprecise consonants present in unilateral upper motor neuron dysarthria.

There are a number of physical symptoms and speech errors more characteristic of unilateral upper motor neuron dysarthria than of the other dysarthrias. When any of the following are noted during the motor speech assessment in Chapter 6, the client may have unilateral upper motor neuron dysarthria:

- Unilateral weakness in the lower face and tongue is common in this dysarthria.
- Oral reflexes usually are within normal limits—absent or hyperactive reflexes are not observed.
- A mild to moderate articulation deficit is the primary deficit in this dysarthria, although mild hypernasality or harsh vocal quality can be noted in a few clients with this dysarthria.
- Muscle atrophy is not observed in unilateral upper motor dysarthria.

Diagnosing Ataxic Dysarthria

The assessment tasks in Chapter 6 that may be particularly useful in detecting key characteristics of ataxic dysarthria include the following:

- *Alternate motion rates* can be particularly effective in diagnosing ataxic dysarthria. Clients with this dysarthria will have significant difficulty maintaining a regular rhythm during their productions. They will tend to speed up and slow down in an irregular pattern during this task. Moreover, they also may demonstrate inconsistent fluctuations in loudness and articulatory accuracy while saying the target syllables.
- *Connected speech* during conversation or reading aloud can reveal the irregular articulatory breakdowns that are common to ataxic dysarthria, especially if there are multisyllabic words in the topic of conversation or reading material.

There are a number of physical symptoms and speech errors more characteristic of ataxic dysarthria than of the other dysarthrias. When any of the following are noted during the motor speech assessment in Chapter 6, the client may have ataxic dysarthria:

- There tends to be a generalized uncoordinated quality to the connected speech, often described as "sounding like being drunk."

- Alternate motion rates and connected speech can evoke irregular articulatory breakdowns and inconsistent difficulties in maintaining consistent loudness.

- Alternate motion rates also can reveal difficulty in maintaining a regular rhythm during productions of the target syllables.

Diagnosing Hypokinetic Dysarthria

The assessment tasks in Chapter 6 that may be particularly useful in detecting key characteristics of hypokinetic dysarthria include the following:

- *Alternate motion rates* can evoke varied articulation rates, imprecise consonants, and blurred syllables.

- *Vowel prolongations* can reveal breathy vocal quality and shallow breath support.

- *Connected speech* in conversation or while reading aloud can highlight the prosodic errors of this dysarthria (monopitch, monoloudness, inappropriate silences, reduced stress) and the presence of increased speech rate.

There are a number of physical symptoms and speech errors more characteristic of hypokinetic dysarthria than of the other dysarthrias. When any of the following are noted during the motor speech assessment in Chapter 6, the client may have hypokinetic dysarthria:

- A resting tremor and reduced facial expression are indicative of hypokinetic dysarthria.

- An increased rate of speech and blurred phoneme production is only found in hypokinetic dysarthria; however, note that these two deficits are not present in the majority of individuals with this dysarthria. Their absence should not be considered evidence against the diagnosis of hypokinetic dysarthria.

Essential Assessment Tasks for Hyperkinetic Dysarthria

The assessment tasks in Chapter 6 that may be particularly useful in detecting key characteristics of hyperkinetic dysarthria include the following:

- During the motor speech assessment, be alert for the particular involuntary movements that are associated with specific hyperkinetic disorders. For example, myoclonic movements tend to be brief muscle contractions of a single muscle or a single body part, and essential tremor is an action tremor that mostly affects the head, arms, and hands.

- *Connected speech* in conversation or while reading aloud may provide the best opportunity to evoke the speech errors of hyperkinetic dysarthria. These tasks can reveal the respiratory, phonatory, articulatory, and prosodic errors that are common to this dysarthria.

- *Vowel prolongations* can demonstrate the harsh vocal quality that is sometimes present in hyperkinetic dysarthria. They also are useful for revealing involuntary contractions of the larynx that do not affect connected speech, such as in mild cases of essential voice tremor or palatopharyngolaryngeal myoclonus.

- *Alternate motion rates* can help identify the speech rate variability and irregular articulatory breakdowns.

There are physical symptoms and speech errors more characteristic of hyperkinetic dysarthria than of the other dysarthrias. When any of the following are noted during the motor speech assessment in Chapter 6, the client may have hyperkinetic dysarthria:

- Duffy (2005) indicated that only essential tremor and palatopharyngolaryngeal myoclonus produce regular muscular contractions; other types of hyperkinetic dysarthria are associated with more sustained or irregular involuntary movements.

- The hyperkinetic movements that cause this type of dysarthria often can be observed even when the client is not speaking. In other types of dysarthria, the motor deficits causing the speech problem are noted only while the client is speaking (Duffy, 2005).

Postassessment Counseling

Conclude the dysarthria assessment with postassessment counseling of the client and family. During this session, the clinician shares the assessment information with the client, accompanying family members, and other caregivers. Subsequent to the postassessment counseling, the clinician makes an analysis of information obtained from the case history and interview, reports from other specialists, clinical assessment results, instrumental evaluations, and results of questionnaires or other tests. Integrating the information collected from all sources and means, the clinician writes a diagnostic report. See Chapter 1 for details on the analysis and integration of assessment data and clinical report writing.

During the postassessment counseling session, the clinician makes a diagnosis, offers recommendations, and suggests a prognosis. The clinician also answers questions from the client and the family members about the disorder and the planned clinical services.

Make a Tentative Diagnosis

Although a final analysis of assessment results may not be completed yet, the clinician nonetheless will have come to tentative but generally valid clinical conclusions at the end of the assessment session. The clinician can make statements about the nature of the speech disorder, its prognosis, and treatment options. The clinician might describe the client's speech characteristics (e.g., imprecise consonants, harsh vocal quality, hypernasality) that justify the diagnosis. The clinician also might point out disorders that are *not* indicated by the assessment. For example, a client may worry that changes in speech are early signs of a degenerative condition such as Parkinson's disease. If the medical reports and the dysarthria assessment rule out this type of disorder, the clinician should share this important information with the client.

Make Recommendations

The clinician may recommend treatment for the dysarthria, depending on the type and severity of the disorder. Whether the client has had a medical evaluation for the speech problem or the SLP is the first professional to be consulted will determine the immediate course of action, however. A client with possible neurological involvement should be referred to a neurologist if this has not already been done.

Suggest a Prognosis

It usually is difficult to make a firm prognosis for improved speech production in clients with dysarthria because of the numerous variables that are involved. A few of these variables include the cause and severity of the dysarthria, the motivation of the client, and the circumstances in which the client needs to communicate. Co-occurring conditions such as aphasia or apraxia of speech also make it difficult to offer an accurate prognosis. In general, individuals with a mild or moderate dysarthria (that is not caused by a degenerative disorder) can expect to show some improved speech production with treatment. The extent of the improvement will not be known during the postassessment counseling session, so it often is wise to avoid specific predictions when discussing the prognosis with the client and family. Some individuals with severe dysarthria also can show improved speech production with treatment, but the gains typically take longer and are less pronounced than for individuals with milder dysarthria. Other individuals with severe dysarthria (or dysarthria due to a degenerative disease) will not show improved speech production, and the treatment options for them might involve alternative and augmentative communication procedures.

Answer the Client's Questions

The client and family members will have questions about dysarthria and its treatment during the postassessment counseling session. They deserve honest and scientifically justified answers. Some commonly encountered questions and their answers are described here, but the clinician should be ready for other questions. Clients with complicated medical conditions will have additional questions specific to those conditions. The clinician also needs to modify the terms to suit the educational level of the client and the accompanying family members.

> ***What causes dysarthria?*** Dysarthria has many causes. In some individuals, it is caused by strokes, physical trauma, degenerative diseases, infections, and a number of other conditions. [*The clinician provides an explanation of dysarthria, give examples.*] An injury that damages the nerve that innervates the tongue is one cause of dysarthria. In other individuals, dysarthria can be the result of a stroke that prevents normal muscle contractions. Treatment in such cases is initially medical, followed by speech therapy once the condition is stabilized. Several neurological diseases that affect the vocal fold functioning are known to cause dysarthria along with other types of communication problems. For example, Parkinson's disease can cause speech and voice disorders. [*The clinician addresses the client's specific type of voice disorder and gives more details.*]

How long does it take to treat dysarthria effectively? It depends on the type of dysarthria. Some take more time than others. In a few conditions, there really is little that can be done to improve a client's speech. Certain types of dysarthria may need medical attention before or during speech therapy; this tends to extend the treatment time. Usually, the progress will be faster if we start the treatment soon and we are consistent than if we delay it or have frequent interruptions. We offer treatment twice a week. [*If not, the clinician gives the actual schedule.*] If you work at home on our assignments and family members offer support, the progress might be even better. As you can guess, more severe problems and a problem with additional medical complications will take more time. [*The clinician expands the answer to give additional information relevant to the client's dysarthria.*]

What are some of the treatment options? There are a great many treatment options for dysarthria. The type of recommended treatment depends on the type of dysarthria and its severity. Some types of dysarthria are primarily managed medically, such as the use of Botox to treat certain movement disorders (e.g., essential voice tremor, spasmodic dysphonia, focal dystonia) and the prescription of levodopa for Parkinson's disease. Other types of treatment use a prosthetic device to compensate for the dysarthria. Examples of this include a portable amplifier to boost loudness in hypokinetic dysarthria, a palatal lift to reduce the hypernasality in flaccid dysarthria, and a bite block to stabilize the jaw in hyperkinetic dysarthria. A third category of treatment is behavioral in nature, meaning that the clinician and client work together to minimize the effects of the dysarthria on speech production and enhance the client's ability to produce the most natural sounding speech possible. These techniques generally are applied to specific speech errors. For instance, minimal contrast drills and phonetic placement tasks are used to treat articulation errors; intonation drills and contrastive stress tasks address prosody errors. In addition, clinicians often use a combination of effective procedures—intelligibility drills are easily combined with phonetic placement tasks during the same treatment activity. [*The clinician expands the answer to give more treatment information relevant to the client's dysarthria.*]

When do we start treatment? It usually is better to start treatment as soon as possible. The sooner we start, the better might be the outcome. [*The clinician gives additional information, depending on whether the client needs to be referred to other specialists before starting treatment; also, depending on the service setting, the clinician tells when and how the treatment might begin.*]

References

Berry, W. R., Darley, F. L., Aronson, A. E., & Goldstein, N. P. (1974). Dysarthria in Wilson's disease. *Journal of Speech and Hearing Research, 17,*169–183.

Darley, F. L., Aronson, A. E., & Brown, J. R. (1969a). Clusters of deviant speech dimensions in the dysarthrias. *Journal of Speech and Hearing Research, 12,* 462–496.

Darley, F. L., Aronson, A. E., & Brown, J. R. (1969b). Differential diagnostic patterns of dysarthria. *Journal of Speech and Hearing Research, 12,* 246–269.

Darley, F. L., Brown, J.R., & Goldstein, N. P. (1972). Dysarthria in multiple sclerosis. *Journal of Speech and Hearing Research, 15,* 229–245.

Drummond, S. (1993). *Dysarthria Examination Battery.* San Antonio, TX: Communication Skills Builders.

Duffy, J. R. (2005). *Motor speech disorders: Substrates, differential diagnosis, and management* (2nd ed.). St. Louis, MO: Elsevier Mosby.

Duffy, J. R., & Folger, N. W. (1986, November). *Dysarthria in unilateral central nervous system lesions.* Paper presented at the annual meeting of the American Speech-Language-Hearing Association. Detroit, MI.

Enderby, P., & Palmer, R. (2008). *Frenchay dysarthria assessment.* (2nd ed.). Austin, TX: Pro-Ed.

Heilman, K. M., Watson, R. T., & Greer, M. (1977). *Handbook for differential diagnosis of neurologic signs and symptoms.* New York, NY: Appleton-Century-Crofts.

Linebaugh, C. W. (1979). The dysarthrias of Shy-Drager syndrome. *Journal of Speech and Hearing Disorders, 44,* 55–60.

McNeil, M. R. (1997) *Clinical management of sensorimotor speech disorders.* New York, NY: Thieme.

Ramig, L. O., Fox, C., & Sapir, S. (2004, May). Parkinson's disease: Speech and voice disorders and their treatment with the Lee Silverman Voice Treatment. *Seminars in Speech and Language, 25*(2), 169–180.

Yorkston, K. M., & Beukelman, D. R. (1981). *Assessment of intelligibility of dysarthric speech.* Austin, TX: Pro-Ed.

Yorkston, K. M., Beukelman, D. R., & Traynor, C. (1984*). Computerized assessment of intelligibility of dysarthric speech: A computerized assessment tool.* Austin, TX: Pro-Ed.

Yorkston, K., Beukelman, D., Hakel, M., & Dorsey, M. (2007). *Speech intelligibility test for windows.* Lincoln, NE: Institute for Rehabilitation Science and Engineering at Madonna Rehabilitation Hospital.

Yorkston, K., Beukelman, D., Strand, E., & Bell, K. (1999). *Management of motor speech disorders in children and adults.* Austin, TX: Pro-Ed.

CHAPTER 6

Assessment of Dysarthria: Protocols

- Overview of Dysarthria Protocols
- Interview Protocol
- Dysarthria Assessment Protocol 1: Orofacial Examination
- Dysarthria Assessment Protocol 2: Respiratory and Phonatory Function
- Dysarthria Assessment Protocol 3: Speech Production (Articulation)
- Dysarthria Assessment Protocol 4: Production of Prosody
- Dysarthria Assessment Protocol 5: Resonance

Overview of Dysarthria Protocols

Assessment protocols provided in this chapter help assess dysarthria in adults in an efficient manner. The protocols offer ready-made formats that clinicians can use in structuring their client and family interviews and assessing various parameters of dysarthria.

The protocols offered in this chapter also are available on the accompanying CD. The clinician may print the needed protocols in evaluating his or her clients. The clinician may combine these protocols in suitable ways to facilitate the evaluation of an adult's dysarthria.

In assessing adults with multiple disorders, the clinician may combine these protocols with protocols from other chapters. For example, the clinician may combine the dysarthria assessment protocols with apraxia of speech assessment protocols (Chapter 4) or aphasia assessment protocols (Chapter 8).

The protocols given in this chapter are specific to dysarthria in adults. To complete the assessment on a given client, the clinician should combine these disorder-specific protocols with the common assessment protocols given in Chapter 2:

- The Adult Case History
- Orofacial Examination and Hearing Screening Protocol
- Diadochokinetic Assessment Protocol for Adults
- Adult Assessment Report Outline

Assessment of Dysarthria: Interview Protocol

Name _____ DOB _____ Date _____ Clinician _____

Individualize this protocol on the CD and print it for your use.

Preparation

- Review the guidelines given under *The Initial Clinical Interview* in Chapter 1.
- Arrange for comfortable seating and lighting.
- Record the interview on audio or video.
- Initially interview the client alone and then have the accompanying person join the interview.
- Review the case history ahead of time and take note of areas you want to explore during the interview.

Introduction

Introduce yourself. Describe the assessment plan and tell the client the time it will take.

> **Example:** "Hello Mr. / Mrs. [*client's name*]. My name is [*your name*] I am the speech-language pathologist who will be assessing you today. I would like to start by reviewing the case history and asking you a few questions. After we finish talking, I will work with you. Today's assessment should take about [*estimate the amount of time you plan to spend*]."

Interview Questions

The questions are generally directed toward the adult client with suspected dysarthria. When interviewing the client and the accompanying person together, it is essential to pose the same, but reworded, question to the accompanying person. A few examples are shown within the brackets; the clinician may use this strategy whenever necessary.

- What is your main concern regarding your speech? [What do you think is his (her) main problem?]
- How would you describe your speech problem? [How would you describe her (his) speech problem?]
- When did you first notice that your speech was different? [When did you notice that his (her) speech was different?
- Has your speech changed over time? If so, how?
- Have you seen your family doctor about your speech?
- Did your family doctor refer you to a specialist?
- What did the doctor(s) tell you?

(continues)

Assessment Dysarthria: Interview Protocol (continued)

- Besides a speech problem, are you concerned with any aspects of your talking?

- How would you describe these other talking problems? [How would you describe his (her) overall speech?]

- Are there times when your speech is better or worse? For example, is it better in the morning than in the evening? [Do you also think her (his) speech varies throughout the day?]

- Do you believe that your speech problem is affecting your social interactions? Would you describe how?

- Do you think that your speech problem is affecting your job performance? How is it affected?

- Has anyone else in your family ever experienced speech problems?

- Do you have any other chronic health conditions or concerns?

- Are you currently on any medications?

- It looks like I have most of the information I wanted from you. Do you have any questions for me at this point?

- Thank you for your information. It will be helpful in my assessment. I will now work with you to better understand your speech problem. When we are done, we will discuss our findings.

Review the case history again and ask additional questions if needed.

Dysarthria Assessment Protocol 1: Orofacial Examination

Name _____ DOB _____ Date _____ Clinician _____

Individualize this protocol on the CD and print it for your use. 💿

Instructions: Answer the following questions about the client's orofacial abilities. The clinician also may make an estimate of severity (0 = *No deficit*, 1 = *Mild*, 2 = *Moderate*, 3 = *Severe*).

Assessment of Face Muscles at Rest	Yes	No	Severity
1. Is the mouth symmetrical while at rest? If there is drooping to one side, which side of the mouth is affected?			
2. Can you separate the client's lips while she (he) tries to keep the mouth closed?			
3. When the client raises the eyebrows, do you observe wrinkling on both sides of the forehead? If not, which side does not show wrinkling?			
4. Are both of the client's eyes fully open? If not, which side is not fully open?			
Assessment of Face Muscles during Movement			
1. Is the client's smile symmetrical? If not, which side is drooping?			
2. When the client puckers the lips, is the "pucker" symmetrical?			
3. When the client puffs out the cheeks, can the lips hold their seal when the clinician squeezes the cheeks?			
Assessment of the Jaw Muscles			
1. Can the client fully elevate the jaw?			
2. Can the client keep the jaw open when the clinician tries to close it?			
3. Can the client keep the jaw closed when the clinician tries to open it?			
4. Can the client move the jaw from side to side?			

(continues)

Dysarthria Assessment Protocol 1: Orofacial Examination (continued)

Assessment of Tongue Muscles at Rest	Yes	No	Severity
1. Is the tongue size normal?			
2. Does the tongue rest symmetrically in the mouth?			
3. Is the shape of the tongue symmetrical? If not, describe how it is asymmetrical.			
4. Are involuntary tongue movements observable? If so, describe them.			
Assessment of Tongue Muscles during Movement			
1. Is the client able to fully protrude the tongue?			
2. Does the tongue deviate to one side when it is protruded? If so, to which side does it deviate?			
3. Can the tongue tip reach the alveolar ridge?			
4. Can the tongue tip reach the upper lip?			
5. When the tongue is protruded, can the client keep it near midline while the clinician tries to move it left or right?			
6. When the tongue tip pushes out the cheek, can the clinician readily push the cheek back in? If so, on which side is it easier to "push in"?			
Assessment of Gross Velar Movement			
1. Each time the client says "Ah," does the velum rise symmetrically?			
Assessment of Basic Laryngeal Function			
1. Can the client produce a sharp cough?			
2. Can the client produce a sharp glottal stop?			
3. When the client inhales quickly, is stridor present?			
Clinician's summative statement			

Dysarthria Assessment Protocol 2: Respiratory and Phonatory Function

Name _____ DOB _____ Date _____ Clinician _____

Individualize this protocol on the CD and print it for your use. 💿

Instructions: Answer the following questions about the client's respiratory and phonatory abilities. The clinician also may make an estimate of severity (0 = *No deficit*, 1 = *Mild*, 2 = *Moderate*, 3 = *Severe*).

Assessment of Respiratory and Phonatory Function	Yes	No	Severity
1. **After taking the deepest breath possible, how long can the client prolong an "Ah"?**			
Duration of trial one:			
Duration of trial two:			
Duration of trial three:			
2. **Judge the loudness of the client's phonation**			
Is loudness normal?			
Is loudness excessive?			
Is loudness reduced?			
3. **Judge the quality of the client's phonation**			
Is the phonation steady and clear?			
Is there evidence of harshness?			
Is there evidence of breathiness?			
Is there evidence of hypernasality?			
Is diplophonia present?			
4. **Judge the pitch of the client's phonation**			
Is the pitch normal?			
Is the pitch too high?			
Is the pitch too low?			
Is a tremor present in the phonation?			
Are there pitch breaks in the phonation?			
Clinician's summative statement			

Dysarthria Assessment Protocol 3:
Speech Production (Articulation)

Name _____ DOB _____ Date _____ Clinician _____

Individualize this protocol on the CD and print it for your use.

Instructions: Answer the following questions about the client's articulation abilities. The clinician also may make an estimate of severity (0 = *No deficit*, 1 = *Mild*, 2 = *Moderate*, 3 = *Severe*). Normal rates for Alternate Motion Rates (AMRs) are approximately 6 productions per second, although "kuh" productions may be slightly slower (Kent, Kent, & Rosenbek, 1987).

Assessment of Alternate Motion Rates (AMRs)	Yes	No	Severity
1. Have the client take a single, deep breath and say "puh-puh-puh" as rapidly and evenly as possible. Demonstrate.			
Duration of trial one:			
Duration of trial two:			
Duration of trial three:			
2. Now have the client say "tuh-tuh-tuh" as rapidly and evenly as possible. Demonstrate.			
Duration of trial one:			
Duration of trial two:			
Duration of trial three:			
3. Now have the client say "kuh-kuh-kuh" as rapidly and evenly as possible. Demonstrate			
Duration of trial one:			
Duration of trial two:			
Duration of trial three:			
4. Judge the quality of the client's AMRs.			
Are the AMRs slower than normal?			
Are the AMRs faster than normal?			
Are the AMRs produced evenly (i.e., rhythmically)?			
Is the client's pitch normal during productions?			
Is the client's loudness within normal limits?			
Is tremor evident in the productions?			

Assessment of Alternate Motion Rates (AMRs)	Yes	No	Severity
Is the articulation clear and precise?			
Is resonation normal?			
Is nasal emission present?			
Is there normal range of movement in the jaw and lips?			
Is articulatory groping present?			
Is an obvious delay evident before the productions?			
Assessment of Sequential Motion Rate (SMR)	**Yes**	**No**	**Severity**
1. Have the client take a single, deep breath and say "puh-tuh-kuh" as rapidly and evenly as possible. Demonstrate.			
Duration of trial one:			
Duration of trial two:			
Duration of trial three:			
2. Judge the quality of the client's SMR.			
Are the productions of each syllable smooth?			
Are there hesitations, substitutions, or omissions of phonemes?			
Are there transpositions of phonemes?			
Clinician's summative statement			

Dysarthria Assessment Protocol 4: Production of Prosody

Name _____ DOB _____ Date _____ Clinician _____

Individualize this protocol on the CD and print it for your use. ⊙

Instructions: Have the client perform the following tasks, and judge the client's ability to accurately produce prosody. The clinician also may make an estimate of severity (0 = *No deficit*, 1 = *Mild*, 2 = *Moderate*, 3 = *Severe*). These tasks have been adapted from Vogel and Cannito (2001).

Assessment of Prosody	Correct	Incorrect	Severity
1. Have the client say each of these sentences with the appropriate rising (question) or falling (statement) intonation.			
She went home?			
She went home.			
We are going to be late?			
We are going to be late.			
The food is in the basket?			
The food is in the basket.			
Oh, you don't like that?			
Oh, you don't like that.			
2. Have the client say each of the following sentences with the correct emotional intonation.			
(Happy) He is coming back today.			
(Happy) I passed the test.			
(Happy) I was so glad to meet her.			
(Sad) I lost all the money.			
(Sad) My car broke down.			
(Sad) I'm feeling pretty sick.			
(Angry) I can't stand it anymore.			
(Angry) You are not going to do it.			
(Angry) Not if I have anything to say about it.			

Assessment of Prosody	Correct	Incorrect	Severity
3. Have the client read the following sentences, adding emphatic stress on the italicized words.			
Jan threw the football to *her*.			
Jan threw the football to her.			
Jan threw the *football* to her.			
Larry bought the best ring.			
Larry *bought* the best ring.			
Larry bought the best *ring*.			
Sam and Jerry *rode* the red bikes.			
Sam and Jerry rode the *red* bikes.			
Sam and Jerry rode the red *bikes*.			
4. Have the client say the following sentences; listen for a pause at the syntactic juncture.			
When we were younger, he was the best.			
If I don't get to work, we will be in trouble.			
The movie started on time, and it was good.			
If he does it again, he will win.			
When I get enough money, I will quit.			
While I washed the car, he cleaned the kitchen.			
Clinician's summative statement			

Dysarthria Assessment Protocol 5: Resonance

Name _____ DOB _____ Date _____ Clinician _____

Individualize this protocol on the CD and print it for your use. 💿

Instructions: Have the client perform the following tasks that assess the ability to maintain normal resonance. The clinician also may make an estimate of severity (0 = *No deficit*, 1 = *Mild*, 2 = *Moderate*, 3 = *Severe*).

Assessment of Resonance	Yes	No	Severity
1. Have the client produce a prolonged /U/. Hold a dental or laryngeal mirror under each nostril. Look for misting of the mirror during the production of the vowel.			
Leakage from the left nostril?			
Leakage from the right nostril?			
Leakage from both?			
2. Have the client produce a prolonged /U/. With your hand, repeatedly squeeze and release both of the client's nostrils while he or she is producing the vowel.			
Is there a change in resonance when both nostrils are closed?			
3. If you detected a change in resonance on the prior task, have the client produce the vowel again, but this time only occlude one nostril at a time.			
Is there a change in resonance when the LEFT nostril is closed?			
Is there a change in resonance when the RIGHT nostril is closed?			
Clinician's summative statement			

References

Kent, R. D., Kent, J. F., & Rosenbek, J. C. (1987). Maximum performance test of speech production. *Journal of Speech and Hearing Disorders, 52,* 367–387.

Vogel, D., & Cannito, M. P. (Eds.). (2001). *Treating disordered speech motor control* (2nd ed.). Austin, TX: Pro-Ed.

PART III
Assessment of Aphasia

CHAPTER 7

Assessment of Aphasia: Resources

- Epidemiology of Aphasia
- Etiology and Neuropathology of Aphasia
- Characteristics of Aphasia
- Types of Aphasia
- Overview of Assessment
- Screening for Aphasia
- Standardized Tests for Aphasia
- Assessment of Speech Production
- Assessment of Narrative and Conversational Skills
- Assessment of Functional Communication
- Quality of Life Assessment
- Assessment of Bilingual or Multilingual Patients
- Analysis and Integration of Assessment Results
- Postassessment Counseling

Epidemiology of Aphasia

Aphasia is a language disorder due to recent brain injury in people who had acquired and produced language prior to its onset. As such, aphasia is a disorder typically diagnosed in adults. The term implies a partial or near-complete *loss* of preexisting language skills due to brain injury. It is not a failure to learn language skills.

Among the varied definitions, some aphasiologists emphasize impairments in the cognitive functions that underlie language (Chapey, 2001; Davis, 2000), although nonlinguistic cognitive skills are thought to be intact. Others suggest that the aphasic impairments are not limited to language and language-related cognitive skills, but include social limitations as the patient may be unable to fully participate in life events (Simmons-Mackie, 2001). But all experts agree that in aphasia, the language impairments are primary.

Classifying aphasia into different types is a common clinical practice, although many patients cannot be precisely classified (Hegde, 2006). If classified, symptoms in some patients may change over time, rendering their initial classification invalid. Some experts believe that different types of aphasia only suggest different *predominant* symptoms, not exclusively different symptoms (Darley, 1982). Some experts believe it is an overclassified disorder (Benson & Ardilla, 1996).

The prevalence of aphasia in the general population varies with the prevalence of diseases that cause brain injury. The most current statistics related to the prevalence of neurological diseases and associated aphasia may be found at the National Center for Health Statistics and the American Stroke Association. Epidemiological observations related to brain injury and aphasia generally include the following:

- **Strokes are a common cause of aphasia and disability.** About 700,000 new cases of stroke are reported each year; of these 327,000 (47%) are males and 373,000 (53%) are females. About two thirds of all strokes occur in patients age 65 and older. Men have a higher risk of stroke than women, but because of their longevity, more women than men have strokes. About 12% of all mortality is due to strokes. Ischemic strokes are more common than hemorrhagic strokes.

- **Prevalence of strokes is different across ethnocultural groups.** African Americans have higher risk of first stroke than whites. Deaths rates related to strokes are also higher in African Americans than in whites. The death rates are roughly comparable in whites and Asian Americans and lower in Hispanics and Native Americans (http//www.americanheart.org; Horner, Swanson, Bosworth, & Matchar, 2003; Payne 1997). Strokes at younger age (22–44 years) are more common among Hispanics and African Americans than whites.

- **Ethnicity and the type of stroke may be related.** Ischemic strokes are more common in whites than in Hispanics. Native Americans, African Americans, Asian Americans, and Hispanics are more prone to have hemorrhagic strokes than whites.

- **Medical risk factors affect the incidence of strokes**. High blood pressure, smoking, high cholesterol levels, obesity, a poor and high-sodium diet, and lack of exercise increase the chances of stroke.

- **Ethnicity may affect the level of disability due to strokes.** African-American females experience greater levels of disability than any other females or males. White males experience the least amount of stroke-related disability.

Etiology and Neuropathology of Aphasia

In general, the main and the proximal cause of aphasia is damage to the language structures of the brain. There is, nonetheless, a chain of events that causes that brain damage, which in turn causes aphasia. Although strokes are a common cause, there are other neurological events that can cause aphasia. Detailed case history and medical test results will often reveal a series of adverse events culminating in aphasia.

- **Vascular disorders are a common cause of strokes and aphasia.** A patient may have had a particular type of vascular disorder:
  - *A thrombosis is a blood clot within an artery.* It can restrict or block the blood supply to the brain structures that lie beyond the clot. The brain tissue that does not receive oxygenated blood is damaged. Formation of blood clots (*thrombi*) are due to a slowly developing disease process known as *atherosclerosis,* which is narrowing and hardening of the artery due mainly to lipid and calcium deposits. A thrombosis causes *ischemic strokes* that are caused by interrupted blood supply.
  - *Embolism is another arterial disease.* An embolus, typically formed elsewhere, travels through an artery, gets lodged as the artery gets smaller, and thus blocks the blood flow. Brain tissue damage follows. Embolism also causes ischemic strokes.
  - *Aneurysm is a swelling in a thinned-out portion of an artery.* This balloon-like swelling eventually bursts resulting in cerebral hemorrhage and brain damage. Aneurysm causes hemorrhagic strokes.
- **Traumatic brain injury (TBI) may cause strokes and aphasia.** Any type of external force acting on the head can cause injury to the brain, resulting in aphasia in some cases. See Chapter 13 for details on TBI.
- **Brain tumors are an infrequent cause of aphasia.** Three common types of tumors (classified as Grade I, II, III, or IV) are *primary tumors* that grow within the brain, *metastatic tumors* that are migrated into the brain from other parts of the body, and *meningiomas* that grow within the meninges.
- **Brain toxicity may cause strokes and aphasia in some cases.** Toxicity from lead and mercury, prescription drug overdose, drug interactions, and illicit drug abuse may all cause strokes.
- **Several types of infections may cause strokes and aphasia.** Bacterial (e.g., meningitis) as well as viral infections (e.g., mumps, measles, or untreated syphilis) may cause aphasia or aphasic-like symptoms. HIV infection and AIDS also may result in aphasia or dementia.

Characteristics of Aphasia

Although each aphasia type has a few distinguishing characteristics, there are several major characteristics that help to diagnose aphasia. Not all symptoms are found in all clients. The symptoms found across clients tend to vary in their severity. Some symptoms may be dominant, others insignificant, thus suggesting a specific type of aphasia (Hegde, 2006). However, in assessing a client with probable aphasia, the clinician keeps in perspective the following kinds of impairments that help diagnose aphasia, while realizing that the severity of the impairments in specific individuals may vary from negligible to significant:

- **Paraphasia is word and sound substitutions.** Considered fundamental to aphasia, such substitutions that impair communication are considered *unintended,* because being aware of their mistakes, many try to correct them. Several types of paraphasic speech have been described:
  - *Verbal paraphasia may be semantic or random.* Semantic paraphasia is word substitutions that are based on similarity in meaning (e.g., *son* for *daughter*). Random paraphasia is inexplicable.
  - *Neologistic paraphasia is invention of meaningless words.* The client who cannot produce a meaningful word in a sentence may invent one (also called *jargon*).
  - *Phonemic paraphasia is sound substitutions or additions.* A client may say *loman* for *woman* or *wolman* for *woman*.

- **Naming problems may be a persistent problem.** Also called anomia, naming or word-finding problems may be fundamental to aphasia, and therefore, not especially useful in distinguishing the different types. A few contexts help assess naming difficulties:
  - *Confrontation naming difficulty is most pervasive.* The client has difficulty naming a stimulus when asked to name it (e.g., showing a pen, and asking "What is this?").
  - *Naming a described object may be impaired.* The client has difficulty naming something the clinician describes (e.g., this is something you use to write with. What is it?").
  - *Supplying a name to complete a sentence may be difficult.* The client may be unable to supply the word pen, when the clinician says "You write with a . . . "
  - *Naming stimuli within a class may be impaired.* The client may have difficulty naming more than a few items of furniture, animals, flowers, and so forth.

- **Speech fluency may be decreased or increased.** Two broad types of aphasia are distinguished on the basis of hypo- or hyperfluency:
  - *Fluency is impaired in four types of aphasia.* Therefore, Broca's, transcortical motor, mixed transcortical aphasia, and global aphasia are classified *nonfluent*. The speech is slow, effortful, uneven in its flow, and may be full of dysfluencies and false starts.
  - *Fluency is unimpaired in four other types.* Fluency may in fact be excessive in clients with Wernicke's aphasia. Those with transcortical sensory, conduction,

and anomic aphasia also have relatively intact fluency in spite of their somewhat paraphasic speech. The speech is generally fast, effortless, and flowing, but may not make much sense because of neologistic expressions.

- **Auditory comprehension problems may be subtle or gross.** Found in most patients, auditory comprehension problems vary across clients and across types of aphasia:
  - *Auditory comprehension problems do not distinguish the types of aphasia.* They are associated with both fluent and nonfluent aphasia types. Generally, clients with Broca's, transcortical motor, conduction, and anomic aphasia have better auditory comprehension than those with Wernicke's, global, and transcortical sensory aphasia.
  - *Difficulty may extend to any response topography.* When the difficulty is moderate to severe, words, phrases, sentences, and discourse may all be difficult to comprehend.

- **Grammatical impairments may be negligible or severe.** Syntactic and morphologic problems are more prominent in some clients than in others, depending on their type of aphasia:
  - *Speech in clients with nonfluent aphasia is generally agrammatic.* Nonfluent aphasic speech is telegraphic and agrammatic. The client may omit such *function* words as articles, prepositions, conjunctions, auxiliary verbs, and plural, possessive, and past tense inflections).
  - *Speech in clients with fluent aphasia is generally grammatic.* Deviations in producing syntactic or morphological features are within normal limits.

- **Speech repetition (imitation) skills may be retained or impaired.** Aphasia may differentially affect a person's imitation of words, phrases, and sentences that are modeled for them. Whether repetition skills are retained or impaired is of differential diagnostic significance:
  - *Some clients have relatively poor repetition skills.* Generally, those with Broca's, Wernicke's, and conduction aphasia have impaired repetition skills.
  - *Others have relatively good repetition skills.* Clients with anomic, transcortical motor, or transcortical sensory aphasia have relatively intact repetition skills.

- **Speech rate may be affected.** Speech rate is a function of such other variables as reduced or increased fluency and naming difficulties. Therefore, speech rate may be affected differentially in different aphasia types:
  - *Clients with nonfluent aphasias generally have reduced speech rate.* A slower speech rate in these clients may be due to their increased dysfluencies and persistent naming problems.
  - *Clients with fluent aphasias have normal or even increased speech rate.* Their increased rate may be due to their hyperfluency and a tendency to create jargon as they continue to speak.

- **Gestural communication may be impaired.** This impairment may not entirely be due to any motor difficulty (e.g., paresis or paralysis of hands). In diagnosing impaired gestural communication, the clinician should rule out motor deficits. A client's difficulty with gestures may parallel his or her oral language problem:

- ○ *Gestures may be absent or few as the client talks.* Few or no gestures may accompany the speech of clients who have aphasia. The clients may have difficulty imitating gestures modeled for them.

- ○ *Gestures of others may be difficult to understand.* Clients with aphasia may fail to respond to gestures that accompany speech that is directed to them.

- **Reading and writing problems parallel verbal language problems.** Reading problems of individuals with aphasia are called *alexia,* and the writing problems are called *agraphia.* Both reading and writing skills may be affected to varying degrees, and reflect the problems in oral communication:

  - ○ *The writing of some clients may be slow, effortful, and agrammatic.* For instance, individuals with Broca's aphasia write (as well as speak) slowly, sparsely, with a great deal of effort, and omit grammatical elements in their sentences.

  - ○ *The writing of other clients may be effortless and copious, but problematic.* For instance, individuals with Wernicke's aphasia may write much, and write easily and grammatically, but their writing may be full of neologistic words, making little sense.

  - ○ *Reading problems may be severe in some cases.* For instance, some clients may not recognize printed words. Others may read word by word.

  - ○ *Some may struggle to read.* Clients may read with great difficulty, read slowly, and make many mistakes in oral reading.

  - ○ *Reading comprehension deficits parallel oral language deficits.* Clients with aphasia may have varying degrees of difficulty in comprehending what they read. This is generally consistent with their difficulty in understanding spoken speech.

- **Bilingual deficits may vary across individuals.** Most bilingual speakers have one dominant language, although some may speak two languages, each with a high level of proficiency. In most bilingual speakers (as in monolingual speakers), it is the left hemisphere that is dominant for both the languages. Therefore, a left hemisphere stroke is likely to affect both the languages. The symptoms and the eventual recovery patterns, however, will depend on the relative proficiency in the two languages. The symptom complex and the types of aphasia in bilinguals is the same as that in monolingual speakers. Therefore, the research interest has been in the patterns of recovery of language skills (Benson & Ardila, 1996; Lorenzen & Murray, 2008; Paradis, 1987, 1998; Roberts, 2008):

  - ○ *Language deficits may be greater in one language.* The other language skills may be near normal.

  - ○ *The patterns of language recovery vary across individuals.* Some individuals may recover both of their languages to varying extents. Other clients with bilingual aphasia recover mostly or only the dominant language; a few may recover their primary (and currently weak) language that has not been spoken for years.

- *One language may be regained first, only to be lost again.* This loss typically follows the regaining of the other language.

- *Recovery of the two languages may be more or less simultaneous.* In some individuals, the recovery of the two languages may be months apart.

- *A loss of one language may be relatively permanent.* Some individuals may never recover one of their languages.

- *An alternate pattern of loss and gain may be evident in some speakers.* Both the languages may be gained as well as lost in an alternating manner.

- *Expressions of the two languages may be mixed.* This language mixing is not code switching, and the patient may be unable to control it.

- *Translation skills may be differentially impaired.* Some patients may *automatically translate* one language expression into another. Some may translate *only one specific language* into the other, but not vice versa. Others may translate, but *may not comprehend* what they translate.

- *A lost accent may be recovered.* The accent of a language not spoken for years may reemerge in some clients.

Types of Aphasia

As noted before, nonfluent and fluent aphasias are the two broad classifications of aphasia. For the clinician concerned with a differential diagnosis of the type of aphasia in a client, it is essential to assess the general characteristics of aphasia as listed in the previous section. Although the symptoms and their severity may vary across clients, the clinician needs to keep in perspective all potential symptoms of aphasia during assessment.

In this section, we will describe the specific characteristics of the major types of aphasia. We will highlight the basic neuropathology as well as the unique features of the different types that should be considered in making a differential diagnosis.

Nonfluent Aphasia

The four types of nonfluent aphasias are all characterized by reduced speech rate, excessive speaking effort, omission of grammatic features, shorter utterances, impaired prosody, limited amount of speech, and difficulty initiating speech (Hegde, 2006). Lesions in the anterior parts of the brain tend to produce nonfluent types of aphasia. Variations in the specific sites of lesion (within the anterior brain) produce the different types of nonfluent aphasia:

- **Broca's aphasia is common and typical of nonfluent aphasia.** This is the classic agrammatic, effortful, nonfluent type of aphasia. In assessing Broca's aphasia, the clinician should consider the following:
  - *The neuroanatomical basis of Broca's aphasia is controversial.* Generally, the area affected is supplied by the middle cerebral artery. Deep cortical damage surrounding Broca's area is essential to produce this type of aphasia (Damasio,

2008). Lesions limited to Broca's area (in the left inferior frontal gyrus) may not necessarily produce aphasia, though it might produce transient mutism and subsequent apraxia. A few clients with symptoms consistent with Broca's aphasia may have intact Broca's area. In a few other cases, damage to Broca's area may produce *transcortical motor aphasia*—obviously a different kind of nonfluent aphasia. Such extensive cortical damage tends to reduce metabolic rates in other, unaffected areas of the brain. Therefore, reduced functional efficiency of areas other than Broca's may be involved in producing the total symptom complex.

○ *Neurological symptoms are obvious.* Clients with Broca's aphasia may have right-sided hemiparesis or hemiplegia. Immediately postonset, they may use a wheelchair, and later, a cane or walker. These are not the features of clients with Wernicke's aphasia.

○ *Language production is nonfluent, limited, agrammatic, effortful, slow, and uneven in its flow.* Utterances are short. Repetition of modeled speech is impaired; the client is especially likely to omit any grammatical features that are a part of modeled speech. Naming the stimuli presented (confrontation naming) is particularly difficult. The speech may be aprosodic and monotonous, lacking in rhythm and intonation. The clients have relatively intact, though rarely completely normal, auditory comprehension of spoken speech or silently read material. Reading and writing difficulties parallel the oral language problems. The client may read slowly and with a great deal of effort, and may fail to understand some or most of what he or she reads. Writing, also slow and effortful, may show poorly formed or omitted letters and omission of grammatical elements.

○ *Articulation may be affected, though not as a feature of aphasia.* Clients with Broca's aphasia may not produce speech sounds correctly, possibly because of an associated but independent apraxia of speech. This is expected, as Broca's area is also considered the motor speech planning area. Distortions of consonants and vowels are common. See Chapters 3 and 4 for assessment of apraxia of speech.

○ *Dysarthria may also be an associated but independent disorder.* Again, this is not a feature of any aphasia, but it may coexist with Broca's aphasia because of the neuromuscular involvement. See Chapters 5 and 6 for assessment of dysarthria.

○ *Paraphasia is not a significant feature of Broca's aphasia.* It is the hallmark of nonfluent aphasias (e.g., Wernicke's aphasia).

○ *A previously diagnosed global aphasia may evolve into Broca's.* It is important during assessment to consider whether a client who now exhibits Broca's aphasia was once diagnosed to have global aphasia (Peach, 2008).

○ *Clients with Broca's aphasia communicate better than those with Wernicke's.* Clients with Broca's aphasia are generally alert and give relevant answers to questions; they are cooperative during assessment. Lacking in meaningless jargon and better preserved auditory comprehension, they can carry on a conversation, even if limited, during assessment. These features contrast with those of Wernicke's aphasia.

- **Transcortical motor aphasia (TMA) is less common than Broca's.** The disorder is not truly *transcortical*, but the term is generally accepted to describe a form of nonfluent aphasia with intact repetition skills. The clinician's concerns during assessment are as follows:
  - *The lesions are often in the anterior superior frontal lobe.* The association pathways are typically affected. The supplemental motor areas may be involved. Broca's and Wernicke's areas are unaffected, but may be disconnected from other areas. The areas of lesion are supplied by the anterior cerebral artery.
  - *Neuromotor symptoms may be obvious.* Impaired movement (akinesia), including slowness of movement (bradykinesia), hemiparesis, and buccofacial apraxia may be evident to varying extents across clients.
  - *Apathy may be a unique feature.* Clients with TMA may be withdrawn and disinterested in communication. They often have to be coaxed to talk, though they may say only a word or two when urged.
  - *Muteness may be an initial symptom.* This speechlessness may be due to the client's akinesia.
  - *Difficulty initiating speech is a significant feature.* Having great difficulty initiating speech, a client may try to get his or her speech initiated by such (self) motor prompts as clapping hands, nodding the head, abruptly rising from a sitting position, and so forth.
  - *Once initiated, such series as numbers may be produced uninterrupted.* They may need some prompts to get started. Continuous and spontaneous speech, however, may still be difficult to both initiate and sustain.
  - *Intact repetition skills are a diagnostic sign.* This feature sets the client apart from those with Broca's aphasia. Even though producing only limited utterances after some coaxing, the client may readily and correctly imitate phrases and sentences, even longer ones.
  - *Echolalia may be another diagnostic feature.* The initial speechlessness may soon give rise to echolalic speech. Clients may repeat what they hear as well as what they themselves are saying (self-echolalia). Self-echolalic responses may be preservative. Intact repetition and echolalia may be related.
  - *Auditory comprehension is relatively good.* Some difficulty may be noted in understanding complex verbal or written material.
  - *Reading skills are better preserved than the writing skills.* Slow reading aloud and impaired comprehension of complex material may be evident.
  - *Writing problems may be significant.* When coaxed, the client may write little, with spelling mistakes, and large and poorly formed letters.
- **Mixed transcortical aphasia (MTA) is rare.** Clients with MTA may have symptoms of nonfluent aphasia, combined with some dominant features of fluent aphasia. When assessing this type of aphasia the clinician should consider the following:
  - *The watershed area of the brain is typically damaged.* Stenosis of the internal carotid artery is the most frequent vascular disease that causes the brain damage.

○ *The brain damage spares Broca's and Wernicke's areas, but isolates them from other areas.* This is the reason why MTA is also called *isolation of the speech area.*

○ *Repetition is well preserved, but all other language skills are severely affected.* Excellent, though nonfunctional, repetition skills of clients with MTA are similar to those with TMA. In response to a question, the client may actually repeat the question. The difference between TMA and MTA is that the latter is associated with profound impairments in most other language skills. Fluency, grammar, naming, and even pointing may be severely affected. Articulation may be good, however, and paraphasia may not be a significant factor, partly because most patients produce little or no spontaneous speech.

○ *Auditory comprehension is affected, often severely.* This is unlike most nonfluent aphasias, and in fact akin to fluent aphasias.

○ *Reading and writing skills may be severely impaired.* Reading aloud, reading comprehension, and writing may all be affected to a significant extent.

• **Global aphasia is the most severe type of nonfluent aphasia.** This type of aphasia affects all aspects of communication, and there are no particularly spared skills (Collins, 2005). In assessing clients with potential global aphasia, the clinician should consider the following:

○ *All language areas of the brain are affected.* In most cases, the entire perisylvian region, including both Broca's and Wernicke's areas, may be damaged. In some cases the lesions may extend to deeper white matter of the brain, the basal ganglia, the internal capsule, and the thalamus. The regions damaged are supplied by the middle cerebral artery.

○ *Neurological symptoms are strong.* Right hemiparesis, hemiplegia, and sensory loss may be evident in most clients. Hemineglect (ignoring a side of the body) may be a feature.

○ *Verbal and nonverbal apraxia may be present.* This is as expected because of extensive damage to speech and language centers of the brain.

○ *All language skills are severely impaired.* Clients with global aphasia may utter a word or two, a few overly learned responses (e.g., How do you do?), and *yes* or *no* responses to questions related to personal information. Some may repeat such consonant-vowel combinations as do-do-do or ma-ma-ma (Peach, 2008). Most clients cannot repeat even simple, single words.

○ *Auditory comprehension may be impaired.* Their understanding may be limited to single words spoken to them, although some clients may exhibit better understanding. They can perform such nonverbal tasks as matching words to pictures, suggesting an understanding of instructions.

○ *Reading and writing skills are affected.* Impairments generally match those found in oral communication.

Fluent Aphasia

The four types of fluent aphasias are characterized by hyperfluency, excessive speech, easy and effortless speech, good articulation, longer utterances, normal prosody, relatively intact grammar, neologism, omission of meaningful words, and generally ineffective communication mostly due to neologism—a profusion of meaningless words (Hegde, 2006)). Lesions in the posterior portions of the brain produce fluent types of aphasia. Variations in the specific lesion sites in the posterior brain cause the differential symptoms of the four major types of fluent aphasia:

- **Wernicke's is a classic form of fluent aphasia.** One of the least controversial syndromes, Wernicke's aphasia is the prototype of fluent aphasia. Impaired auditory comprehension and paraphasic hyperfluency are the main features of Wernicke's aphasia. In assessing this type of aphasia, the clinician should consider the following:
  - *Wernicke's area is typically damaged.* The lesion or lesions may be found on the posterior portion of the superior temporal gyrus in the dominant hemisphere. The second temporal gyrus, the surrounding parietal region, the angular gyrus, and the supramarginal gyrus may be involved. The damaged areas are supplied by the posterior branches of the left middle cerebral artery.
  - *Neuromotor impairments may be absent.* This contrasts with Broca's aphasia. Clients with Wernicke's aphasia may appear physically normal with no paresis or paralysis because of the spared motor centers of the brain.
  - *Psychiatric symptoms may be evident and misleading.* Clients may appear confused because of incessant speech that does not make sense. They also may entertain paranoid, suicidal, or homicidal thoughts. Depression may be an additional feature. A mistaken diagnosis of schizophrenia should be avoided.
  - *Normal or hyperfluency is the main distinguishing feature.* The clients are so prolific in their word output, that their fluency is often described as *press of speech* or *logorrhea* (an irresistible urge to keep talking). Incessant and effortless, their speech moves ahead with a rapid rate with normal phrase length (five to eight words or more).
  - *Articulation is unaffected.* Wernicke's aphasia is not associated with the same type of speech production difficulty found in Broca's aphasia.
  - *Repetition skills are impaired.* Clients with more severe auditory comprehension deficits also show more severe impairment in repeating modeled speech.
  - *Grammar is better preserved than in Broca's aphasia.* Although their sentences appear grammatical, clients with Wernicke's aphasia make some special kinds of grammatical errors called *paragrammatism* (Goodglass, Kaplan, & Barresi, 2001). They may substitute, omit, or excessively use grammatical morphemes in their speech.
  - *Word-finding problems may be severe.* Nonetheless, they will manage to maintain their fluent speech because of their tendency to create new words as they speak. Neologistic content words will replace the actual words they cannot say. The grammatical morphemes, however, may be produced correctly, except for paragrammatism.
  - *Communication is poor, in spite of incessantly fluent speech.* Much of what the clients with Wernicke's aphasia say may be meaningless or empty because of their paraphasic and paragrammatic speech. Such nonspecific words as this, that, stuff, and thing are copious in their speech. Consequently, they communicate much less effectively than those with Broca's aphasia.

○ *Impaired auditory comprehension is a diagnostic feature.* Though the extent may be variable across clients, most clients with Wernicke's aphasia have a significant deficit in auditory comprehension of spoken speech. Some may get the gross message, but not the details or nuances. Some may have such profound impairment that they fail to understand the simplest of directions or commands.

○ *Lack of concern distinguishes Wernicke's clients from Broca's.* In spite of their ineffective communication, clients with Wernicke's aphasia tend to be unconcerned about their language deficits.

○ *Reading and writing skills are affected.* Clients may fail to recognize the sounds of written words. They may not recognize the letters of the alphabet and may not comprehend what they read. Their writing will parallel their speech: neologistic, copious, effortless, and misspelled.

- **Transcortical sensory aphasia (TSA) is distinguishable by echolalic repetition.** Other than good repetition and echolalic responses, the symptoms of TSA are similar to those of Wernicke's aphasia. In assessing TSA, clinicians should consider the following:

  ○ *Lesions are often found in the temporoparietal area of the brain.* Wernicke's and Broca's areas are typically unaffected. The damaged parts of the brain are typically in the watershed area of the middle cerebral artery.

  ○ *Hemiparesis may be an initial symptom.* The recovery from hemiparesis present at onset is common. Therefore, clients in the latter stages of TSA may not have obvious neurological symptoms.

  ○ *Speech fluency and articulation are unimpaired.* Fluency of speech and speech production skills in TSA are similar to that of Wernicke's aphasia.

  ○ *Syntactic skills are generally good.* Grammar and morphologic productions are comparable to those found in Wernicke's aphasia, and are contrasted with those of Broca's aphasia.

  ○ *Paraphasia and empty speech are a common feature.* Once again, these features are similar to those found in Wernicke's aphasia. Press of speech or logorrhea may be infrequent, however.

  ○ *Naming problems may be prominent.* This might explain their paraphasic and empty speech.

  ○ *Repetition is good, but echolalia may be significant.* Good repetition skills in TSA are a contrast to Wernicke's aphasia, with its impaired repetition. Echolalia is also a contrast to Wernicke's aphasia, in which it is absent. Clients may repeat a clinician's questions before responding to them.

  ○ *Auditory comprehension is impaired.* Paradoxically, many clients may exhibit severe difficulty in responding to simple commands or instructions, though they can repeat them.

  ○ *Serial (automatic) speech may be normal.* Although they may have difficulty initiating serial speech, they continue with no difficulty once they get initiated with the clinician's help. The may automatically complete a poem or a sentence the clinician begins to say.

○ *Reading comprehension may be poor and writing may be difficult.* Their oral reading skills may be normal or nearly so, however. Their writing problems are similar to those with Wernicke's aphasia.

- **Conduction aphasia is distinguishable by near-normal auditory comprehension.** A rare and controversial syndrome, conduction aphasia is similar to Wernicke's in most symptoms. In contrast to those with Wernicke's aphasia, clients with conduction aphasia comprehend spoken speech much better. In assessing conduction aphasia, clinicians should consider the following:

  ○ *Brain lesion sites vary in conduction aphasia.* Often, damage may be evident in the lower portions of the left parietal lobe. Other sites of lesion include the upper portions of the temporal lobe, the insula, and the arcuate fasciculus. Wernicke's and Broca's areas are unaffected.

  ○ *Neurological symptoms vary across clients.* Some clients may experience no neurological symptoms. Others may have mild to severe paresis of the right upper extremity (including the face). Motor recovery is common, although some may continue to have oral and limb apraxia.

  ○ *Fluency is variable across clients.* Although some are more fluent than others, clients with conduction aphasia are generally less fluent than those with Wernicke's aphasia. Their fluency is often interrupted by pauses (hesitations) and self-corrections.

  ○ *Repetition is impaired.* A notable difficulty in repeating modeled words, phrases, and sentences is a major distinguishing feature of conduction aphasia. The clients may have difficulty repeating words and phrases they routinely produce in their speech.

  ○ *Speech may be paraphasic.* Literal paraphasia is more common than the semantic or neologistic variety.

  ○ *Word-finding problems may be significant.* For clients with conduction aphasia, content words may be more elusive than function words.

  ○ *Naming problems may be mild to severe.* Clients with conduction aphasia may point to the object names, but may not name the object when asked to. Some patients may produce multiple paraphasic responses when asked to name an object.

  ○ *Articulation is mostly normal.* Sound substitutions (literal paraphasia), especially the substitution of simpler phonemes for complex ones, are common. This may not be a strict speech sound production problem, however.

  ○ *Syntactic and prosodic features may be normal.* These aspects are similar to Wernicke's aphasia and stand in contrast to Broca's.

  ○ *Auditory comprehension tends to be good.* Clients with conduction aphasia comprehend typical conversations. Some may have difficulty comprehending grammatically more complex speech, however.

  ○ *Reading and writing problems may be evident.* Paraphasias characterize oral reading, although silent reading comprehension tends to be good. Misspelling and omissions, reversals, and substitutions of letters characterize the client's writing.

  ○ *Attempts at self-correction are common.* Their attempts tend to be unsuccessful, however.

- **Anomic aphasia is the most controversial of the fluent types.** While anomia (naming difficulty) is a symptom of most types of aphasia, anomic aphasia is a syndrome in which the naming difficulties exceed other language problems (Hegde, 2006). Anomia is found in such other disorders as dementia, increased intracranial pressure, traumatic brain injury, and right-hemisphere injury. Existence of anomic aphasia has been questioned, and some consider it akin to transcortical sensory aphasia (Benson & Ardila, 1996). In assessing anomic aphasia, clinicians should consider the following:

  ○ *Neuroanatomical sites of lesion are varied.* In some cases, the site of lesion may be unclear. Lesions may be found in the angular gyrus and the second temporal gyrus.

  ○ *Word-finding difficulty far exceeds all other impairments.* While most other language skills are better preserved or nearly normal, the pervasive word-finding difficulty (anomia) is severe enough to be debilitating to the client.

  ○ *Fluency is good, but affected by word-finding problems.* Persistent naming difficulty interrupts the flow of speech. While speaking, the clients with anomic aphasia tend to pause and repeat themselves. Their fluent speech may be empty because their circumlocution and production of nonspecific words (e.g., *this, that stuff,* and *thing*). This verbal paraphasia limits fluency.

  ○ *Syntax may be within normal limits.* Serious impairments in grammar and morphological productions are not characteristic of anomic aphasia.

  ○ *Auditory comprehension is good.* They can comprehend typical conversation without much difficulty. Subtle problems may exist with complex verbal material, however.

  ○ *Repetition is normal.* The clients with anomic aphasia have no significant problem repeating after the clinician.

  ○ *Speech articulation is good.* Anomic aphasia generally does not affect speech sound production.

  ○ *Reading and writing problems are not typical.* Clients with anomic aphasia read and write normally. Their reading comprehension is good.

As the previous description makes clear, different types of aphasia share many features because they all are aphasias; most types differ by a few specific features. Therefore, in diagnosing each client with aphasia, the clinician should take into consideration the entire range of symptoms associated with aphasia.

Overview of Assessment

Assessment of aphasia has multiple concerns. The clinician needs to understand the client's (a) current and projected health condition, (b) current communication deficits and needs, (c) overall quality of life, (d) strengths and family and social support systems, (e) expected return to the previous or a new employment setting, (f) what the client and the caregivers expect from treatment and rehabilitation, and (g) the cultural and verbal background of the client and the family. Much information on these variables may be obtained from a detailed case history, reports from the medical and rehabilitation professionals, and a carefully conducted interview of the client and the caregivers. Specific assessment procedures, when completed, will help build a profile of the client and the family.

Assessment includes both standard and special procedures specific to aphasia. To complete a thorough assessment, the clinician will:

- Have the client or the family fill out a case history form
- Hold an interview with the client and the caregiver
- Administer a hearing screening test
- Complete an orofacial examination and assess diadochokinetic rates
- Administer selected standardized tests
- Assess speech production
- Assess narrative and conversational skills
- Assess functional communication skills
- Assess communication-related quality of life
- Analyze and integrate the assessment results
- Offer postassessment counseling

The clinician can use the standard case history form given in Chapter 2. During the interview, the clinician may ask specific questions about the onset of stroke or other events that triggered aphasia, subsequent medical management, current health status of the client, cultural and verbal background of the client and the family, and so forth. The clinician may use additional protocols given in Chapter 2 to make an orofacial examination, assess the diadochokinetic rates, and screen the client's hearing. The clinician will then proceed to collect diagnostic data from a conversational speech and language sample, standardized tests, or other nonstandardized procedures. To assess aphasia, clinicians usually assess a variety of skills that are either impaired or preserved in clients. These include fluency of speech, naming, repetition, syntactic and morphologic skills, conversational speech, speech sound production, serial speech and singing, auditory comprehension, reading and writing, and nonverbal communication. The degree to which each of these and other skills are assessed will depend on the individual client and the apparent severity of symptoms. Not all skills necessarily need to be assessed in-depth in all clients.

At the end of the assessment, the clinician will counsel the client and the caregivers about the assessment results, discuss speech-language treatment options, suggest a prognosis, and answer any questions the client and the caregivers may ask.

Screening for Aphasia

Clinicians working in hospitals and other medical settings may need to screen specific patients for aphasia. It is prudent to screen patients before embarking on a time-consuming diagnostic assessment. Clinicians may use their own established procedures or one of the available aphasia screening tests to determine if an individual should be assessed further.

Experienced clinicians may use quick procedures based on their own clinical expertise. Patients recently admitted to hospitals for a cerebrovascular accident or other neurological problems that may be associated with aphasia are candidates for a quick bedside screening. The clinician may screen patients by having them perform a few standard tasks. For instance, the clinician may not only engage the patient in conversation for a few minutes, but also ask the client to point to, name, and describe a few objects or pictures; count numbers, recite the names of months and days of the week; repeat a few words, phrases, and sentences; and answer a few questions about orientation to time, space, and person. The patient's responses may be sufficient to determine whether more in-depth assessment is necessary.

If preferred, several screening tests are available. Table 7–1 lists a few commonly used aphasia screening tests. Clinicians may administer one of these tests to screen a patient in 10 to 15 minutes.

Standardized Tests for Aphasia

There are three main varieties of standardized tests for diagnosing aphasia. The first variety is the classic type of general aphasia diagnostic tests. Some of these tests help assess aphasia in general, whereas others seek to diagnose specific types of aphasia. The second variety is the nontraditional functional communication assessment tools. These tools are designed to overcome some of the limitations of standardized tests. (See Table 7–2 for a sample listing of general aphasia diagnostic tests and functional communication assessment tools.) The third variety is bilingual tests designed to assess aphasia in English and another language.

Aphasia affects multiple skills, and an assessment of most if not all skills requires multiple subtests. Consequently, several standardized tests are long and take several

Table 7–1. Selected screening tests of aphasia

Screening Test	Author and Reference
Aphasia Language Performance Scales (ALPS)	Keenan and Brassell (1975)
The Boston Diagnostic Aphasia Examination (BDAE) (3rd ed.)—the short form	Goodglass, Kaplan, & Barresi (2001)
Sklar Aphasia Scale (SAS)	Sklar (1983)
Acute Aphasia Screening Protocol (AASP)	Crary, Haak, and Malinsky (1989)
Aphasia Screening Test	Whurr (1996)
Bedside Evaluation Screening Test, Second Edition (BEST)	Fitch-West and Sands (1998)
Quick Assessment for Aphasia	Tanner and Culbertson (1999)

hours to administer. To complete the tasks on the same test, some clients take twice as much time as others. This variability is mostly due to the physical condition of the clients at the time of examination. Clients in poorer health who are fatigued easily take more time than those with better health and alertness. Patients who are depressed, talk excessively during assessment, and are otherwise distracted, might also need extra time to complete a test.

The *Minnesota Test for Differential Diagnosis of Aphasia* (MTTDA; Schuel, 1972) is a classic test, as it is one of the earliest published. MTTDA, perhaps used more frequently in the past than at present, contains subtests to assess the following five types of impairments: auditory, speech and language, visual and reading, visuomotor and writing, and numerical and arithmetic. A practical difficulty with this test is its length of administration: The 47 subtests take 3 to 6 hours to administer and score. Consequently, some clinicians

Table 7–2. General Diagnostic and Functional Communication Assessments

General Diagnostic Tests	
Test Name	**Author and Reference**
The Minnesota Test for Differential Diagnosis of Aphasia (MTDDA)	Schuell, 1973
The Boston Diagnostic Aphasia Examination (BDAE-3)	Goodglass, Kaplan, & Barresi, 2001
Boston Assessment of Severe Aphasia (BASA)	Helm-Estabrooks, Ramsberger, Morgan, & Nicholas, 1989.
The Western Aphasia Battery-Revised (WAB-R)	Kertesz, 2006
The Porch Index of Communicative Ability (PICA)	Porch, 2001
The Neurosensory Center Comprehensive Examination for Aphasia (NCCEA)	Spreen & Benton, 1977
Functional Communication Assessment	
Functional Communication Profile	Sarno, 1969
Communication Abilities of Daily Living, Second Edition	Holland, Frattali, & Fromm, 1998
The Communicative Effectiveness Index (CETI)	Lomas, et al., 1989
Communication Profile: A Functional Survey	Payne, 1994
Functional Assessment of Communication Skills for Adults (ASHA FACS)	Frattali, Thompson, Holland, Wohl, & Ferkietic, 1995.
Amsterdam Nijmegan Everyday Language Test (ANELT)	Blomert, Kean, Koster, & Schokker, 1994.

may administer only selected subtests. The test results do not permit a classification of aphasia into types, but they help assign a patient into one of five groups: (1) simple aphasia; (2) aphasia with visual involvement; (3) aphasia with sensorimotor involvement; (4) aphasia with scattered findings; and (5) irreversible aphasic syndrome.

The *Boston Diagnostic Aphasia Examination—Third Edition* (BDAE-3; Goodglass, Kaplan, & Baresi, 2001) is a commonly used test that is designed to classify a patient into one of the major aphasia types, although in practice, the type of aphasia may not be clear in many patients. With 27 subtests, BDAE is another fairly long test. It takes 1 to 5 hours to administer, with an average of 2 hours per patient (Brookshire, 2007). The test results are suggestive of the site of brain lesion or lesions.

BDAE helps assess most skills that are impaired in aphasia, including articulation, fluency, word-finding difficulty, repetition, serial speech, grammar, paraphasia, auditory comprehension, oral reading and reading comprehension, writing, and singing. The client's performance on the test may be rated on a 5-point rating scale to evaluate the severity of the symptoms. The test offers a separate naming test that may be administered with it or independently.

The *Boston Assessment of Severe Aphasia* (BASA; Helm-Estabrooks, Ramsberger, Nicholas, & Morgan, 1989),which contains 15 subtests and 61 items, targets for assessment auditory comprehension, repetition, social greetings and simple conversation, *yes/no* questions, orientation to time, signing one's name, buccofacial or limb apraxia, gestural recognition, oral and gestural recognition, reading comprehension, writing, and visuospatial skills. Because it can be administered in less than 40 minutes in most cases, it may be administered relatively soon after a stroke, and may be a useful bedside assessment tool.

The Western Aphasia Battery (WAB; Kertesz, 1982) is another widely used test. Comprehensive in its coverage of impaired skills, the test can be administered in 1 to 2 hours. The skills the test evaluates include speech content, fluency, auditory comprehension, repetition, naming, reading, writing, calculation, drawing, nonverbal thinking, and performance on block designs.

The WAB seeks to classify patients into one of the major aphasia types, although a classification based on this test may not be consistent with the classification based on other tests, such as the BDAE (Wertz, Deal, & Robinson, 1984). Another difficulty with the WAB is that its classification may be inconsistent with clinical judgment of aphasia types in given clients (Swindell, Holland, & Fromm, 1984). Furthermore, the test results do not allow for unclassifiable patients as the scores force all into one or the other type.

The Porch Index of Communicative Ability (PICA; Porch, 2001) has some unique features. For instance, its earlier items are more difficult than the later items; it uses the same set of stimuli in all of its subtests; instructions to the patients are specified word-by-word; when and how to give a prompt or cue also are specified. The clinician uses the following 10 stimuli to assess the various skills: pen, pencil, matches, scissors, key, quarter, toothbrush, comb, fork, and knife.

PICA's 18 subtests and 181 test items help assess auditory comprehension by pointing to objects; reading printed words; oral expressive language mainly through object descriptions, naming, sentence completion, and repetition; pantomime to demonstrate functions of objects; visual matching of pictures to objects or objects to pictures; writing names and functions of objects, writing words when spelled, and writing to dictation; and copying names and geometric forms. This comprehensive test may be administered in an hour. There is some concern that the test measures speech and language skills to a limited extent, and that the test scores may not be relevant to communication in everyday situations (Davis, 2000). Clinicians who wish to administer PICA should undergo intensive training. A complex response scoring system ranges from 1 (*no response*) through 16 (*complex*, described as spontaneous, accurate, fluent elaboration about the test item). The PICA has been found useful in predicting and assessing improvement with and without treatment in aphasic patients.

The Neurosensory Center Comprehensive Examination for Aphasia (NCCEA; Spreen & Benton, 1977) contains 20 language subtests as well as additional tests for visual and tactile functions. The NCCEA may be used to assess language comprehension and production, reading, writing, copying, word fluency, digit and sentence repetition, visual object naming, sentence construction, and articulation. The scoring system takes into consideration the age and education of the patient.

The NCCEA has a low ceiling because it contains only the easy test items. Therefore, the test may more effectively assess patients with severe impairment than those with milder deficits. The scores on the test reflect both the weaknesses as well as the strengths of the patient.

The Kentucky Aphasia Test (KAT; Marshall & Wright, 2007) is a newer test designed to overcome some of the weaknesses of the previously described tests, chiefly among them, impractical administration time that most of them require. Described as a user-friendly test, the KAT has undergone some preliminary standardization and an experimental version is now available (Marshall & Wright, 2007). It simplifies initial assessment by including only an orientation test, a picture description task, and six 10-item subtests to assess expressive and receptive language skills. The authors avoided the reading and writing subtests because the main concern in the initial assessment and treatment is functional oral communication. Three forms of the test, KAT-1, KAT-2, and KAT-3 are designed to assess clients with severe, moderate, and mild forms of aphasia, respectively.

Assessment of Speech Production

Aphasia, although a language disorder, is often associated with speech production problems. Apraxia of speech (AOS) or dysarthria may be a coexisting motor speech disorder, especially in patients with anterior brain lesions. As noted previously, Broca's aphasia may be associated with AOS. A persistent dysarthria may be an associated speech problem especially in clients with bilateral brain damage (Duffy, 2005; Freed, 2000). Speech production (articulation) may also be impaired in clients with global aphasia. Fluent aphasias, caused by the more posterior brain lesions are not typically associated with speech production problems. In assessing motor speech disorders associated with aphasia, the clinician may consider the following:

- **A conversational speech sample will be useful.** An extended interview with the client, adequately recorded, may be used to assess speech production skills and analyze the speech sound error patterns.

- **Several aphasia tests have items to assess speech production.** These subtests may be adequate to diagnose a coexisting motor speech disorder. If a more detailed assessment of speech production is considered essential, the clinician may analyze the recorded speech sample.

- **Apraxia of speech and dysarthria assessment procedures may be used.** For an in-depth assessment of motor speech disorders, the clinician may consult Chapters 3 and 4 (AOS) and Chapters 5 and 6 (dysarthria). The clinician may administer standardized tests described in those chapters and use the protocols given in Chapter 4 for AOS, and Chapter 6 for dysarthria.

Assessment of Narrative and Conversational Skills

An assessment of narrative (discourse) and conversational skills is important for targeting more elaborate language skills during treatment. This assessment goes beyond an evaluation of discrete confrontation naming, isolated sentence productions, analysis of grammaticality, speech repetition, and so forth. The clinician needs to evoke connected and extended speech to analyze discourse and conversation. Several strategies are available:

- **Picture description is a standard procedure.** Having the client describing a story-telling type of picture is a simple method of evoking narration from the client. Many standardized tests of aphasia include subtests or specific test items to evoke such narrations. For instance, the *Boston Diagnostic Aphasia Examination* has the well-known "cookie theft" picture that helps evoke a narrative story from a client. Clinicians may present not one, but a series of pictures, all tied thematically—telling an extended story through them. In this case, the clinician may select pictures that are especially relevant to a client's interest, hobby, or ethnocultural background.

- **Story telling is a spontaneous method.** The clinician may evoke a narrative by simply asking the client to tell a story he or she knows. If this strategy fails, the clinician can tell a story and ask the client to retell it. The clinician also may ask the client to read a story silently and retell it. These latter strategies allow the clinician to select a story that matches the client's interests, hobbies, or ethnocultural background. For instance, the clinician may ask a client to narrate an interesting episode that occurred during a fishing trip, knowing that the client had taken many such trips.

- **Holding a conversation is essential.** To assess conversational skills, the clinician should engage the client in conversation; no standardized procedure will help. The interview the clinician holds with the client is essentially a conversation. This task can be valuable in assessing various conversational (pragmatic skills).

In clients with nonfluent aphasia, word-finding problems and limited fluency are significant variables that affect narrative and conversational skills. In clients with fluent aphasia, narratives may be profuse, but meaning may be limited. Such other variables as fatigue and the general health conditions may make it difficult for the client to sustain a conversation for an extended period of time. Premorbid language and literacy skills also are important variables to consider.

Analysis of narrative skills, even with some specified procedures, tends to be subjective. No single method of analysis has been agreed upon by clinicians. Such concepts as *lack of cohesion, limited range of information offered, missing the details, failure to convey the idea, poverty of expression, sparseness of speech,* and so forth involve judgments the clinician may differ making. Some missing details in a narrated story may be obvious, however, and the chronology of events the client narrates may be different from what is depicted in the picture. Within a broad range, the amount of information offered may be judged as *inadequate, adequate, profuse and meaningful,* and *profuse but meaningless.*

Analysis of conversational skills is somewhat better handled than the analysis of narrative skills, even though this analysis also requires some judgment. During the interview, the clinician can take notes on various conversational behaviors of the client:

- **Frequency of topic initiation may be noted.** The clinician can record the frequency with which the client spontaneously (without a prompt) initiated conversation on a topic. That the client spoke only when spoken to is another good measure of diminished spontaneous speech.

- **The duration for which the client spoke on a topic may be measured.** Frequency with which the client abruptly changed topics of conversation is also an indirect measure of topic maintenance.

- **The number of inappropriate comments and interruptions may be noted.** The clinician may take note of such comments and interruptions while engaging the client in conversation.

- **The appropriateness of eye contact may be judged or measured.** During conversation, the clinician may periodically sample the durations for which the client maintained eye contact or make global judgments as to their seeming appropriateness.

- **Conversational repair strategies may be noted.** The number of times the client asked for clarification when the clinician purposefully made a few ambiguous statements may be noted. The clinician also can make such statements as "I don't understand," "I am not sure what you mean," to assess the frequency with which the client rephrases or elaborates his or her statements.

Assessment of Functional Communication

Functional communication assessment is an approach to assessing clients to find out how their communication disorders affect their everyday communication, typically with an emphasis on evaluating how well they meet their basic communication needs. The approach is valid in assessing any disorder of communication. Several functional assessment tools are available for clients with aphasia.

A major assumption of functional communication assessment approach is that the standardized tests place perhaps too much emphasis on syntactic, morphologic, phonologic, and other structural accuracy of communication, not necessarily whether the communication attempts are effective in naturalistic contexts (e.g., the hospital ward or the home of the client). It is more important to find out if, in natural settings, a client can request food or water, express pain, indicate such needs as going to the bathroom, than grammatical accuracy of his or her production in a test situation. Excessive reliance on testing repetition skills, grammatical correctness, and responses to somewhat artificial test stimuli under highly controlled conditions do not assess effective communication in everyday situations. Clients who are more effective in functional communication skills when they return to their home and workplace may enjoy a better quality of life than those who lack such skills. Such concerns have led to the development of functional communication skills in patients with aphasia.

Functional assessment tools may not be as rigidly standardized nor administered as the tests described in the previous section. Functional approaches allow for observation of the client's communication skills in naturalistic settings (e.g., the hospital's cafeteria, a typical dialogue with a healthcare provider, conversation with a family member). Clinicians evaluate their observations for effectiveness of communication, not necessarily grammatical accuracy, although the degree of such accuracy may be noted as well. Functional assessment tools typically require the clinician to rate the client's behaviors being observed.

It is not suggested here that functional assessment approaches replace other, more traditional approaches, including standardized tests. In many clients, it may be important to assess phonologic, syntactic, and morphologic accuracy of their language productions. After good recovery and effective speech-language treatment, some clients may be in a position to return to their jobs that require correct and accurate oral and written communication. Others may want to achieve, and may have the potential to achieve, more than the basic functional communication; more formal and appropriate communication, including conversational skills, may enhance their personal and social lives (Kagan & Gailey, 1993). Therefore, clinicians should consider all assessment approaches and develop a comprehensive and client-specific assessment procedure that best serves the communication needs of the individual.

Several functional assessment tools are currently available. Clinicians may use them in addition to standardized tests and other procedures. A brief description of the major functional assessment tools follows.

Functional Communication Profile (Sarno, 1969) represents an early attempt at assessing functional communication skills of patients with aphasia. It is designed to assess behaviors in five categories: movement, speaking, understanding, reading, calculation, and writing. In following this protocol, clinicians will observe the patients' interactions to judge the adequacy and appropriateness of their communicative behaviors. To build an adequate communication profile of the client, the clinician is required to interview family members and examine the case history to fully understand the premorbid language skills of the patient. Using a 9-point rating scale, the clinician rates such communicative skills as indicating *yes* or *no*, reading newspaper headlines, and making change.

Communication Abilities of Daily Living, Second Edition (Holland, Frattali, & Fromm, 1998) is foremost among functional assessment tools that sample daily communication in everyday situations. The skills evaluated include reading, writing, and using numbers; social interaction; divergent communication; contextual communication; nonverbal communication; sequential relationships; and humor/metaphor absurdity. The test contains 50 items. To assess representative communication in everyday situations, the test helps arrange simulated interaction with others (e.g., a receptionist or a physician). Communication related to such daily activities as driving, shopping, and making phone calls may be assessed. Specific tasks designed to assess communicative effectiveness include reading a map, telling how he or she might get from point A to point B, listing items found in a grocery store, and so forth. Italian and Japanese versions also are available.

The Communicative Effectiveness Index (CETI; Lomas, Pickard, Bester, & Associates, 1989) targets four domains of functional communication skills for assessment: basic needs (e.g., toileting, eating, grooming); life skills (e.g., shopping, understanding traffic signals, using the telephone); social needs (e.g., playing cards, writing to a friend); and health threat (e.g., calling for help, letting someone know about one's own medical condition). The authors consulted stroke survivors and their spouses in selecting the functional skills for assessment. The clinician rates such skills as giving yes/no answers, expressing physical pain or discomfort, and starting a conversation as "not at all able" to "as able as before the stroke." In the client's home or other naturalistic setting, a family member, a friend, or a neighbor may be requested to rate the skills.

Communication Profile: A Functional Survey (Payne, 1994) is a unique instrument in that its standardization included ethnic minority patients from African-American, American Indian/Alaska Native, Asian-American/Pacific Islander, and Asian-American ethnic groups. Different living conditions, employment history, and income levels also have been sampled. It helps construct communication profile of patients by rating their skills on a 5-point scale. The patient or a caregiver also may rate the everyday communication skills, including speaking, reading, writing, and understanding spoken speech.

The *Functional Assessment of Communication Skills for Adults* (ASHA FACS; Frattali, Thompson, Holland, Wohl, & Ferketi, 1995) is a rating scale that the clinician or a caregiver might use to rate behaviors in four domains: social communication (e.g., use of familiar names, understanding of TV/radio, explanation of how to do something); communication of basic needs (e.g., expression of likes and dislikes, request for help); reading, writing, and number concepts (e.g., following written instructions, completion of forms); making money transactions; and daily planning (e.g., telling time, following a map). The behaviors are rated for their *independence* on a 7-point scale. The higher the rating, the lesser the dependence on others (the greater the independence from others) for a particular skill to be performed. In rating the skills, the clinician also takes into consideration the adequacy, appropriateness, promptness, and communication sharing. The tool helps assess the effectiveness of aphasia rehabilitation programs.

Several other assessment tools, used perhaps less frequently, but useful nonetheless, are available. For instance, the *Amsterdam Nijmegan Everyday Language Test* (ANELT; Blomert, Kean, Koster, & Schokker, 1994) may be used to assess various pragmatic (everyday) language skills. The test items describe various communicative situations (e.g., changing a doctor's appointment) and asks the client how he or she would handle it.

The *Pragmatic Protocol* (Prutting & Kirschner, 1987) is another assessment protocol that requires the clinician to record a sample of conversation to analyze and rate such skills as requests, commands, and topic maintenance. The clinician calculates a *percentage correct* for each skill observed. Another functional communication assessment protocol is the *Everyday Communicative Needs Assessment* (Worrall, 1992) in which an interview and specific speech tasks help evaluate how a patient with aphasia is able (or not able) to handle financial tasks (e.g., writing checks, reading bank statements), using the telephone (e.g., dialing emergency numbers, writing down phone messages), preparing food (e.g., following recipes, reading food package labels), and general household activities (e.g., setting washing machines, directing workmen).

It is obvious that functional communication skill assessment goes beyond the traditional assessment of impaired speech and language skills. When combined with the more traditional assessment tests and conversational speech samples, the functional assessment tools generate valuable information about the client's everyday communication capabilities as well as needs. Such a comprehensive assessment of clients with aphasia can help generate client-specific treatment approaches. The results of assessment can provide good pretreatment measures against which treatment progress can be measured and compared.

Quality of Life Assessment

A measure related to functional assessment is the quality of life (QOL) assessment. This also goes beyond the traditional measures of speech and language skills. The main concern in QOL is the degree to which a disorder or an impairment interferes with the daily living activities, participation in the social milieu, and the subjectively felt satisfaction with one's own life. The World Health Organization's (1992) *International Classification of Impairments, Disabilities, and Handicaps* (ICIDH) and the *World Health Organization Quality of Life* (WHO-QOL) (2004) measure have influenced clinical assessment across disciplines. The degree to which a clinical condition creates impairments, disabilities, and handicaps to an individual determines that individual's QOL (World Health Organization, 1992). *Impairments* are defined as structural or functional abnormality, *disability* is the effects of impairments on behavior, and *handicaps* are the negative effects of disabilities on daily life. In a later revision of the classification, newer terms, presumably less negative in their connotations, replace the older ones. The term *body functions and structures* means the same as impairment, *activity restriction* is the same as disability, and *participation restriction* replaces handicap (World Health Organization, 2001). The need to make such distinctions between impairments, disabilities, and handicaps may be questioned because the effects a clinical condition has on a person's behavior under specified environmental conditions may be directly measured without intervening concepts. However, clients and clinicians agree that a clinical condition affects how a person lives; performs daily activities; participates in social, occupational, and leisure activities; and enjoys life. It is important to measure such effects to design an effective treatment or rehabilitation program for clients.

Measures of QOL tend to be more subjective than most other measures clinicians might obtain from their clients. QOL is a global concept that is difficult to define in operational (measurable) terms. Consequently, QOL measures are often responses given to a series of printed questions presented to clients. There are several questionnaires that measure QOL, but most, like the WHO-QOL-BREF (World Health Organization, 2004), tend to be general in their orientation or place heavy emphasis on physical health and mobility. Some examples of general (as well as communication-specific) QOL questions are given in Table 7–3. Such general measures of QOL may not be sensitive to the particular kinds of effects communication impairments have on a person's QOL. Nonetheless, clinicians may administer such general questionnaires as the WHO-QOL, as a supplement to one that is specific to aphasia.

Table 7–3. Examples of questions on QOL questionnaires

General	Communication-Specific
How satisfied are you with your life?	I have trouble understanding what others say.
How satisfied are you with your personal relationships?	I remain mostly silent in group interactions.
How healthy is your physical environment?	People have trouble understanding me.
How well are you able to get around?	I avoid social events.
How satisfied are you with your sleep?	I enjoy talking with people.
The conditions in my life are excellent.	I am able to do most of the things I did in the past.
I stay at home most of the time.	I use the telephone as usual.
I am doing fewer social activities with groups of people.	I enjoy reading books.
I stand up only with someone's help.	I am able to write as usual.

Obviously, measures that are specific to aphasia are more useful than general QOL questionnaires. Functional communication measures, described in the previous section, generally seek to evaluate how a client communicates in his or her natural environment. Clinicians can infer that clients who are generally more effective in social communication enjoy a better QOL than those who are socially ineffective in their communication. Some questionnaires, going beyond just functional communication, seek to assess the overall QOL that include other variables not usually sampled in functional assessment procedures; see Table 7–3 for examples of communication-specific (as well as general) questions that may help assess the QOL.

A communication-specific measure is *Communication Quality of Life Scale* (ASHA-CQL), sponsored by the American Speech-Language-Hearing Association (Paul, et al., 2004). It includes 17 communication-specific questions of the kind shown in Table 7–3. The questions are simple and short, so the clients with brain injury can understand and respond with little or no difficulty.

Assessment of Bilingual or Multilingual Patients

Clinicians face an increasing demand for services to be offered to clients who are bilingual or multilingual. It is difficult to make reliable and valid assessment of such patients unless the clinician is bilingual, and speaks the same two languages as the client. This situation is not often realized. Therefore, the clinician has to use a variety of tactics to make a reasonable assessment of bilingual patients (Roberts, 2008).

Interviewing the family and the client may pose a particular challenge to the clinician who does not speak the client's (and the family's) primary language. One solution is to refer the client to a clinician who speaks the client's language and specializes in assessing bilingual or multilingual clients. Such clinicians, however, are not always available. Therefore, the next option for the clinician is to enlist the help of an interpreter who has some professional training and experience in assisting SLPs make a valid assessment. To the extent possible, the clinician should avoid the assistance of a family member in translating or interpreting the interview questions and answers. Even so, enlisting the help of a family member who is bilingual may be unavoidable. In such cases, the clinician has to emphasize the family member to translate the questions, answers, and other information as objectively as possible. The clinician may ask the family member or a professionally trained interpreter to say in English what he or she asks the client. The clinician will follow the ASHA guidelines on serving the linguistic minority clients (American Speech-Language-Hearing Association, 1985).

A monolingual English-speaking clinician who needs to administer standardized tests to bilingual clients whose English is inadequate to understand the test items faces additional challenges. Although a few aphasia diagnostic tests are now available in different languages, the monolingual English-speaking clinician, or a bilingual clinician who does not speak the language of the client, will be unable to administer any of them. Once again, a professionally trained interpreter might be helpful. When no test that is relevant to the client's first language is available, some clinicians may administer an English test with the help of an interpreter. Translating test items to another language, however, raises questions of reliability and validity. In such cases, a more client-specific, functional communication approach may be preferable.

Only a few tests are now available to assess individuals who speak English and another language, as listed in Table 7–4. The *Multilingual Aphasia Examination* (Benton & Hamsher, 1978) is one of the few tests that are available in multiple languages. The test may be administered in English, French, German, Italian, and Spanish versions. In each language, the test may be used to evaluate naming, repetition, fluency, auditory comprehension, spelling, and writing. The same patient may be tested in two or more languages using the alternate forms.

The *Bilingual Aphasia Test* (BAT; Paradis, 1987). A comprehensive test that measures all aspects of language, BAT has parallel forms in more than 60 languages (Roberts, 2008). The clinician also can assess patients' skill in translating from one to the other language they spoke premorbidly. The clinician also can compare the relative performance on any two languages. Items to assess phonologic, morphologic, syntactic, lexical, and semantic aspects of the languages are included in each test. Language may be assessed in auditory, visual, oral, and manual modalities.

Some English tests have been translated into a few other languages. The Boston Diagnostic Aphasia Examination (BDAE; Goodglass, Kaplan, & Barresi, 2001), the Boston Naming Test (Kaplan, Goodglass & Weintraub, 2001), and Communication Abilities in Daily Living (Holland, Frattali, & Fromm, 1998) are available in various languages including Spanish, Italian, and Chinese. There are questions about the validity of translated tests, and the test items translated from one language to the other may or may not be appropriate for patients with a different cultural and linguistic background. A test standardized on the population from which the clients are drawn for diagnostic assessment

Table 7–4. Bilingual tests of aphasia

Bilingual Aphasia Tests	
Multilingual Aphasia Examination	Benton and Hamsher (1978)
Bilingual Aphasia Test (BAT)	Paradis (1987)
Boston Diagnostic Aphasia Examination (Translated)	Goodglass, Kaplan, and Barresi (2001)
Boston Naming Test (Translated)	Kaplan, Goodglass, and Weintraub (1983)
Communication Abilities in Daily Living (Translated)	Holland, Frattali, and Fromm (1998)
Western Aphasia Battery (Spanish)	Kertesz, Pascual-Leone, and Pascual-Leone (1990)

will be more valid than translated tests. Being aware of these limitations; clinicians may administer a translated test when no other more relevant assessment tools are available. In such cases, the clinicians will interpret the results cautiously and avoid making normative comparisons in favor of a client-specific analysis.

Analysis and Integration of Assessment Results

An overall analysis and integration of assessment results is essential to make valid clinical decisions. Assessment of aphasia is more continuous than it is for some of the other disorders of communication (e.g., fluency disorders). The client's health status might improve or deteriorate, depending on disease complications that are associated with aphasia. With such changes, the severity of aphasia will also change for the better or for worse. The type of aphasia might also change due to improvement or deterioration in the client's general health status. To track these changes, the clinician needs to make periodic, even if brief, assessments to ascertain the client's communication skills at different points during treatment and rehabilitation.

The clinician might take the following steps to analyze and integrate the assessment results before writing a diagnostic report:

- **The case history and interview information should be summarized.** The time and the conditions of the onset of aphasia and the symptoms that preceded and followed the onset may be summarized as reported by the caregivers and the client. The client's family constellation and the ethnocultural (including verbal) background should be described. History of the client's health, education, occupation, hobbies, literacy skills, and interests should be summarized.

- **Medical assessment and treatment should be summarized.** The medical procedures (e.g., neurological examinations, imaging) done on the client, specific neurological and medical diagnosis made on the client (e.g., stroke, tumor, traumatic brain injury) should be summarized. The current medical treatment the client is undergoing should be noted. The current physical condition of the client (e.g., stable, deteriorating, improving) should be described. The recommendation of medical specialists for rehabilitation, including speech-language treatment should be specified.

- **Aphasia assessment results should be described.** The clinician should analyze all the assessment procedures performed on the client, including the interview, observations, standardized tests, and any client-specific or criterion-referenced measures. This analysis may help summarize the client's:
  - *Overall communication skills.* A summary of the client's overall communication skills will help build a profile of the client.
  - *Auditory comprehension of spoken speech.* Interview, case history, and the standardized test results relative to the client's auditory comprehension of spoken speech may be summarized to help make a differential diagnosis of the aphasia type.
  - *Speech fluency.* Because of its importance in make a differential diagnosis of the type of aphasia a client may have, it is essential to summarize the assessment results relative to speech fluency. Among other features, reduced speech rate (less than 50 wpm), excessive speaking effort, limited phrase length (less than 5 words), sparseness of speech, difficulty initiating speech, and frequent pauses and uneven flow may be highlighted.
  - *Syntactic and morphological skills.* The kinds of sentences the client produces, omission of grammatic morphemes, excessive use of content words, and unfinished (incomplete sentences) may be described. These observations also help make a differential diagnosis of the type of aphasia.
  - *Naming skills.* A more general impairment of aphasia, the naming skills may be summarized as evidenced on the naming subtests of standardized aphasia tests and as noted during the interview.
  - *Repetition skills.* Another differential diagnostic feature of the different types of aphasia, repetitions skills, as noted on the administered standardized tests and as observed by the clinician, should be highlighted.
  - *Narrative and conversational skills.* Narrative skills, as revealed by picture description and story telling or retelling should be described. Conversational skills (e.g., topic initiation, topic maintenance, conversational repair) as observed during the interview and throughout the assessment may be summarized.
  - *Speech production skills.* Clients with nonfluent aphasia may have an independent motor speech disorder. Therefore, the analysis and summary should include statements about speech production and the error patterns found during the interview and on standardized tests.
  - *Automatic and echolalic speech.* Because these two may be of differential diagnostic significance, the clinician should highlight their presence.
  - *Reading and writing skills.* Errors in oral reading and comprehension of both orally and silently read material may be summarized. Errors noted on writing samples should be summarized as well.

○ *Nonverbal communication.* The client's production of gestures that accompany speech or gestures that serve as independent means of communication may be described.

○ *Bilingual and bicultural skills.* If the client is bilingual and bicultural, relative deficits in the two languages should be noted. Assessment results of primary language and that of the secondary language should be summarized. Translational problems (e.g., automatic translation, one-way translation, translation without comprehension) may be noted.

• **A diagnosis and differential diagnosis may be made.** The diagnosis of aphasia will be made based on the features described in the earlier sections of the chapter and summarized under the previous list. A differential diagnosis of the type of aphasia may be made based on:

○ *Broca's aphasia.* Agrammatic, nonfluent, hesitant, and limited speech; impaired naming and repetition, better speech comprehension than expression; impaired reading aloud and writing; paraphasia, not a major symptom; possibly an independent speech production problem; right hemiparesis or hemiplegia.

○ *Transcortical motor aphasia.* Good speech comprehension, initial muteness and impaired fluency, some paraphasia, mildly impaired naming, good articulation, good repetition but echolalia and perseveration, good reading comprehension, impaired writing, possible right hemiparesis or hemiplegia.

○ *Mixed transcortical aphasia.* Impaired speech comprehension, fluency, grammar, naming skills, reading aloud, reading comprehension, writing; nonsignificant paraphasia, good articulation, good (but parrot-like and nonfunctional) repetition.

○ *Global aphasia.* Severely impaired speech comprehension, fluency, articulation, grammar, naming, reading, and writing. Severe deficits in all aspects of language.

○ *Wernicke's aphasia.* Normal or hyperfluency (100 to 200 wpm), severely impaired speech comprehension, good grammar (with pseudogrammatical sentences), severely impaired naming, semantic and neologistic paraphasia, impaired repetition, impaired reading and writing, good articulation, absence of paresis or paralysis; may sound confused.

○ *Transcortical sensory aphasia.* Impaired speech comprehension, impaired naming, fluent but paraphasic and echolalic speech, good grammar, good articulation, good but echolalic repetition, good reading aloud but poor comprehension, impaired writing, an initial hemiparesis that clears, and unilateral neglect.

○ *Conduction aphasia.* Mild (if present) speech comprehension deficit, good fluency (with some pauses), good grammar, normal articulation, severely impaired repetition, impaired naming, literal paraphasia, impaired reading aloud with good reading comprehension, and impaired writing.

○ *Anomic aphasia.* Severely impaired naming, against the background of mostly well-preserved language, reading, and writing skills.

- **Recommendations may be specified.** The analysis and integration of assessment data will result in the clinician's recommendations for the client, the family members, and other caregivers. Language treatment for clients with aphasia is known to be effective, and typically recommended (Chapey, 2008; Davis, 2000; Hegde, 2006; Martin, Thompson, & Worrall, 2008).

Postassessment Counseling

After completing the assessment, the clinician discusses the results of the assessment with the client and the family members. The clinician summarizes the main findings for them, suggests a diagnosis, recommends treatment, and answers their questions about aphasia, its treatment, prognosis, and so forth.

Make a Tentative Diagnosis

Even though the results of assessment will not have been made, the clinician will have judged the nature of the language disorder. Therefore, the clinician can suggest the diagnosis of aphasia to the client and the attending caregivers. The communication deficits that support the diagnosis of aphasia then will be described to them.

If the assessment results support a particular type of aphasia, the clinician might specify it. The clinician will then describe the key language impairments that suggest the diagnosis of a particular type of aphasia. Although the clinician will avoid making any kind of neurological diagnosis, he or she might support the diagnosis with the obvious neurological symptoms that are a part of the symptom complex. For instance, the clinician might add that the client's Broca's aphasia and the right paralysis or paresis are associated conditions.

Make Recommendations

Most aphasiologists recommend treatment, even in cases of such severe forms as global aphasia (Brookshire, 2007; Chapey, 2001; Martin, Thompson, & Worrall, 2008). Treatment may be offered at least on a trial basis to evaluate the benefits to the client and the family. The clinician might give a brief description of the recommended treatment procedure.

Suggest Prognosis

The clinician will suggest a prognosis based on the assessment results, the type of aphasia diagnosed, and the knowledge of treatment outcome research for aphasia. As always, the prognosis is suggested in probabilistic terms and the conditions under which certain outcomes may be expected. For instance, the clinician might contrast potential outcomes of treatment versus no treatment.

Answer the Client's and the Caregivers' Questions

Aphasic clients and their families probably will have a number of questions about aphasia. The amount of information they desire usually depends on how much they have received from other medical professionals. Usually it is best to assume that clients and families would like to know more about the disorder, even if they are not actively asking questions. To encourage the family, the clinician can ask a general question such as, "Do you have any questions about aphasia?" during the postassessment counseling session. This open invitation can help the client and family feel comfortable to seek more information. Here is a sample of questions that may arise at the end of the assessment:

- What is aphasia?—It is an acquired disorder that occurs when the brain's language centers are damaged. It affects speaking, listening, reading, and writing in varying amounts. The client's intelligence and personality are generally not affected.

- How many people have aphasia?—There are about a million people in the United States with aphasia.

- What are the physical problems associated with aphasia?—It depends on the type of aphasia. Clients with Broca's, global, and perhaps conduction aphasia may have weakness or paralysis on the right side of their bodies. They also may have numbness on the right side as well. Clients with a fluent aphasia, such as Wernicke's aphasia, usually do not demonstrate weakness or paralysis. A few clients with aphasia will experience seizures after their stroke or head injury.

- What is the typical recovery time for someone with aphasia?—This varies significantly from person to person, depending on how severe the brain damage was. If the damage was mild, a good outcome may be evident in several months. But even then, the client still may have some residual problems with word finding, spelling, and reading. In cases of more severe damage, a full recovery probably is not possible, although slow improvements in language abilities can occur for years after the onset of the disorder. Treatment can help many clients recover as much of their language abilities as possible and learn compensatory techniques for sharing information.

- What is the best way to speak to a person with aphasia?—If you are asking the aphasic person a question, speak slightly slower than normal and avoid using long, complicated sentences; give them extra time to process what you are saying. If they are trying to say something to you, give them extra time to get the words out. Do not try to complete words or sentences for the person; let him or her have the opportunity to finish the utterance independently. Only if the person asks for help should you fill in the missing words.

- What is the most common cause of aphasia?—Most cases of aphasia are caused by a stroke, but other conditions such as a head injury, infection, and tumor can cause it as well.

References

American Speech-Language-Hearing Association. (1985). Clinical management of communicatively handicapped minority language populations. *Asha, 27,* 57–60.

Benson, D. F., & Ardila, A. (1996). *Aphasia: A clinical perspective.* New York, NY: Oxford University Press.

Benton, A. L., & Hamsher, K. (1978). *Multilingual aphasia examination* (rev. ed.). Iowa City, IA: University of Iowa.

Blomert, L., Kean, M. L., Koster, C., & Schokker, J. (1994). Amsterdam-Nijmegen everyday language test: Construction, reliability, and validity. *Aphasiology, 8*(4), 381–407.

Brookshire, R. (2007). *An introduction to neurogenic communication disorders* (7th ed.). St. Louis, MO: Mosby Year Book.

Chapey, R. (2001) (Ed.). *Language intervention strategies in adult aphasia and related neurogenic disorders* (4th ed.) Baltimore, MD: Lippincott Williams & Wilkins.

Collins, M. J. (2005). Global aphasia. In L. L. LaPointe (Ed.), *Aphasia and related neurogenic language disorders* (3rd ed.,pp. 186–198). New York, NY: Thieme Medical.

Crary, M. A., Haak, N. J., & Malinsky, A. E. (1989). Preliminary psychometric evaluation of an acute aphasia screening protocol. *Aphasiology, 3*:611-618.

Damasio, H. (2008). Neural basis of language disorders. In R. Chapey (Ed), *Language intervention strategies in aphasia and related neurogenic communication disorders* (pp. 20–43). Philadelphia, PA: Lippincott Williams & Wilkins.

Darley, F. L. (1982). *Aphasia.* Philadelphia, PA: W. B. Saunders.

Davis, G. A. (2000). *Aphasiology: Disorders and clinical practice.* Needham Heights, MA: Allyn & Bacon.

Duffy, J. R. (2005). *Motor speech disorders* (2nd ed.). St. Louis, MO: Elsevier Mosby.

Fitch-West, J., & Sands, E. (1998). *Bedside Evaluation Screening Test* (2nd ed.). Austin, TX: Pro-Ed.

Frattali, C. M., Thompson, C. K., Holland, A. L., Wohl, C. B., & Ferkietic, M. M. (1995). *Functional assessment of communication skills for adults* (ASHA FACS). Rockville, MD: American Speech-Language-Hearing Association.

Freed, D. (2000). *Motor speech disorders: Diagnosis and treatment.* Clifton Park, NY: Cengage Delmar.

Goodglass, H., Kaplan, E., & Baressi, B. (2001). *The Boston diagnostic aphasia examination* (3rd ed.). Austin, TX: Pro-Ed.

Hegde, M. N. (2006). *A coursebook on aphasia and other neurogenic language disorders* (3rd ed.). Clifton Park, NY: Cengage Delmar.

Helm-Estabrooks, N., Ramsberger, G., Nicholas, M., & Morgan, A. (1989). *Boston Assessment of Severe Aphasia.* Austin, TX: Pro-Ed.

Holland, A. L., Frattali, C. M., & Fromm, D. (1998). *Communication activities in daily living, Second Edition.* Austin, TX: Pro-Ed.

Horner, R. D., Swanson, J. W., Bosworth, H. B., & Matchar, D. B. (2003). Effects of race and poverty on the process and outcome of inpatient rehabilitation services among stroke patients. *Stroke, 43*(4), 1027–1038.

Kaplan, E., Goodglass, H., & Weintraub, S. (2001). *The Boston naming test* (2nd ed.). Philadelphia, PA: Lippincott Williams & Wilkins.

Kagan, A., & Gailey, G. (1993). Functional is not enough. Training conversation partners for aphasic adults. In A. Holland & M. Forbes (Eds.), *Aphasia treatment: World perspectives* (pp. 199–225). San Diego, CA: Singular.

Keenan, J. S. and E. G. Brassell (1975). *Aphasia language performance scales.* Murfreeboro, TN: Pinnacle Press.

Kertesz, A. (2006). *Western Aphasia Battery-Revised.* San Antonio. TX: Pearson.

Kertesz, A., Pascual-Leone, P., & Pascual-Leone, G. (1990). *Western Aphasia Battery en versión y adaptación castellana.* Valencia, Spain: Nau Libres.

Kertesz, A. (1982). *Western aphasia battery.* New York, NY: Grune & Stratton.

Lomas, J., Pickard, L., Bester, S., & Associates (1989). The communicative effectiveness index: Clinical and research assessment of head injury outcome. *International Rehabilitation Medicine, 7,* 145–149.

Lorenzen, B. L., & Murray, L. L. (2008). Bilingual aphasia: A theoretical and clinical review. *American Journal of Speech-Language Pathology, 17,* 299–317.

Marshall, R. C., & Wright, H. H. (2007). Developing a clinician-friendly aphasia test. *American Journal of Speech-Language Pathology, 16,* 295–315.

Martin, N., Thompson, C. K., & Worrall, L. (Eds.). (2008). *Aphasia rehabilitation: The impairment and its consequences.* San Diego, CA: Plural.

Paradis, M. (1987). *Bilingual aphasia test.* Hillsdale, NJ: Lawrence Erlbaum Associates.

Paradis, M. (1998). Acquired aphasia in bilingual speakers. In M. Taylor-Sarno (Ed.), *Acquired aphasia* (3rd ed., pp. 531–540). New York, NY: Academic Press.

Paul, D. R., Frattalli, C. M., Holland, A. L., and Associates (2003). *Quality of communication life scale.* Bethesda, MD: American Speech-Language-Hearing Association.

Payne, J. C. (1994). *Communication profile: A functional skills survey.* Tucson, AZ: Communication Skill Builders.

Payne, J. C. (1997). *Adult neurogenic language disorders: Assessment and treatment.* San Diego, CA: Singular.

Peach, R. (2008). Global aphasia: Identification and management. In R. Chapey (Ed), *Language intervention strategies in aphasia and related neurogenic communication disorders* (pp. 565–594). Philadelphia, PA: Lippincott Williams & Wilkins.

Porch, B. E. (2001). *Porch index of communicative ability* (4th ed.). Palo Alto, CA: Consulting Psychologists Press.

Prutting, C. A., & Kirschner, D. M. (1987). A clinical appraisal of the pragmatic aspects of language. *Journal of Speech and Hearing Disorders, 52,* 105–119.

Roberts, P. M. (2008). Issues in assessment and treatment of bilingual and culturally diverse patients. In R. Chapey (Ed.), *Language intervention strategies in aphasia and related neurogenic communication disorders* (pp. 245–275).Philadelphia, PA: Lippincott Williams & Wilkins.

Sarno, M. T. (1969). *The functional communication profile: Manual of directions.* New York, NY: New York University Medical Center, Institute of Rehabilitation Medicine.

Schuell, H. M. (1972). *Differential diagnosis of aphasia with the Minnesota Test* (2nd ed., revised by Sefer, J. W.). Minneapolis, MN: University of Minnesota Press.

Simmons-Mackie, N. (2008). Social approaches to aphasia intervention. In R. Chapey (Ed.), *Language intervention strategies in aphasia and related neurogenic communication disorders* (5th ed., pp. 290–318). Philadelphia, PA: Wolter Kluver/Lippincott Williams & Wilkins.

Sklar, M. (1983). *Sklar Aphasia Scale-Revised.* Los Angles, CA: Wester Psychological Services.

Spreen, O., & Benton, A. L. (1977). *Neurosensory center comprehensive examination for aphasia.* Victoria, BC: University of Victoria.

Swindell, C. S., Holland, A. L., & Fromm, D. (1984). Classification of aphasia: WAB type versus clinical impressions. In R. H. Brookshire (Ed.), *Clinical aphasiology conference proceedings* (pp. 48–54). Minneapolis, MN: BRK Publishers.

Tanner, D. & Culbertson, W. (1999). *Quick assessment for apraxia of speech.* Oceanside, CA: Academic Communication Associates.

Wertz, R. T., Deal, J. J., & Robinson, A. J. (1984). Classifying the aphasias: A comparison of the Boston diagnostic aphasia examination and the western aphasia battery. In R. H. Brookshire (Ed.), *Clinical aphasiology conference proceedings* (pp. 40–47). Minneapolis, MN: BRK Publishers.

World Health Organization. (1992). *The ICD-10 classification of mental and behavioral disorders.* Geneva, Switzerland: Author.

World Health Organization. (2001). ICIDH-2. *International classification of impairments, disabilities, and handicaps.* Geneva, Switzerland: Author.

World Health Organization Quality of Life (WHOQOL-BREF) (2004). Geneva, Switzerland: Author.

Worrall, L. (1992). Functional communication assessment: An Australian perspective. *Aphasiology, 6,* 105–110.

Whurr, R. (1996). *The Aphasia Screening Test* (2nd ed.). London, UK: Harcourt.

CHAPTER 8

Assessment of Aphasia: Protocols

- Overview of Aphasia Protocols
- Aphasia Interview Protocol
- Auditory Comprehension Assessment Protocol
- Connected Speech and Grammatical Skills Assessment Protocol
- Repetition and Echolalia Assessment Protocol
- Naming and Word Finding Assessment Protocol
- Fluency Assessment Protocol
- Reading, Writing, and Calculations Assessment Protocol
- Aphasia Summative Diagnostic Protocol

Overview of Aphasia Protocols

Assessment Protocols provided in this chapter help assess aphasia in adults in an efficient manner. The protocols offer ready-made formats that clinicians can use in structuring their client and family interviews and assessing various parameters of communication impaired in aphasia.

The protocols offered in this chapter also are available on the accompanying CD. The clinician may print the needed protocols in evaluating their clients. The clinician may combine these protocols in suitable ways to facilitate the evaluation of an adult's aphasia.

This chapter offers assessment protocols that are specific to aphasia. To complete the assessment on a given client, the clinician should combine these disorder-specific protocols with the common assessment protocols given in Chapter 2:

- The Adult Case History
- Orofacial Examination and Hearing Screening Protocol
- Diadochokinetic Assessment Protocol for Adults
- Adult Assessment Report Outline

In assessing adults with aphasia who have other disorders of communication, the clinician may combine these protocols with protocols from other chapters. For example, the clinician may combine apraxia of speech assessment protocols given in Chapter 4 and dysarthria assessment protocols given in Chapter 6.

Beginning With the Common Protocols

The protocols given in this chapter are specific to aphasia in adults. To complete the assessment on a given client, the clinician should combine these disorder-specific protocols with the common assessment protocols given in Chapter 2:

- The Adult Case History
- Orofacial Examination and Hearing Screening Protocol
- Functional Communication Assessment Protocol
- Quality of Life Assessment Protocol
- Diadochokinetic Assessment Protocol for Adults
- Adult Assessment Report Outline

Aphasia Interview Protocol

Client's Name _____ Age _____ DOB _____

Diagnosis _____ Date _____ Clinician _____

Note that your interview of the client and caregivers is concerned with getting additional information on the client's current health, communication skills and impairments, certain premorbid information, information on the family constellation and support for the client, reasons for seeking help, and so forth.

Individualize this protocol on the CD and print it for your use.

Prepare Yourself for the Interview

☐ Review the *Interview Guidelines* presented in Chapter 1.

☐ Arrange for comfortable seating and adequate lighting.

☐ Conduct the interview in a quiet room.

☐ Record the interview whenever possible.

☐ Review the case history ahead of time, noting areas about which you want to review or obtain more information.

☐ Review all the medical reports that are available to you; try to get the missing reports before you see the client, if this is practical.

Greet and Introduce Yourself

☐ Greet the client and the accompanying persons.

☐ Introduce yourself. Briefly review your assessment plan for the day and give an estimate of the duration of assessment.

> **Example:** "Hello Mr./Mrs. [*the client's name*]. How are you today? [I am glad you are doing fine.] My name is [*your name*], and I am the speech-language pathologist who will be assessing you today. I would like to start by reviewing the case history and asking you a few questions. After we finish talking, I will work with you. Today's assessment should take about [*estimate the amount of time you plan to spend*]."

Use Discretion in Asking the Interview Questions

The following kinds of questions are generally appropriate to ask clients with aphasia or their caregivers who accompany them. Depending on the client's education, judged sophistication, as well as the current communication and auditory comprehension skills, you may have to rephrase

(continues)

Aphasia Interview Protocol (continued)

the questions, simplify them when necessary, skip certain questions, add new questions, ask more follow-up questions to ones suggested here, and so forth. The questions that follow are written such that they are directed to the clients themselves. Some clients, however, may not be in a position to answer them. For instance, many with a severe form of any type of aphasia may not be good candidates for a valid source of case history information, though the interaction may still provide important diagnostic information. Generally, clients with profound auditory comprehension deficits and empty speech (e.g., those with Wernicke's aphasia) as well as those with global aphasia may not be good sources of information. In such cases, the clinician needs to put the questions to the family members or other caregivers. If so, the questions need to be rephrased to properly address the actual informant, who may be a family member or another caregiver. Although the outline shows the questions that need to be asked and answered, avoid relentless questioning. Frequently, paraphrase what the informants' answers to your questions. Ask about the informants' views, thoughts, or feelings. If appropriate, express approval of what they say. Note that it is not just the clinician who asks questions; clients, family members, or other informants will have questions that the clinician needs to answer. If they have questions about the typical features of aphasia, causes of the problem, treatment and rehabilitation options, and so forth, answer briefly and promise more detailed information later.

Questions about the Current Communication Problem

☐ What are you mostly concerned with your speech and language skills?

☐ Would you please describe the problem? *[Ask or skip the following questions depending on how well the client describes his or her problems.]*

☐ Do you have difficulty expressing your basic needs?

☐ At home, are you able to talk in sentences like you did before?

☐ Are you able to talk smoothly and fluently, or do you have to pause and think of words?

☐ Do you think you are able to hold a conversation with someone, like you did before your illness?

☐ Do you have problems remembering names of people and things?

☐ Are you reading and writing like you did before your illness?

☐ Do you have difficulty understanding what others say to you?

☐ What do you do when you don't understand someone?

☐ Do you think people have difficulty understanding what you say to them?

☐ What do you do when others don't understand your speech?

☐ When did you start having difficulty with your speech?

☐ Now I would like you to tell me about the circumstances under which you started having speech difficulties. For instance, what were you doing and what time was it? *[Most patients may describe the symptoms of a stroke; ask follow-up questions about the stroke onset.]*

☐ Did you have any muscle or movement problems at the time of onset? For example, any paralysis?

☐ Did you go to the hospital right away?

☐ How was your speech before you went to the hospital? [*Ask follow-up questions on the speech around the time of the onset of aphasia*]

☐ Were you awake and alert when you arrived in the hospital?

☐ How was your speech when you arrived in the hospital?

☐ What kind of treatment did you receive there?

☐ For how long did you stay in the hospital?

☐ Was there an improvement in your speech and physical condition when you left the hospital?

☐ In the past did you have any other kind of speech problem? [*Give examples of stuttering or voice disorders if the client is unsure.*]

Questions about Previous Speech-Language Services

☐ Have you received speech or language therapy before? [*Skip the rest if the answer is negative.*]

☐ When and where did you receive such therapy?

☐ Was it for aphasia or some other problem?

☐ Do you remember what kind of therapy it was? What did you do in the therapy sessions?

☐ What were the results? Were you satisfied with the outcome?

Questions about General Health

☐ Now I want to know your general health history. How was your health in the previous years? [*Ask follow-up questions about previous strokes or other neurological diseases, their consequences, and treatment and rehabilitation.*]

☐ Are there any medical or surgical treatments scheduled for you?

☐ What kinds of medications are you on?

☐ Are you able to eat and drink normally? [*Ask follow-up questions if the client mentions swallowing problems; ask for descriptions of problems and how they are being managed.*]

☐ Do you sleep well? [*Ask follow-up questions on their management if the client mentions sleep problems.*]

☐ Are you seeing other specialists these days? [*Ask follow-up questions if the answer is affirmative; find out who is offering what kinds of services.*]

(continues)

Aphasia Interview Protocol (continued)

Questions about Hearing

- ☐ Are you concerned with your hearing? *[Skip the rest if the answer is negative.]*
- ☐ When did you get your hearing tested? Where and when?
- ☐ What were the results and recommendations?
- ☐ Do you use a hearing aid? How regularly?
- ☐ Is your hearing aid helping you hear better? Are you satisfied with it?

Questions about Occupation and Hobbies

- ☐ I want to know something about your occupation. What kind of work did you do?
- ☐ Have you returned to your job? Do you plan to?
- ☐ Do you think your communication problems will make it difficult to return to your job?
- ☐ I want to know a little bit about how you spend time now. How would you describe your daily activities?
- ☐ What kind of hobbies did you enjoy before your illness?
- ☐ Do you still do those things?

Questions about Family History of Communication Disorders

- ☐ I would like to ask you a few questions about your family. With whom do you live?
- ☐ Is there any family history of strokes or other kinds of neurological problems? *[Skip the rest if the answer is negative]*
- ☐ Are there any other members of your family that have the kinds of speech and language difficulties you have? *[Ask follow-up questions if the answer is positive; ask about the treatment received and their current communication status.]*
- ☐ Are there any other type of communication problems in any of your relatives? *[If necessary, give such examples as* stuttering *or* voice *problems; ask about the current communication status.]*

Questions about Bilingualism

- ☐ I want to know if you speak another language. Do you? *[Skip the rest if the answer is negative.]*
  [Ask follow-up questions if the answer is positive; ask about the language or languages spoken; whether English is the first or second language; the sequence with which they were learned; competency in each language.]

☐ What is your first or primary language?

☐ Your second language?

☐ When did you learn your second language?

☐ Which is your dominant language?

☐ Which language do you speak at home? And at work?

☐ In your home, who else speaks the same two languages as you do? [*Ask follow-up questions about the spouse's or other primary caregiver's bilingual status.*]

☐ Do you read and write in both the languages?

☐ Do you think your communication is affected in both the languages to the same extent? If not, which language is now better?

☐ Assuming you would like therapy, in which language do you prefer it?

Questions about Behavioral Health

☐ How do you rate your overall mood these days? [*If the client suggests an unfavorable mood or mood swings, ask follow-up questions to find out more about what triggers the negative emotions and what is being done about it.*]

☐ Do you feel depressed or lonely?

☐ Are you able to handle your everyday activities? [*If the answer suggests problems, explore them further; find out what kinds of activities are more difficult and why.*]

☐ Are there any other kinds of concerns you have about your speech or anything else in your life now?

☐ Is there anything else you want to tell me about your speech-language difficulty? [*Ask follow-up questions about any other problem the client or the informant may mention.*]

Ask additional questions as needed to make sure all the information needed has been obtained.

Close the Interview

Before you close the initial interview and begin your assessment, summarize the major points you have learned from the interview. Allow the client and the accompanying caregivers an opportunity to interpret or correct information. Close the interview with the following:

☐ You have been very helpful in providing good information that will be helpful in my assessment. I think I have learned much about you and your family. Now, do you have any questions for me at this point?

☐ Thank you very much for you input. Now, I will work with you. When we are finished, we will discuss the findings. I will then answer your questions about aphasia and its treatment.

Auditory Comprehension Assessment Protocol

Client's Name _____ Age _____ DOB _____

Diagnosis _____ Date _____ Clinician _____

Yes – No Questions

Ask the following questions. A correct response requires a "yes" or "no" verbal response or an unambiguous head nod for "yes" and head shake for "no." If a response is unclear, repeat the question once.

Clinician asks	Correct Response	Correct After Repeat	Incorrect Response
Is your name Robert (or Roberta)?			
Is your name _____?			
Are you sitting in a chair?			
Are you married?			
Do you have two arms?			
Are you eating dinner right now?			
Are there trees in a forest?			
Are you standing in the corner?			
Do cows live in the water?			
Is 6:00 AM early in the morning?			
Is New York in Germany?			
Is cement used in laying bricks?			
Are all soldiers brave?			
Does everyone drive a car to work?			
Does the sun set in the west?			

Identifying Pictured Objects (in a field of three)

Using color photographs of common objects, place three photographs in front of the client. Ensure that no items are from the same semantic category (e.g., sponge, shirt, hamburger). Ask the client to point to one of the three items. Repeat the name of the target item once if requested.

Clinician asks	Correct Response	Correct After Repeat	Incorrect Response
Show me the "eggs."			
Show me the "wheel."			
Show me the "television."			
Show me the "toaster."			
Show me the "desk."			
Show me the "shoes."			
Show me the "cheese."			
Show me the "sink."			
Show me the "bus."			
Show me the "fence."			

Following Directions

Ask the client to point to the following items in the room. A correct response requires an unambiguous gesture that indicates the item. If a response is unclear, repeat the command once.

Clinician asks	Correct Response	Correct After Repeat	Incorrect Response
Point to me.			
Point to yourself.			
Point to a chair.			
Point to the ceiling.			
Point to me and then to the table.			
Point to my pencil and then to the floor.			
Point to something made of metal.			
Show me two fingers, then "thumbs up."			
Show me the table, floor, and chair.			
Show me your head, neck, and arm.			

(continues)

Auditory Comprehension Assessment Protocol (continued)

Comprehending a Narrative

Read the following paragraph to the client at a normal rate of speed. Ask the following questions. Repeat a question once if requested.

One December night, a family had gathered round their hearth. Up the chimney roared the fire, brightening the room with its broad blaze. The faces of the father and mother had a sober gladness; the children laughed; the eldest daughter was the image of happiness at 17. The cold wind rattled the door with a sound of wailing. For a moment it saddened them, but they were glad again when they saw that the latch was lifted by some traveler, whose footsteps had been unheard amid the dreary blast of winter. (Adapted from Hawthorne's "The Ambitious Guest.")

Clinician asks	Correct Response	Correct After Repeat	Incorrect Response
Is the weather warm in the story?			
Is there a father and mother in the story?			
Is the daughter 17 years old?			
Do they have a fireplace?			
Did the wind make them happy?			
Is there more than one child in the story?			
Did the story happen in January?			
Was the family alarmed by the visitor?			

Connected Speech and Grammatical Skills Assessment Protocol

Client's Name _____ Age _____ DOB _____

Diagnosis _____ Date _____ Clinician _____

Description of a Picture

Show the client the picture on the next page, and say, "Tell me everything that is happening in this picture." Prompt the client for more information if the description is extremely brief. If possible, make an audio recording. Mark the "Score" column for the description that most accurately reflects the client's narrative.

The Client's Description	Score
The description is within normal limits—with normal sentence structure, correct grammatical morphemes (e.g., plurals, possessives, present progressive -*ing*), and fluent verbalizations without word-finding difficulties.	
The description is nearly normal—with occasional hesitations and revisions, accurate articulation, but perhaps a slightly slower than the normal rate of speech.	
Fluent description with normal sentence structure—but with word-finding problems, occasional paraphasic errors, and revisions and pauses.	
Some evidence of agrammatism, but mostly normal or near-normal sentence structure; accurate production of most grammatical morphemes; evident are word-finding errors.	
Primarily agrammatic description, consisting primarily of nouns and verbs, with missing function words (e.g., articles, conjunctions, prepositions) and bound morphemes; noted are pauses, hesitations, and word-finding difficulties.	
Fluent but primarily semantic jargon-filled description; normal utterance length; mostly English words, but at least half of them unintelligible; normal intonation; fluent articulation with few or no pauses or hesitations.	
Fluent description, with neologistic jargon; normal utterance length; all words unintelligible; normal intonation; fluent articulation with few or no pauses or hesitations.	
Single word descriptions with paraphasic errors; labored and halting articulation; word-finding difficulties with frequent, prolonged pauses.	
Short and halting description, primarily filled with repeated, stereotypic utterances.	
No intelligible utterances, though attending to the picture.	

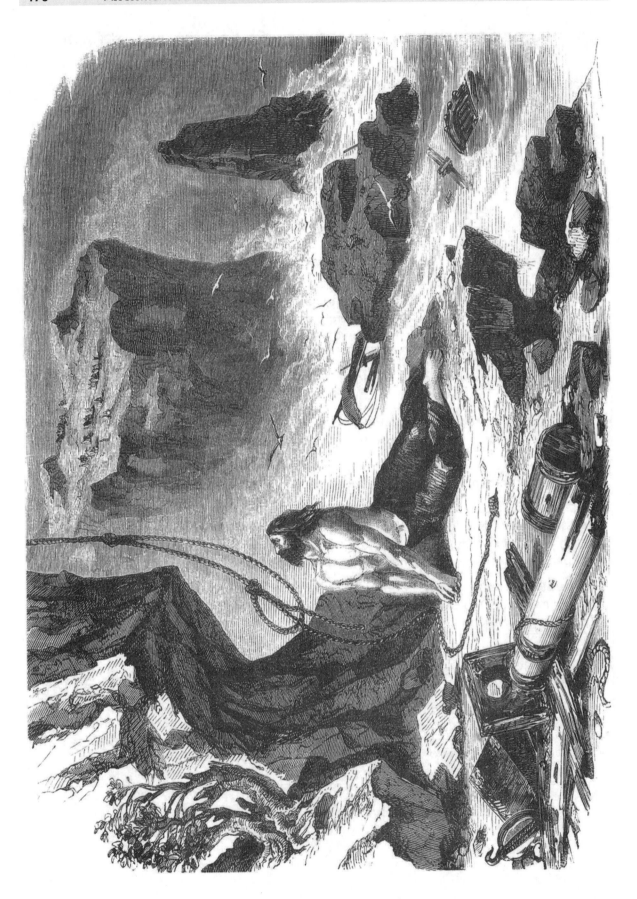

Repetition and Echolalia Assessment Protocol

Client's Name _____ Age _____ DOB _____

Diagnosis _____ Date _____ Clinician _____

Score: Correct (C) Partially Correct (PC) Incorrect (IC)

Repetition of Single Words			
Clinician Models	*Client's Responses*		
Say *"chair"*	C	PC	IC
Say *"spoon"*	C	PC	IC
Say *"run"*	C	PC	IC
Say *"mine"*	C	PC	IC
Say *"sock"*	C	PC	IC
Say *"book"*	C	PC	IC
Say *"fireplace"*	C	PC	IC
Say *"penmanship"*	C	PC	IC
Say *"conditioner"*	C	PC	IC
Say *"examination"*	C	PC	IC
Repetition of Sentences			
Clinician Models	*Client's Responses*		
Say *"I am fine."*	C	PC	IC
Say *"How are you?"*	C	PC	IC
Say *"It's getting cloudy."*	C	PC	IC
Say *"I think it will rain today."*	C	PC	IC
Say *"Let's go to downtown and see a nice movie."*	C	PC	IC
Say *"I'm not sure I can do it, but I'm willing to give it a try."*	C	PC	IC
Say *"Why do you say we don't have milk, when we bought a gallon yesterday?*	C	PC	IC
Say *"The man who was only a spectator of the game was hit by the ball."*	C	PC	IC

(continues)

Repetition and Echolalia Assessment Protocol (continued)

Echolalic Repetition: Exemplars Observed During Assessment
1. _____
2. _____
3. _____
4. _____
5. _____

Naming and Word Finding Assessment Protocol

Client's Name _____ Age _____ DOB _____

Diagnosis _____ Date _____ Clinician _____

Assess Responsive Naming

Ask questions with no physical stimulus presentation. Write down the incorrect responses.

Clinician asks	Correct response	Incorrect response
What do people wear to see better?	"Glasses"	
What is that you are sitting on?	"Chair"	
What do you use to unlock a door?	"Key"	
What do you use to cut vegetables?	"Knife"	
What do you do when you are tired?	"Sleep" or "Rest"	
What do you use to write?	"Pen" or "Pencil"	
What do you want when you are thirsty?	"Water"	
What do you want when you are hungry?	"Food"	

Assess Confrontation Naming

Ask questions after presenting a picture. Write down the incorrect responses; take note of the missing article. Score the self-corrections as:

No = *No attempt*   S = *Successful*   UnS = *Unsuccessful*

Clinician asks	Correct response	Incorrect	Self-corrections		
What is this?	"A dog"		No	S	UnS
What is this?	"A book"		No	S	UnS
What is this?	"A pen"		No	S	UnS
What is this?	"A house"		No	S	UnS
What is this?	"A spoon"		No	S	UnS
What is this?	"A tree"		No	S	UnS
What is this?	"A glass"		No	S	UnS

(continues)

Naming and Word Finding Assessment Protocol (continued)

Assess Categorical Naming (Word Fluency Test)

Give one minute for each category. Write down the responses or the number of responses given. Norms for non-brain-damaged individuals: 17 animals in one minute. For words beginning with F, A, and S, they average 37 total items (FAS scores combined) (Tombaugh, Kozak, & Rees, 1999).

Clinician asks	Client's responses
"Tell me the names of all the animals you can think of."	
"I will say a letter of the alphabet. I want you to tell me all the words you can think of that start with that letter. Ready? Let's start with the letter 'F.'"	
"Now the letter 'A.'"	
"The last one is letter 'S.'"	

Assess Naming to Complete Incomplete Models (Sentence Completion)

Write down the responses given.

Clinician's questions	Client's responses
"You write with a . . . "	
"You eat with a . . . "	
"You can fly in an . . . "	
"You sleep in a . . . "	
"You drive a . . . ."	
"A man will go to a barber for a . . . "	
"You drink water from a . . . "	
"People buy food at a . . . "	
"On a nice day, the sky is . . . "	
"She cut the paper with a pair of . . . "	

Assess Serial Naming

Write down the responses given.

Clinician asks	Client's responses
"Please name the days of the week."	
"Please name the months in a year."	
"Please count to 20."	
"Please say all the letters of the alphabet."	

Fluency Assessment Protocol

Client's Name _____ Age _____ DOB _____

Diagnosis _____ Date _____ Clinician _____

The analysis was based on at least two of the following three (Check all that apply):

☐ Interview (recorded or judged live)

☐ Picture description sample (recorded or judged live)

☐ A conversational speech sample (recorded or judged live)

Use this *Fluency Assessment Protocol* on the CD to individualize it for printing. 💿

Parameters of Fluency in Aphasia	Evaluation
Phrase length per utterance	☐ Normal ☐ Limited ☐ Extremely Limited (5–8 words) _____ _____
Paraphasia	☐ Mild ☐ Moderate ☐ Severe *Observed types:* ☐ Phonemic ☐ Semantic ☐ Neologistic
Dysfluencies	☐ Mild ☐ Moderate ☐ Severe *Observed types:* ☐ Pauses ☐ Repetitions ☐ Interjections ☐ Revisions (False starts) ☐ Sound prolongations Others (specify):
Ease of speech production	☐ Normal (easily initiated, flowing, effortless) ☐ Effortful (slow to initiate, halting, aprosodic, sparse)
Rate of speech	☐ Normal (more than 50 wpm) ☐ Slow (less than 50 wpm)
Smoothness of articulation	☐ Normal (smooth, easy, accurate) ☐ Impaired (effortful, groping, inaccurate)
Meaningfulness of fluency (empty speech)	☐ Normal fluency and meaningful speech ☐ Limited fluency and meaningful speech ☐ Normal (or near-normal) fluency and meaningless speech ☐ Hyperfluency and meaningless speech
Overall Evaluation:	☐ Normal fluency ☐ Below normal fluency ☐ Hyperfluency ☐ Mostly meaningful ☐ Mostly meaningless

Diagnosis: _____ Clinician: _____

Reading, Writing, and Calculation Assessment Protocol

Client's Name _____ Age _____ DOB _____

Diagnosis _____ Date _____ Clinician _____

Assessment of Reading Skills: Matching Letters and Numbers

Show a single letter or number, and ask the client to point to the same item in a field of three choices.

Letter or Number	Correct	Incorrect
C		
B		
H		
W		
P		
9		
8		
2		
5		
7		

(continues)

Reading, Writing, and Calculation Assessment Protocol (continued)

Matching Pictures to Written Words

Show a picture of an object and ask the client to match it to the correct written word in a field of three choices. Use the same color photographs you used for the *Identifying the Picture Objects* task.

Word	Correct	Incorrect
Eggs		
Wheel		
Television		
Toaster		
Desk		
Shoes		
Cheese		
Sink		
Bus		
Fence		

Reading Aloud (Single Words)

Show a single written word and ask the client to read it aloud. Score intelligible responses with no phonemic substitutions or omissions as correct. *Also score as* correct *intelligible responses though containing distorted phonemes.*

Word	Correct	Incorrect
Grass		
Light		
Rug		
Run		
Money		
Hungry		
Driveway		
Football		
Combination		
Timekeeper		

Reading Aloud (Sentences)

Show a printed sentence and ask the client to read it aloud. Score as correct *intelligible response with no phonemic substitutions or omissions. Also score as* correct *words with distorted phonemes that are still intelligible.*

Sentence to be read aloud	Correct	Incorrect
It is easy.		
The clothes are dirty.		
Open the door.		
Fit the piece in there.		
It moved quickly.		
Open the door.		
Let him do it on his own.		
The music was far too loud.		
My hand got burned on the stove.		
What is the best thing to do in that situation?		

(continues)

Reading, Writing, and Calculation Assessment Protocol (continued)

Reading Comprehension (Single Sentences)

Show a printed sentence with the final word omitted and ask the client to read it and complete the sentence by choosing the correct missing word from a field of three (A, B, C).

Sentences	A	B	C
Put the key in the _____.	cover	candy	door
I enjoyed reading the _____.	book	shoes	cotton
He plays music on his _____.	tooth	guitar	lamp
While sleeping, he often will _____.	run	snore	flower
The boy missed school because he was _____.	cable	picture	sick
The old movie was in black and _____.	purple	red	white
My doctor is a general _____.	practitioner	contractor	military
Why save money for a rainy _____?	morning	night	day
It is hard to learn a new _____.	language	day	friend
When I was gone, she cleaned the _____.	bathroom	event	better

Reading Comprehension (Paragraph)

Ask the client to read the following paragraph and then answer multiple choice questions about it. Accept correct verbal or nonverbal (e.g., gestural) responses. Do not show the paragraph while the client answers the questions.

A fox was taking her babies out for a walk one beautiful morning. As she came to a stream, the fox encountered a lioness with her cub. "Why such airs over one solitary cub?" sneered the fox, "Look at my healthy and numerous litter of five, and imagine, if you are able, how a proud mother should feel." The lioness gave her a squelching look, and lifting up her nose, walked away, saying calmly, "Yes, just look at that wonderful collection. What are they? Foxes! I've only one, but remember that one is a lion." Quality is better than quantity.

Clinician asks	Choice A	Choice B	Choice C
What time of day were they out walking?	morning	afternoon	evening
Which animal had only one baby?	fox	lion	rabbit
The fox had how many babies?	three	four	five
What was the weather like in the story?	hot	cold	nice
Where did the fox encounter the lion?	on the grass	near the hill	at the stream

Writing Letters and Numbers to Dictation

Say the names of letters and numbers and ask the client to write them on paper.

Letters and numbers	Correct	Incorrect
J		
E		
U		
P		
Q		
5		
7		
2		
9		
4		

Copying Text

Present the following letters and words to the client, one at a time, and ask him or her to copy them onto a separate piece of paper.

Target Items	Correct	Incorrect
A		
M		
B		
fan		
wall		
hand		
light		
carpet		
telephone		
wooden desk		

(continues)

Reading, Writing, and Calculation Assessment Protocol (continued)

Functional Writing

Ask the client to write personal, functional information. Score as correct *if the response is fully legible and spelled accurately. Also score as* correct *is the word is legible, even with distorted letters.*

Clinician's Request	Correct	Incorrect
Write your first name.		
Write your last name.		
Write your phone number.		
Write your street and city address.		
Write your birthday.		
Write the numbers 1 to 10.		
Write the name of your _____ (spouse).		
Write the name of your _____ (child, friend).		
Write the name of the city where you were born.		
Write the first names of your parents.		

Writing the Names of Pictured Items

Present color photographs of single objects or demonstrate actions, and ask the client to write the name of what you just presented or demonstrated.

Pictures or Actions	Correct	Incorrect
book		
bed		
shirt		
sleeping		
clock		
running		
lighthouse		
ironing board		
traffic sign		
watermelon		

Writing Sentences

Ask the client to "Watch me carefully as I perform an action. Then please write a complete sentence that describes my action."

Score a response as correct *if all words are spelled correctly and it is a grammatically complete sentence* (e.g., the client should write for the first action, *You snapped your fingers.*).

Clinician's actions	Correct	Incorrect
Snaps her fingers		
Rubs her chin		
Knocks once on the table		
Clears her throat		
Rubs her hands together as if feeling cold		
Stretches her arms and yawns		
Stands up and sits down		
Looks at her watch		
Writes something on a piece of paper		
Reads a book		

(continues)

Reading, Writing, and Calculation Assessment Protocol (continued)

Writing a Narrative

Present the previous "Shipwreck picture" and ask the client to write a story about what is happening in it. Place a check mark in the "Score" column that best reflects the client's narrative.

Client's Written Narrative	Score
The written narrative is within normal limits, includes all important details of the picture; punctuation and sentence structures are normal, and all words are legible.	
The narrative is nearly normal, with relevant content; some less important details may be missing; letters are all legible, but their form may be awkward.	
The narrative contains complete sentences, but at least one important detail is missing; the written letters are legible, grammatical morphemes are used correctly, and there are no spelling errors.	
The narrative contains at least two complete sentences, but other sentences contain syntactic errors; at least two important details are missing from the narrative; and all words are relevant and legible.	
The narrative contains at least one complete sentence; other words, fully legible and relevant to the picture, may be grouped into phrases; important details are missing; bound morphemes may be missing in some words, and spelling errors are present.	
There are difficulties in forming letters; words are all relevant, but some related words may be grouped into phrases; there are no complete sentences; revisions and spelling errors are noted.	
The narrative consists of single words, all of which are legible and most are relevant to the picture; errors in grammatical morphemes are common.	
The narrative consists of single words, which are mostly legible; at least four words are relevant to the picture.	
Most of the letters are legible but only one or two of the words are relevant to the picture; some words are incomplete.	
The narrative is illegible.	

Assessment of Calculation Skills

Ask the client to perform the basic tasks described. Score whether the client performed the task (Yes) or failed to (No).

Calculation Tasks	Score	

Adds correctly:
    single numbers
    double numbers
	☐ Yes ☐ No
	☐ Yes ☐ No	

Subtracts correctly:
    single numbers
    double numbers
	☐ Yes ☐ No
	☐ Yes ☐ No	

Multiplies correctly:
    single numbers
    double numbers
	☐ Yes ☐ No
	☐ Yes ☐ No	

Divide correctly:
    single numbers
    double numbers
	☐ Yes ☐ No
	☐ Yes ☐ No	

Correctly matches a coin to its value (e.g., a dime = 10 cents)	☐ Yes ☐ No	
Determines equivalents of coin values (e.g., two dimes and a nickel = a quarter).	☐ Yes ☐ No	
Accurately "pays for" an item using paper money.	☐ Yes ☐ No	
Accurately makes change using paper money.	☐ Yes ☐ No	
Accurately "pays for" an item using coins and paper money.	☐ Yes ☐ No	
Accurately makes change using coins.	☐ Yes ☐ No	
Accurately makes change using coins and paper money.	☐ Yes ☐ No	
Determines common fluid value equivalents (e.g., four quarts = one gallon).	☐ Yes ☐ No	
Finds a specific page number in a phone book.	☐ Yes ☐ No	
Matches a digital time display to its equivalent on an analog clock.	☐ Yes ☐ No	

Aphasia Summative Diagnostic Protocol

Client's Name _____ Age _____ DOB _____

Diagnosis _____ Date _____ Clinician _____

Summarize the results of all assessment protocols on this master diagnostic protocol.

	Degree of Impairment			
	None	Mild	Moderate	Severe
Fluency	☐	☐	☐	☐
Agrammatism	☐	☐	☐	☐
Sentence structure	☐	☐	☐	☐
Morphologic features	☐	☐	☐	☐
Paraphasia	☐	☐	☐	☐
Anomia	☐	☐	☐	☐
Confrontation	☐	☐	☐	☐
Spontaneous	☐	☐	☐	☐
Repetition	☐	☐	☐	☐
Of self-productions	☐	☐	☐	☐
Echolalia	☐	☐	☐	☐
Speech production	☐	☐	☐	☐
Apraxia of speech	☐	☐	☐	☐
Dysarthria	☐	☐	☐	☐
Speech comprehension	☐	☐	☐	☐
Simple material	☐	☐	☐	☐
Complex material	☐	☐	☐	☐
Oral Reading	☐	☐	☐	☐
Misreading of words	☐	☐	☐	☐
Omission of words	☐	☐	☐	☐
Reading comprehension	☐	☐	☐	☐
Simple material	☐	☐	☐	☐
Complex material	☐	☐	☐	☐
Writing	☐	☐	☐	☐
Simple writing	☐	☐	☐	☐
Writing to dictation	☐	☐	☐	☐
Text copying	☐	☐	☐	☐

	Degree of Impairment			
	None	Mild	Moderate	Severe
Nonverbal communication	☐	☐	☐	☐
Hand gestures	☐	☐	☐	☐
Facial expressions	☐	☐	☐	☐
Understanding gestures and expressions	☐	☐	☐	☐
Functional communication	☐	☐	☐	☐
Quality of life	☐	☐	☐	☐
Client's rating	☐	☐	☐	☐
Caregiver rating	☐	☐	☐	☐
Diagnosis	*Nonfluent aphasia* Broca's (BA) ☐ Transcortical Motor (TMA) ☐ Mixed Transcortical (MTA) ☐ Global ☐		*Fluent aphasia* Wernicke's (WA) ☐ Transcortical Sensory (TSA) ☐ Conduction (CA) ☐ Anomic (AA) ☐	

Clinician: _____ Date: _____

Reference

Tombaugh, T. N., Kozak, J., & Rees, L. (1999). Normative data stratified by age and education for two measures of verbal fluency: FAS and animal naming. *Archives of Clinical Neuropsychology, 14,* 167–177.

PART IV

Assessment of Right-Hemisphere Syndrome

CHAPTER 9

Assessment of Right-Hemisphere Syndrome (RHS): Resources

- Functions of the Left and the Right Hemispheres
- Epidemiology of RHS
- Etiology and Neuropathology of RHS
- Neurological and Neuromotor Consequences of RHS
- Overview of Assessment
- Screening for RHS
- Standardized Tests for RHS
- Analysis and Integration of Assessment Results
- RHS Assessment Tasks in Chapter 10
- Postassessment Counseling

Functions of the Left and the Right Hemispheres

Although there are many examples of how the two hemispheres of the brain divide their duties, one particularly interesting interpretation is this: The left hemisphere works at a detailed and literal level; it is very proficient at formulating language and providing a focused view of what we are doing at any given moment. The right hemisphere, in turn, is better at making a broader analysis of the world; it lets us see our circumstances in a wider context. Put differently, the left hemisphere lets us concentrate on the trees, while, at the same time, the right hemisphere lets us still be aware of the forest. When it comes to our language abilities, the two hemispheres also have divided responsibilities. Current research says that the left hemisphere tells us *what* to say, and the right hemisphere seems to tell us *how* to say it.

The lateralization of brain function has been known since 1861, which is when Paul Broca presented his famous paper on a patient named Tan to the French Anthropological Society and later to the Anatomical Society of Paris. As a young man of 21, Tan had developed right-side paralysis and a significant language disorder. Although he seemed to demonstrate normal intelligence, he was unable to verbally produce any words other than "tan-tan," hence his nickname. Over a number of years, his condition gradually worsened with changes in his paralysis and cognition becoming especially obvious. He died at the age of 51 in April 1861. Broca's autopsy revealed major lesions in Tan's left cerebral hemisphere, with the oldest and one of the largest clearly evident in the frontal lobe. The right hemisphere appeared to be unaffected. Based on his observations of Tan while he was alive and on the findings of the autopsy, Broca developed the hypothesis that the left hemisphere is responsible for language abilities. Several months later, he was able to perform another autopsy on an individual with language deficits similar to Tan's. He again saw comparable lesions in the left hemisphere that confirmed his theory about language and the left hemisphere.

The Left Hemisphere

Since Broca's discovery, many other researches have contributed to our understanding of hemisphere lateralization, perhaps most notably by Karl Wernicke, who showed that there was at least one other language center in the brain, and by Penfield and Jasper, who mapped specific areas of the cortex during their surgical treatments for epilepsy. Cerebral hemisphere lateralization remains a rich area of research even today, as researchers continue to study how the brain functions. It is well known, for example, that the language centers of most individuals are in the left hemisphere. About 95% of right-handers and 82% of left-handers are "left-hemisphere dominant," meaning that the formulation, integration, and interpretation of language is controlled by the left hemisphere. The left hemisphere also controls the planning and sequencing of muscular movements needed to produce speech, a task performed by a poorly understood part of the left hemisphere called the motor speech programmer. Other left-hemisphere responsibilities include these processes:

- Abstraction and reasoning abilities
- The sequential analysis of data

- The systematic, logical interpretation of information
- Mathematical skills
- Perception of the right visual field
- Sensation from the right side of the body
- Appreciation of sound from the right ear

The Right Hemisphere

Compared to the left, the right hemisphere seems to be more diffusely organized. Its responsibilities are quite varied and include many aspects of attention, memory, perception, and language. When an individual experiences damage to the right hemisphere, any or all of these processes can be impaired. The term *right-hemisphere syndrome* (RHS) is used to describe individuals with this type of injury. The following paragraphs describe most of the normal functions of the right hemisphere, listing the language-related responsibilities first (emotional prosody, discourse, humor, indirect requests, nonliteral language) and the cognition-related functions second (arousal and vigilance, attention, music appreciation, constructional abilities). While reading these descriptions of the right hemisphere's language and cognitive responsibilities, the reader should keep in mind that an examination of one hemisphere in isolation is a bit of an academic exercise, something done for the sake of clarity. In reality, both hemispheres constantly work together, with the functions of one being moderated and enhanced by the functions of the other.

Emotional Prosody

Emotional prosody is the emotional content of a verbal message. The ability to comprehend emotional prosody is essential for understanding the emotional state of others. Likewise, the ability to produce emotional prosody is essential for expressing your own emotional state. Often, it is not the words of a spoken message that convey the speaker's true intent; it is the prosody of the message that tells the real story. For example, when first greeting a coworker in the morning with "How are you?," the verbal response probably will be "I'm fine." If only the words of the spoken response are examined, it would appear that the coworker is doing well. However, if those words are actually spoken with stress and pitch that indicate anger, distress, or sadness, we realize that something is wrong. We know that the coworker really is not fine because we understand the meaning of the response's prosodic content. The right hemisphere seems to be responsible for much of our ability to express and comprehend emotional prosody. This has been confirmed by instrumental and clinical studies. For example, Wada tests, which anaesthetize one hemisphere of the brain, have shown that normal, healthy individuals have difficulty producing emotional prosody when the right hemisphere is deadened. Dichotic listening tests reveal that judgments about the emotional content of speech are quicker and more accurate when the message is sent only to the left ear (which has crossed connections primarily to the right hemisphere). Finally, PET and functional MRI studies indicate right hemisphere function when individuals are asked to comprehend spoken emotional prosody.

Producing and Understanding Discourse

Although engaging in a conversation may appear to be a simple skill that is learned early in life, it actually is a remarkably complicated process with many subtle expectations of both the speaker and listener. When we engage in a conversation, we typically follow rules of how the interaction should proceed. For example, we maintain the topic of the conversation, shifting it only when appropriate. We provide just enough information to keep the conversation progressing and do not leave out significant information or bog it down with extraneous details. We make inferences about the intended meaning of what is being said. We present our part of the conversation in a logical, easy-to-follow manner. We also understand that the context of the conversation must be taken into consideration; conversing with a judge in a courtroom is different than chatting with a friend in a restaurant. Studies have suggested that these discourse skills are heavily dependent on the proper functioning of the right hemisphere (Myers, 1999). For example, the right hemisphere is involved in understanding the communicative context in which we are speaking. It also lets us know when we are providing appropriate amounts of communicative content during a conversation, and it helps us produce and comprehend central concepts. Lastly, it allows us to make correct inferences about what is said in our conversations.

Humor

The appreciation of certain types of humor and the understanding of sarcasm depend on our abilities to integrate context and make accurate inferences about what is said. They also sometimes require that we revise our original assumptions. For example, the following joke expects the reader to infer what is absurd about the punch line:

> A man goes into a casino and sees a guy playing poker with a cat. After watching for a while, he is completely amazed and says, "This is incredible. That's the smartest cat in the world!" The guy says, "Oh, she's not that smart. I've won four of the last six hands!"

The response of the man playing poker is a surprise, but the humor of it only can be understood by integrating it with the whole context of the joke. Research suggests that the appreciation of this type of joke is dependent on the right hemisphere's ability to combine new, unexpected information with our original interpretations of the context (Bihrle, Browell, Powelson, & Gardner, 1986). Without this ability, we may recognize the surprise element of the punch line but not the absurdity that makes it funny.

Indirect Requests

Indirect requests are statements that ask the listener to respond to the nonliteral meaning of the request and disregard the literal meaning. For example, if a wife says to her husband, "It has been a long time since you washed the car," she is indirectly asking him to actually wash the car because it is dirty. She really is not interested in how long it has been since it was washed; only that it is needs washing now. This type of request requires the listener to be sensitive to the nonliteral elements if it is to be interpreted accurately. Research indicates that the right hemisphere plays an important role in allowing us to understand the intended meaning of indirect requests (Foldi, 1987), and it has shown that individuals with damage to the right hemisphere often have difficulty understanding the implied meaning of these statements.

Comprehension of Nonliteral Language

Our capability to comprehend nonliteral language like metaphors and idioms is closely related to the ability to understand indirect requests. To interpret these sayings correctly, the listener must determine the nonliteral meaning of the words and disregard the literal meaning. These "figures of speech" are used surprisingly often in daily conversations. Metaphors are words used to facilitate the understanding of one thing in terms of something else; they create an implied analogy between two objects or ideas. Examples include, "Her hair was a fierce lion's mane," and "School is a gateway to adulthood." Idioms are a phrase whose nonliteral meaning is different from the normal meaning of the words. The nonliteral meaning of an idiom cannot be interpreted by the literal meaning; users must learn the meaning from the context in which it is used. For example, a common American idiom is "Spill the beans." It has a literal meaning that is easy to interpret, but the nonliteral meaning must be derived by hearing it used in the proper context. This is why idioms from other cultures or countries can be impossible to understand if you have not been exposed to them in their original context. For example, most American readers will not understand the meaning of the Chinese idiom "Black is derived from blue but is darker." We do not understand its nonliteral meaning because we have not heard it used contextually or had it explained to us. (By the way, it means that the student has surpassed the teacher.) Studies by several researchers have indicated that understanding the nonliteral meanings of these sayings is dependent on the right hemisphere's ability to use contextual cues to determine the intended usage (Bryan, 1988; Winner & Gardner, 1977).

Arousal and Vigilance

These two important processes are associated with right-hemisphere function. Arousal is physical and mental alertness, often indicated by increased blood pressure and heart rate and a generalized quickness of response. Vigilance, also known as sustained attention, is a person's ability to monitor the immediate surroundings for long periods, always being ready to react to certain stimuli when they appear. A good example of arousal is the increased alertness and heart rate that a college student feels just before a final examination. An example of vigilance is a duck hunter who must wait for long periods for the infrequent duck to fly within range of a shotgun, yet be immediately ready to shoot the instant it happens. Instrumental research has indicated that when individuals experience arousal and vigilance, the right hemisphere has significantly increased metabolic activity and blood flow compared to the left hemisphere. Clinical studies of right-hemisphere-damaged patients indicate that many of them have reduced arousal and vigilance, which is known as being hyporesponsive. These patients demonstrate diminished responsivity to stimuli with slow initiation and reaction times.

Attention

Other attention processes also are strongly influenced by the right hemisphere. *Selective attention* is the ability to screen out or ignore a distracting or competing stimulus and concentrate on the task at hand. A classic example of selective attention is the ability to conduct a conversation with another person during a loud party. Because of selective attention, we can concentrate on the speech of our conversational partner and disregard the noise from the other conversations and music in the room. Selective attention gives us freedom from distractibility. *Orienting* is yet another type of attention. It is the shifting of attention toward the direction of a stimulus. Orienting usually is indicated by the movement of the head and eye, although it can be demonstrated by hand, arm, and other movements. Looking toward a person who says your name is an example of this ability. *Alternating attention* (having the mental flexibility to shift your attention between tasks that have different conditions) and *divided attention* (responding simultaneously to multiple tasks, where two or more stimuli need to be observed or where two or more responses are necessary) are two final types of attention. An example of alternating attention is looking at a recipe (reading) and then completing that step (cooking). An example of divided attention is driving while talking on a cell phone. These four complex mental processes are not exclusively under the control of the right hemisphere, but clinical studies have clearly shown that when the right hemisphere is damaged, all or some of them are impaired, often significantly.

Music Appreciation

Damage to the right temporal lobe has been linked to problems with such musical abilities as remembering pitch, keeping time, loudness, and timbre (Tompkins, 1995), but it is possible that the right hemisphere only has dominance for music skills in those of us with little musical talent. Research has indicated that the right hemisphere is dominant for musical perception in people with minimal musical knowledge, but for those with sophisticated musical skills, the left hemisphere has dominance. It may be that as a person gains musical knowledge, hemisphere dominance gradually shifts from the right to the left hemisphere (Critchley & Henson, 1977).

Constructional Abilities

The right hemisphere is essential for our ability to assemble objects from a collection of parts, such as putting together a model car, matching scraps of cloth to that in a quilt pattern, and taking apart and reassembling a kitchen appliance. This skill is sometimes called *constructional praxis*. Individuals with right-hemisphere damage can demonstrate obvious deficits in this ability, a condition that many sources incorrectly call *constructional apraxia* (Brookshire, 2007).

Epidemiology of RHS

The prevalence of RHS in the general population is unknown, but it is safe to assume that it varies with the prevalence of diseases that cause brain injury. Any condition that has the potential to cause focal lesions in one hemisphere can cause RHS. The most current statistics related to the prevalence of neurological diseases and associated RHS may be found at the National Center for Health Statistics and the American Stroke Association.

Epidemiological observations related to brain injury and RHS generally include the following:

- **Strokes are a common cause of RHS and disability.** About 700,000 new cases of stroke are reported each year; of these, 327,000 (47%) are males and 373,000 (53%) are females. About two thirds of all strokes are associated with people age 65 and older. Men have a higher risk of stroke than women, but because of their longevity, more women than men have strokes. About 12% all mortality is due to strokes. Ischemic strokes are more common than hemorrhagic strokes.

- **Prevalence of strokes is different across ethnocultural groups.** African Americans have a higher risk of a first stroke than whites. Deaths rates related to strokes are also higher in African Americans than in whites. The death rates are roughly comparable in whites and Asian Americans and lower in Hispanics and Native Americans (http//www.americanheart.org; Horner, Swanson, Bosworth, & Matchar, 2003; Payne 1997). Strokes at younger age (22–44 years) are more common among Hispanics and African Americans than whites.

- **Ethnicity and the type of stroke may be related.** Ischemic strokes are more common in whites than in Hispanics. Native Americans, African Americans, Asian Americans, and Hispanics are more prone to have hemorrhagic strokes than whites.

- **Medical risk factors affect the incidence of strokes.** People with high blood pressure, smoking, high cholesterol levels, obesity, poor and high-sodium diet, and lack of exercise increase the chances of stroke.

- **Ethnicity may affect the level of disability due to strokes.** African American females experience a greater level of disability than any other females or males. White males experience the least amount of stroke-related disability.

Etiology and Neuropathology of RHS

In general, the main and the proximal cause of RHS is damage to the parietal, frontal, and temporal lobes of the brain. There is, however, a chain of events that causes that brain damage that in turn causes RHS. Although strokes are a common cause, there are other neurological events that can result in RHS. Detailed case history and medical test results will often reveal a series of adverse events culminating in RHS.

- **Vascular disorders are the most common cause of RHS.** A patient may have had a particular type of vascular disorder:
  - *A thrombosis is a blood clot within an artery.* It can restrict or block the blood supply to the brain structures that lie beyond the clot. The brain tissue that does not receive oxygenated blood is damaged. Formation of blood clots (*thrombi*) are due to a slowly developing disease process known as *atherosclerosis*, which is narrowing and hardening of the artery due mainly to lipid and calcium deposits. A thrombosis causes *ischemic strokes* that are caused by interrupted blood supply.

○ *Embolism is another arterial disease.* An embolus, typically formed elsewhere, travels through an artery, gets lodged as the artery gets smaller, and thus blocks the blood flow. Brain tissue damage follows. Embolism also causes ischemic strokes.

○ *Aneurysm is a swelling in a thinned-out portion of an artery.* This balloon-like swelling eventually bursts resulting in cerebral hemorrhage and brain damage. Aneurysm causes hemorrhagic strokes.

- **Traumatic brain injury (TBI) may cause RHS.** Any type of external force acting on the head can cause injury to the brain, resulting in RHS if the damage is restricted to the right hemisphere. See Chapter 13 for details on TBI.

- **Brain tumors may cause RHS.** There are three common types of tumors (classified as Grade I, II, III, or IV): *primary tumors* that grow within the brain, *metastatic tumors* that are migrated into the brain from other parts of the body, and *meningiomas* that grow within the meninges.

- **Brain toxicity may cause strokes and RHS in some cases.** Toxicity from lead and mercury, prescription drug overdose, drug interactions, and illicit drug abuse may all cause strokes.

- **Several types of infections may cause strokes and RHS.** Although rare, bacterial (e.g., meningitis) as well as viral infections (e.g., mumps, measles, or untreated syphilis) may cause RHS if the infection only affects the right hemisphere.

Prevalence of RHS Symptoms

Information on the prevalence of RHS symptoms among stroke survivors is limited, and there is a fair amount of variability in that which is available. For example, Myers (1999) reported that estimates of neglect in right-hemisphere-damaged individuals ranged from 31% to 66%. Stone, Halligan, and Greenwood (1993) discovered many characteristics of RHS in their stroke patients. They examined 171 right- and left-hemisphere patients 2 to 3 days poststroke for evidence of neglect and similar disorders. Following are the results for their 69 patients with right-hemisphere stroke:

- Visual neglect was present in 82%.
- Hemi-inattention was present in 70%.
- Tactile extinction was present in 65%.
- Allaesthesia (sensations are felt at a point different than the source) was present in 57%.
- Visual extinction was present in 23%.
- Anosognosia (denial of deficits) was present in 28%.
- Anosodiaphoria (indifference to a deficit) was present in 27%.
- Nonbelonging (belief that a body part, such as an arm, belongs to someone else) was present in 36%.

Although these findings were collected very early postonset, they suggest that a significant number of patients with right-hemisphere damage experience RHS deficits, at least initially.

A similarly high number of RHS symptoms results were reported by Blake, Duffy, Myers, and Tompkins (2002) when they reviewed the medical charts of 123 right-hemisphere-damaged adults. They found these RHS deficits in their participants:

- Attention deficits—difficulty concentrating on stimuli—67.5%
- Neglect—unconscious perceptual omission—65.9%
- Perception—visual and tactile perception and construction—63.4%
- Learning and memory deficits—63.4%
- Reasoning and problem-solving deficits—61.0%
- Other cognitive deficits—organizing, sequencing, categorization, integrating—52.0%
- Awareness deficits—lack of insight into deficits and their consequences—43.9%
- Orientation deficits—to self, time, and place—43.1%
- Hyperresponsive—verbosity, impulsiveness, disinhibition—41.5%
- Hyporesponsive—reduced speech, slowness in responding, lack of initiation—39.0%
- Calculation deficits—30.9%
- Hypoaffective—reduced emotional responses—30.1%
- Linguistic deficits—reduced language functions—26.0%
- Aprosodia—deficit in producing or comprehending emotional prosody—19.5%
- Interpersonal interaction deficits—pragmatic language problems—16.3%
- Hyperaffective—emotional lability, pseudobulbar affect—15.4%

Both of these studies (Stone, Halligan, & Greenwood,1993; Blake, Duffy, Myers, & Tompkins, 2002) suggest that neglect and attention problems are the most commonly encountered RHS deficits, although a significant number of additional deficits occur nearly as frequently.

Neurological and Neuromotor Consequences of RHS

There can be many consequences of right-hemisphere damage. Not only in the number of problems that can occur, but also in their scope. Many elements of attention, language, movement, perception, and memory can be affected in cases of RHS. The following paragraphs do not examine all the impairments associated with RHS; they concentrate primarily on those that are of interest to the speech-language pathologist.

Hemispatial (Unilateral) Neglect

This is one of the nonlinguistic deficits associated with RHS. It is a common problem in many individuals with RHS. Right-hemisphere-damaged clients with this deficit do not respond to stimuli on the left side of their bodies or within the left side of their environments. For example, they will leave food on the left side of a plate and disregard words on the left side of a page. Neglect is not just evident in how these clients manipulate objects in front of them; it also can affect how they perceive their bodies. It is not uncommon for a (male) client to shave only the right side of his face and comb his hair on the right side of his head, leaving the left side untouched. Left-side neglect also includes these characteristics:

- It can affect tactile, auditory, and visual stimuli that are present on the left side of the client's space.

- The "dividing line" of where the neglect begins can shift depending on how items are presented—oddly shaped, asymmetrical items tend to draw attention leftward, as do overlapping or connected objects.

- There can be enhanced, "magnetic" attention to items in the right hemispace.

- Affected clients will copy or draw only the right side of an item.

- Affected clients may have difficulty walking or navigating a wheelchair through an open door because they will unknowingly collide with the left side of the opening.

- Even when they have normal sensation in a left-side limb, they will not react to touch or a pinprick to that body part.

Individuals with left-side neglect most commonly have damage to the right parietal lobe, although it can be present when there is damage to other parts of the right hemisphere as well. The reason why right-hemisphere damage causes this neglect is unclear, but it seems that individuals with left-side visual neglect have a problem with *attending* to objects in their left visual fields. Research has shown that individuals with this disorder can, in fact, subconsciously see their left visual fields, but they fail to respond to it. They may read only the letters on the right half of a word, but if cued enough times to look again at the left half of the word, they usually will "see" all the letters. A student clinician of one of the authors had a surprising interaction with a patient with left-side visual neglect. The patient was very puzzled by the student's nametag that had "Speech Therapist" written on it. He looked at the nametag and said, "You're a rapist?" Of course, the student was completely baffled by this question, and asked him what he meant. He said with complete sincerity, "Your nametag says, 'rapist.'" She immediately understood what had happened, and after cueing him to look at all the letters on the left side of the name tag, he was able to read both words. Significantly, throughout the session he needed continual cueing to look to the left whenever he was asked to read or find objects on his left side.

Left-Side Neglect versus Homonymous Hemianopia (left)

Left-side neglect can sometimes be confused with a visual disorder called *homonymous hemianopia (left)*. Individuals with homonymous hemianopia (left) have damage along the optic pathway that extends from the retina of the eye to the occipital lobe of the brain, usually in the right optic tract or geniculorcalcarine tract. Clients with left-side neglect and homonymous hemianopia (left) can superficially appear to demonstrate identical problems when looking for things in their left visual field. Both conditions seem to result in the same kind of left-side visual deficits, but in reality, there are significant differences. Here are several distinguishing characteristics that can help clinicians tell these two conditions apart:

- Site of lesion—Individuals with homonymous hemianopia have damage to the optic pathway; individuals with left-side neglect have damage to the right hemisphere that spares the optic pathway.

- Type of problem—Homonymous hemianopia is an optic pathway deficit; left-side neglect probably is an attentional deficit.

- Ability to compensate—Individuals with homonymous hemianopia often show awareness of their deficit fairly quickly and can learn to compensate for it; individuals with left-side neglect show little awareness of the problem and usually have great difficulty learning to "look to the left."

- Internal representation of the world—Individuals with homonymous hemianopia do not have a disrupted mental representation of the world. If they are asked to draw or describe something, they will not omit the parts of it they cannot see. On the other hand, individuals with left-side neglect show evidence of disrupted left-side mental representations. For example, when asked to verbally describe an imaginary tour through their home, going front to back, they will often fail to mention objects or rooms on the left side of the building. When asked later to describe a tour from the back of the house to the front, they will again fail to mention objects or rooms on the left side of the building— objects or rooms they *did* describe on the initial front to back tour.

Severe visual neglect is most evident in the immediate postlesion period, and it frequently improves with time, although long-term treatment is often needed to help these clients increase their awareness of the problem. Note that right-side visual neglect can occur following left-hemisphere damage, but it is less common and typically less severe than left-side neglect.

Attention Deficits

As Blake, Duffy, Myers, and Tompkins (2002) reported, problems with attention are common in clients with RHS. They will have difficulty maintaining, shifting, and dividing their attention. Each of these problems can pose real challenges for the client because attention is such an important element of daily life. When it is impaired, tasks such as reading, writing, engaging in conversation, watching television, and cooking can become confusing and frustrating. Myers and Blake (2008) described the types of attention that can be affected by right-hemisphere damage:

- Arousal and orienting—Clients with RHS can demonstrate decreased amounts of alertness (hypoarousal). They need extra time and cues to get ready to pay attention to a stimulus. They may not pick up on activities in their surrounding environment and demonstrate a narrow center of attention.

- Vigilance (sustained attention)—Vigilance is being prepared for an upcoming event or stimulus and having an ongoing readiness for activity. Clients with RHS can demonstrate significant problems with this attentional skill. Their impaired readiness affects their ability to fully participate in activities of daily living. Clinicians must be aware of this deficit because it can significantly hinder their progress in therapy.

- Selective attention—This is the ability to maintain attention even when there are interfering and distracting stimuli. As selective attention tasks become more difficult, clients with RHS will show longer reaction times and increased neglect during ongoing tasks.

Emotional Prosody Deficits

Accurately producing and understanding speech with emotional content (emotional prosody) seems to be primarily a right-hemisphere responsibility. We tend to forget that that "reading" another person's emotional state by what we hear is actually a very complicated process. Sometimes it is difficult because the spoken words may not always accurately reflect the person's emotional state. It also can be a challenge because the listener has to make numerous inferences about the context and pitch of the speech and must attend to extralinguistic indicators of what the person is actually feeling, such as facial expression. Numerous studies have suggested that clients with RHS have problems expressing and comprehending emotional prosody. For example, they have difficulty identifying the emotional tone of another person's voice (Schmitt, Hartje, & Willmes, 1997), and they can have difficulty putting emotional prosody into their own utterances (Pell, 1999). Moreover, they can have difficulty recognizing the emotions in the facial expressions of other individuals (Adolfs, Damasio, & Tranel, 2002). Blake, Duffy, Myers, and Tompkins (2002) reported that 19.5% of their 123 right-hemisphere-damaged participants had emotional prosody deficits.

Linguistic Prosody Deficits

Many individuals with RHS demonstrate a flattening of their spoken prosody and difficulty comprehending the prosodic features in another person's speech. Although these linguistic prosody problems generally are not as severe as those with emotional prosody, they can contribute to the discourse and pragmatic difficulties experienced by RHS clients.

- Their connected speech may have reduced intonation. House, Rowe, and Standen (1987) suggested it sounds similar to patients with clinical depression.

- They may have difficulty producing emphatic stress on key words. For example, an RHS client's production of two identical sentences with different emphatic stress ("The boy is playing *football*." and "The *boy* is playing football.") may sound very similar.

- The RHS client's expressive prosody problems can be exacerbated by a co-occurring dysarthria.

- They may demonstrate difficulty comprehending linguistic prosody, but how this affects day-to-day conversation is unknown. Studies have suggested that they can understand prosody for selecting words (e.g., *record* vs. re*cord*) and distinguishing questions and answers (Walker, Daigle, & Buzzard, 2002; Heilman, Bowers, Speedie, & Coslett, 1984).

Discourse Deficits

Discourse is the comprehension and production of conversations and narratives. Many studies have shown that RHS clients can have significant problems with this important language skill (Blake, Duffy, Myers, & Tompkins, 2002).

- Difficulties determining the main point or theme of a conversation or narrative.

- Problems with integrating information into a meaningful whole. For example, RHS clients' comprehension of a conversation may only consist of isolated details; they can have difficulty combining those details into the main point of the discussion.

- Conversational speech may contain excessive, tangential details, such as the RHS client who, when asked about his car, described the items in the trunk, including what tools he had for changing tires.

- Conversational speech may contain too few details. Information critical for fully understanding a point can be omitted from the RHS client's portion of a conversation, leaving the listener confused. Moreover, the RHS client may not attend to the listener's signs of confusion or attempt to repair the breakdown.

- The topic of conversation can change inappropriately. For example, during the assessment interview with one RHS client, the clinician asked if he was right- or left-handed. He answered that he used his right hand for everything and then immediately mentioned that he was good at his job and that he got flowers from friends in Seattle.

- Topic shading may occur, in which the RHS client subtly changes the emphasis of one topic to another without indicating that the topic has shifted. Tompkins (1995) indicated that this usually occurs in informal situations. It can be particularly disruptive when a conversation is exploring a topic or when it happens after a direct question.

- They can have difficulty identifying relationships within a narrative or discussion. For example, while listening to a story about two people working on a project independently, RHS clients may fail to grasp that the two individuals are friends, even if that relationship is stated fairly explicitly in the story.

- RHS clients can be impulsive in their responses, answering questions or making comments with little apparent regard for the stimuli or context. One client with left-side neglect was asked to read the word *authoritarian* aloud. He quickly looked at the word and immediately said, "Mary Ann, a girl's name."

- RHS clients can have difficulty revising their initial understanding of a topic of conversation, even when it is clearly incorrect. For example, in a conversation with a spouse about someone going on a trip, the client may mistakenly assume a son or daughter is taking the trip. He or she will maintain this assumption even when it is obvious that it actually is a neighbor or a friend who is taking the trip.

Reading and Writing Deficits

Many RHS clients will demonstrate reading and writing deficits. Ardila and Rosselli (1993) found that 40% to 73% of RHS clients had writing difficulties. These disorders are especially evident in RHS clients with neglect.

- When reading, RHS clients with neglect may omit the leftward letters of single words, especially in compound words like *baseball.*
- They may omit the words on the left side when reading sentences. Myers (1999) noted that they tend to scan to the left until they discover a meaningful phrase and start reading from there. For example, for a sentence like, *She did her best, and then she went home.*, the client will only read, "She went home."
- Reading paragraphs can be especially difficult for RHS clients with neglect. As when reading individual sentences, they will scan leftward only until they identify a phrase that has meaning and begin reading there.
- Writing deficits also can be evident in RHS clients (Myers, 1999). At the single word level, they may omit or repeat (perseverate) a line in a letter and fail to dot the "i" or cross the "t." When writing sentences, they can omit punctuation marks and words. At the paragraph level, they can leave a large left margin, resulting in sentences that are crowded into the right half of the page. The lines of a paragraph can slant excessively. RHS clients with attention deficits can have difficulties maintaining their concentration while writing a paragraph, demonstrated by losing their place or train of thought during the task.

Pragmatic Deficits

These deficits affect the social use of language and are seen frequently in RHS clients. Not all clients will demonstrate each of the following deficits, but they are a representative sample of what can occur after right-hemisphere damage.

- They may have difficulty maintaining appropriate eye contact during conversation.
- RHS clients may dominate conversations by ignoring normal turn-taking rules and by interrupting other speakers.
- Conversation may be excessively egocentric, keeping the topic constantly on themselves or on subjects of interest to them.
- They may fail to respond to a conversational partner's verbal or nonverbal requests for clarification.
- RHS clients can have difficulty determining which topics of conversation are appropriate for different situations. For example, they may make an off-color or personal comment during a formal social gathering.

- They may have difficulty knowing that a conversation has ended. Even when the conversational partner is standing to leave, RHS clients may continue talking.

- As listeners in a conversation, they may fail to indicate their interest in the speaker's utterances by nodding their heads or smiling.

- Clinical reports indicate that some RHS clients have difficulties with proxemics. They may stand too close to a communication partner during a conversation.

Other Deficits Associated with RHS

- Prosopagnosia—This is a rare condition where individuals have difficulty recognizing the faces of famous or familiar people, even very close family members. It has been associated with several types of acute brain injury, including RHS. Typically, clients with prosopagnosia can successfully recognize objects (e.g., shoes, food, cars) but have great difficulty identifying faces. Interestingly, they can use other sensory inputs to assist in distinguishing one person from another, such as hearing a familiar voice or recognizing a particular piece of clothing.

- Anosognosia—RHS clients with anosognosia seem to be unaware of their deficits, or they deny that they exist. It probably is related to neglect and may be caused by the inability to integrate the body's sensations with the cognitive processes that monitor body and space representations.

- Anosodiaphoria—This condition is somewhat similar to anosognosia and probably also is related to neglect. RHS clients with anosodiaphoria do not deny their disorders; rather, they demonstrate an indifference to them. The clients recognize that the problems are present, but they do not seem particularly upset or worried about them. This term is mostly used in reference to a client's indifference to paralysis.

- Constructional impairments—These are problems with organizing and performing complicated actions in the person's immediate surroundings, such as drawing a complex pattern or building a small object from parts. In psychological testing, this skill often is assessed by having the individual organize blocks into a specific arrangement. Clients with RHS can demonstrate difficulties on these types of building or organizing tasks. They tend to produce distorted, fragmented, and rotated versions of the target patterns (Tompkins, 1995).

- Dysarthria—A co-occurring dysarthria is possible in RHS clients. Upper motor neuron damage in the right hemisphere can cause unilateral upper motor neuron dysarthria. This type of dysarthria is primarily a mild to moderate articulation disorder, and it can contribute to the difficulties RHS clients have in producing appropriate prosody.

- Memory—Several memory deficits have been associated with RHS. Tompkins (1995) mentions difficulties with verbal memory (retaining linguistic information that is presented verbally) and working memory (the active storing and managing of information temporarily while carrying out such other cognitive tasks as reasoning and learning). For example, Tompkins, Bloise, Timko, and

Baumgaertner, (1994) found that participants with RHS had reduced working memory capacity compared to normal participants in a task that required the concurrent processing and storage of verbal information.

- Topographical and geographical disorientation—Both of these disorders have been linked to RHS (Tompkins, 1995). Topographical disorientation is a problem with internal representations of the external environment. Individuals with this condition tend to get lost easily, have difficulty following a map, and misjudge distances. It is often associated with neglect. Individuals with geographical disorientation understand their immediate surroundings (e.g., I'm in a house or hospital, etc.) but be confused about where they are in the world. For example, they may correctly realize they are at a university speech clinic but will state that the university is in the wrong state or country.

- Planning, problem solving, organizing—Although more research into these deficits is needed, clients with RHS can demonstrate difficulties with following sequential directions; organizing daily, weekly, or monthly schedules; keeping a checkbook current; and time management.

Overview of Assessment

Assessment of RHS can be challenging because of the high probability of co-occurring conditions and the diverse collection of RHS symptoms. Before beginning the specifics of an RHS assessment, the clinician needs to understand the client's (a) current and projected health condition, (b) current communication deficits and needs, (c) overall quality of life, (d) strengths, and family and social support systems, (e) expectations on returning to the previous or a new employment setting, (f) expectations of treatment and rehabilitation, and (g) cultural and verbal background. Much information on these variables may be obtained from a detailed case history, reports from the medical and rehabilitation professionals, and a carefully conducted interview of the client and the caregivers. Specific assessment procedures, when completed, will help build a profile of the client and the family.

Assessment includes both standard and special procedures specific to RHS. To complete a thorough assessment, the clinician will:

- Have the client or the family fill out a case history form
- Hold an interview with the client and the caregiver
- Administer a hearing screening test
- Complete an orofacial examination and assess diadochokinetic rates
- Possibly administer a standardized test
- Assess speech production
- Assess narrative and conversational skills
- Assess functional communication skills
- Assess communication-related quality of life

- Analyze and integrate the assessment results
- Offer postassessment counseling

The clinician can use the standard case history form given in Chapter 2. During the interview, the clinician may ask specific questions about the onset of stroke or other events that caused the RHS, subsequent medical management, current health status of the client, cultural and verbal background of the client and the family, and so forth. The clinician may use additional protocols given in Chapter 2 to make an orofacial examination, assess the diadochokinetic rates, and screen the client's hearing. The clinician will then proceed to collect diagnostic data from a conversational speech and language sample and nonstandardized assessment procedures. To assess RHS, clinicians usually assess a variety of skills that are either impaired or preserved in clients. These include reading, writing, drawing, conversational skills, recognizing emotional prosody, and interpreting figurative language. The degree to which each of these and other skills is assessed will depend on the individual client and the apparent severity of symptoms. Not all skills necessarily need to be assessed in depth in all clients. At the end of the assessment, the clinician will counsel the client and the caregivers about the assessment results, discuss speech-language treatment options, suggest a prognosis, and answer any questions the client and the caregivers may ask.

Screening for RHS

Clinicians working in hospitals and other medical settings may need to screen specific patients for RHS. It is prudent to screen patients before embarking on a time-consuming diagnostic assessment. Clinicians may use their own established procedures or an informal screening test to determine if an individual should be assessed further.

Experienced clinicians may use quick procedures based on their own clinical expertise. Patients recently admitted to hospitals for a cerebrovascular accident or other neurological problems that may be associated with RHS are candidates for a quick bedside screening. The clinician may screen patients by having them perform a few standard tasks. For example, the clinician may not only engage the patient in conversation for a few minutes, but also ask the client to describe objects or pictures; count numbers, recite the names of months and days of the week; repeat a few words, phrases, and sentences; and answer questions about orientation to time, space, and person. The patient's responses may be sufficient to determine whether more in-depth assessment is necessary.

Standardized Tests for RHS

Only a handful of published, standardized tests for RHS is currently available. Each is described in this section of the chapter. They are designed to identify the presence of RHS deficits in adult clients and, if present, make an estimate of severity.

Burns Brief Inventory of Communication and Cognition (Burns, 1997). As its name suggests, this is a screening test for RHS. The Burns is unique in that it also includes sections for screening clients with TBI and aphasia. It is a standardized, criterion-referenced instrument that is most appropriate for clients with moderate impairments. The Right Hemisphere Inventory of the test is divided into five sections:

1. Scanning and tracking—examines scanning and tracking of objects and words.

2. Visuospatial skills—assesses attention, recognition of faces, writing, and drawing.

3. Prosody—examines expressive and receptive prosody abilities.

4. Inferences—assesses understanding of implied meanings.

5. Metaphorical language—examines comprehension and interpretation of nonliteral language such as idioms.

The client's performance on each of these tasks is rated according to severity—severe, moderate, mild, or no deficit. Error of measurement data allow clinicians to determine if a client makes significant improvements when the test is retaken. The total administration time is about 30 minutes.

Mini Inventory of Right Brain Injury-Second Edition (MIRBI-R; Pimental & Knight, 2000). This is another screening test for clients with RHS. The standardization sample was a total of 251 individuals—128 with RHS, 45 with left-hemisphere damage, and 78 without brain damage. They ranged in age from 20–80. Pimental, Knight, and Allen (1999) indicated that the MIRBI-R has significantly better psychometric data than did the first edition, with improved normative data, reliability, content validity, criterion prediction validity, concurrent validity, as well as for other measures. The four broad domains of this test (visuospatial/visuoperceptual and attentional processing, lexical knowledge processing, affective processing, and behavior processing) are subdivided into 10 categories:

1. Visual scanning

2. Integrity of gnosis

3. Integrity of body image

4. Visuoverbal processing

5. Visuosymbolic processing

6. Integrity of visuomotor praxis

7. Higher-level language skills

8. Expressing emotion

9. General affect

10. General behavior

Because there are only 27 individual test items on this test, the administration time is short—only about 30 minutes. Raw scores can be converted to percentiles and standard scores, but clinicians need to be aware that the MIRBI-R is only a screening test. If the results suggest that a client may have symptoms of RHS, further assessment will be needed to confirm the diagnosis and develop treatment goals.

Protocole Montreal d'Evaluation de la Communication (Joanette, Ska, & Côté, 2004). This standardized test was designed primarily for assessing clients with RHS, but the authors also recommend it for evaluating conditions such as aphasia, traumatic brain injury, and dementia. It is a comprehensive assessment tool with 14 subtests that assess oral communication abilities, including conversational speech, providing a narrative, comprehension and expression of emotional prosody, and interpreting indirect requests. The administration time is about 2 hours, usually completed over 2 separate sessions. The standardization sample was collected using 180 non-brain-damaged controls, ranging in age from 30 to 85. These data are stratified by age and education. A small number of participants with RHS (n = 15 and 28) were included in the psychometric data. At the current time, this test is available only in French, but translated versions are available in Brazilian Portuguese and Spanish.

Rehabilitation Institute of Chicago Clinical Management of Right Hemisphere Dysfunction-Second Edition (RICE-R; Halper, Cherney, & Burns, 1996). The RICE-R is a comprehensive tool for clinicians working with clients with RHS. The beginning chapters provide an overview of brain function including hemisphere specialization and the characteristics of RHS. There also is a chapter on designing and implementing treatment plans. The assessment tasks of the RICE-R are found in an appendix in the manual. These are divided into five categories:

1. Behavioral observation profile—the clinician interviews and converses with the client.

2. Visual scanning and tracking—assesses visuospatial skills; includes cancellation tasks.

3. Pragmatic rating scale—examines a variety of verbal and nonverbal pragmatic behaviors (e.g., conversational turn taking, maintaining eye contact) and the ability to retell a story.

4. Analysis of writing—assesses the client's spontaneous writing and copying abilities.

5. Metaphorical language—examines the client's understanding of proverbs.

The RICE-R was standardized on 36 participants without brain damage and 40 with RHS. It can provide an estimate of severity for each subtest. Procedures for transferring assessment results into a treatment plan are provided.

Right Hemisphere Language Battery-Second Edition (RHLB-2; Bryan, 1995). This test of language function in clients with RHS was standardized on non-brain-damaged (n = 30), RHS (n = 40), and aphasic (n − 40) participants, ranging in age from 20–80. It contains 7 subtests that assess the language abilities typically associated with the right hemisphere: metaphor-picture matching, written metaphor choice, comprehension of inferred meaning, humor appreciation, lexical semantic recognition, prosody, and discourse production. An Italian version of the RHLB-2 was developed by Zanini, Bryan, De Luca, and Bava (2005). Currently, this test appears to be out of print, but it is available from secondary retailers.

Analysis and Integration of Assessment Results

An overall analysis and integration of assessment results is essential to make valid clinical decisions. Assessment of RHS can be more of an "ongoing" process than it is for other communication disorders because the client's health status might improve or deteriorate, depending on conditions that are associated with RHS. With such changes, the severity of the RHS will also change for the better or for worse. The assessment of RHS sometimes can be complicated by the common co-occurrence of dysarthria, which can contribute to problems with prosody. To track these changes and situations, the clinician needs to make periodic, even if brief, assessments to ascertain the client's communication skills at different points during treatment and rehabilitation.

The clinician might take the following steps to analyze and integrate the assessment results before writing a diagnostic report:

- **The case history and interview information should be summarized.** The time and the conditions of the onset of RHS and the symptoms that preceded and followed the onset may be summarized as reported by the caregivers and the client. The client's family constellation and the ethnocultural (including verbal) background should be described. The history of the client's health, education, occupation, hobbies, literacy skills, and interests should be summarized.

- **Medical assessment and treatment should be summarized.** The medical procedures (e.g., neurological examinations, imaging) done on the client, and specific neurological and medical diagnoses made on the client (e.g., stroke, tumor) should be summarized. The current medical treatment the client is undergoing should be noted. The current physical condition of the client (e.g., stable, deteriorating, improving) should be described. The recommendation by medical specialists for rehabilitation, including speech-language treatment, should be specified.

- **RHS assessment results should be described.** The clinician should analyze all the assessment procedures performed on the client, including the interview, observations, standardized test (if done), and any client-specific or criterion-referenced measures. Assessment of RHS usually does not concentrate on making a differential diagnosis. A neurological evaluation and neuroimaging usually provide definitive information on the presence of a right-hemisphere lesion. Rather, the assessment of a client with right-hemisphere damage should concentrate on finding which characteristics of RHS are present, and if they are, determining their severity. For example, the clinician will want to determine if neglect is present. Although this deficit is found in most RHS clients immediately postonset, not all clients have it. For those showing evidence of neglect, an estimate of severity must be determined. The clinician can determine the presence of many RHS characteristics and make estimates of their severity by administering the assessment tasks in Chapter 10, conducting a standardized test, or both.

- **Recommendations may be specified.** The analysis and integration of assessment data will result in the clinician's recommendations for the client, family members, and other caregivers. Treatment for clients with RHS can be effective and typically is recommended (Lehman-Blake, 2007).

RHS Assessment Tasks in Chapter 10

Because of the unique characteristics of RHS, some clinicians may be unacquainted with the assessment tasks in Chapter 10. For example, unlike many other adult communication disorders, RHS includes attentional and perceptual disorders, such as neglect and visuospatial deficits. These disorders are usually assessed by psychologists using specialized tests that may not be familiar to speech-language pathologists. The following pages provide brief explanations and rationales for the assessment tasks in Chapter 10, as well as suggestions for scoring the client's performance.

Visual Neglect and Visuospatial Skills

- Line cancellation—This is a simple line cancellation task where the client is asked to "cancel out" each line on the page by drawing a line through it. The degree of visual neglect is measured by comparing the number of lines cancelled on the right side of the page to those cancelled on the left side.

- Letter cancellation—The client is asked to cancel out items (the Qs) on the page by drawing a line through them. This task is more difficult than the line cancellation task. First, there are the foils (the Os) on the page that tax selective attention skills. Second, the Qs and Os are placed randomly on the page, not in rows as in the line cancellation task. Third, the Qs are widely spaced on this task; target items that are far apart *do not* tend to draw the client's attention more to the left, making this task harder than the line cancellation task.

- Copy a drawing—Most of the objects on this drawing task are symmetrical, with equal numbers of lines on each half. The presence and severity of neglect is determined by comparing the number of missing or distorted lines for the left half of the objects to those on the right half.

- Line bisection—The client is asked to draw a line through the middle of the two long lines. Although some deviation from the exact middle is normal, clients with neglect will likely place their bisecting line significantly toward the right ends of the lines.

- Reading multisyllabic words—These items become more difficult toward the bottom of the page, with letters that are widely spaced apart. Look for substitutions, omissions, and additions of letters in the left half of the words.

- Reading sentences—This task will be more difficult than the previous one for several reasons. First, there are more words. Second, there are phrases within the right halves of several sentences than can appear to be complete sentences (e.g.,

" . . . it is hot.") if the client does not attend to all of the text. Third, there is not a straight left margin; the client must adjust his or her attention leftward to find the beginning of each sentence. Measure the presence and severity of neglect by the number of words omitted, substituted, or added to the sentences.

- Reading a paragraph—This also is a difficult task. It contains a number of long, multisyllabic words; variable left-side margins, and sentences with embedded phrases that can be read as a complete sentence. Measure neglect by the number of lines in which the client did not begin reading from the left side of the paragraph.

- Copying sentences—On this task, measure neglect by (a) the number of omitted words or letters, (b) missing punctuation, (c) writing that begins in the middle of the page and runs out of room at the right edge of the paper, (d) missing parts of letters (e. g., no crossing of "t"), and (e) slanted lines.

Communication Skills

- Understanding a narrative—This task requires the client to make inferences and choose the best moral of the story from a field of four choices. Many clients with RHS will tend to choose the most literal or concrete answer, not the more abstract but correct choice.

- Producing a narrative—As the client describes the picture, analyze the description for (a) a logical presentation of the pictured event, (b) the appropriate amount of detail (not describing tangential details or providing too little information), (c) making correct inferences (the storm caused a shipwreck; the man survived it; someone seems to have lowered a rope), (d) describing the emotional state of the man, and (e), as an additional assessment of neglect, including details from the left side of the picture.

- Receptive emotional prosody—Record the number of correct choices the client makes on these items. Note if the client looks at the clinician's face for extralinguistic cues about the emotion that is being demonstrated.

- Pragmatics and expressive prosody—This is an assessment of the client's ability to produce normal prosody during a conversation and also demonstrate correct pragmatic skills. The clinician is asked to subjectively judge the client's performance on 12 pragmatic or prosodic behaviors.

Abstract Language

- Understanding idioms—These items assess the client's ability to correctly interpret nonliteral statements. Some RHS clients will tend to provide only the literal meaning of the items (e.g., "'Spill the beans' means someone is messy.")

- Understanding proverbs—These items also assess the client's ability to correctly interpret nonliteral statements. Some RHS clients will tend to provide only the literal meaning of the items (e.g., "'Birds of a feather flock together' means that birds fly together in flocks.)

- Detecting verbal absurdities—These items require the client to evaluate and integrate all the elements of the sentences to determine how they are illogical. Tasks of this sort may highlight problems with integration and analysis that are not apparent on more straightforward tasks.

Postassessment Counseling

The clinician concludes the assessment session with a postassessment counseling. The clinician shares the assessment information with the client, accompanying family members, and other caregivers. Subsequent to the postassessment counseling, the clinician makes an analysis of information obtained from the case history and interview, reports from other specialists, clinical assessment results, instrumental evaluations, and results of questionnaires or other tests. Integrating the information collected from all sources and means, the clinician writes a diagnostic report. See Chapter 1 for details on the analysis and integration of assessment data and clinical report writing. During the postassessment counseling, the clinician makes a diagnosis, offers recommendations, and suggests a prognosis. The clinician also answers questions from the client and the family members about the disorder and the planned clinical services.

Make a Tentative Diagnosis

Although a final analysis of assessment results has not been made, the clinician nonetheless will have come to tentative but generally valid clinical conclusions at the end of the assessment session. The clinician can make statements about the nature of RHS, its prognosis, and treatment options. The clinician might describe the client's language, cognitive, and visuospatial deficits (e.g., problems with understanding prosody, left-side neglect, anosognosia) that justify the diagnosis. The clinician also might describe in general terms the overall functions of the right hemisphere. For example, the clinician might describe how the right hemisphere seems to help us understand the context of a speaking situation and how it assists in the integration of information.

Make Recommendations

The clinician may recommend treatment for the RHS deficits. Whether the client has had a medical evaluation for the voice problem or the SLP is the first professional to be consulted will determine the immediate course of action, however. The client with a voice disorder but has no other complicating medical conditions needs to be referred to a laryngologist if no prior laryngeal consultation has taken place. A client with possible neurological involvement should be referred to a neurologist. Other professionals, including an audiologist, a psychologist, or a psychiatrist may need to be consulted before starting voice therapy. The clinician may schedule for voice treatment when the laryngologist or other medical specialists recommend it.

Suggest a Prognosis

Although treatment for RHS is not nearly as well documented in the research literature as such disorders as aphasia or dysarthria, the general consensus is that improved language and cognitive functioning is possible with effective treatment (Lehman-Blake, 2007). Several other factors, however, may affect the rate and degree of improvement, even with therapy. The type and the severity of the disorder need to be considered. For example, although left-side visual neglect tends to improve spontaneously during the early weeks postonset, much time and effort in treatment are needed to extend these initial gains. Likewise, clients with severe RHS deficits are unlikely to make as much progress in treatment as someone with mild deficits. Other variables that affect prognosis include the motivation of the client and family members and resources to support prolonged therapy, if needed.

Answer the Client's Questions

Not only the client, but also their spouses or other family members will have several questions about RHS and its treatment. They deserve honest and scientifically justified answers. Some commonly encountered questions and their answers are described here; but the clinician should be ready for other questions. Clients with complicated medical conditions will have additional questions specific to those conditions. The clinician also needs to modify the terms to suit the educational level of the client and the accompanying family members.

What causes RHS? The language and cognitive deficits of RHS can be caused by any condition that damages the right hemisphere of the brain. In most individuals, this damage is caused by a stroke, but physical trauma, infections, and a number of other conditions also can cause these problems. [*The clinician provides an explanation of RHS, give examples.*] For example, a stroke that affects the parietal lobe in the right hemisphere can lead to problems with attention. Treatment in such cases is initially medical, followed by speech therapy once the condition is stabilized. In a few individuals, RHS can be the result of a degenerative disease that causes the loss of neurons only in the right hemisphere, at least for a significant period of time. [*The clinician addresses the client's specific cause of RHS and gives more details.*]

How long does it take to treat RHS effectively? It depends on the deficits and their severity. Some deficits take more time than others. Some may need medical attention before or during therapy; this tends to extend the treatment time. The progress will be faster if we start the treatment soon and we are consistent than if we delayed it or have frequent interruptions. We offer treatment twice a week. [*If not, the clinician gives the actual schedule.*] If you work at home on our assignments, and the family members offer support, the progress will be even better. As you can guess, more severe problems and a problem with additional medical complications will take more time. [*The clinician expands the answer to give additional information relevant to the client's RHS disorder.*]

What are some of the treatment options? There are two general categories of treatment for RHS. The first is the facilitation approach. Here the clinician and client work to stimulate the recovery of damaged brain structures by actively engaging in treatment activities. By actively addressing the client's deficits, it is hoped that the treatment will restore some degree of brain function or reallocate impaired brain function to an undamaged area of the brain. The other approach is compensation, where the clinician and client explore ways to work around the deficits. For example, to help the client remember to look all the way to the left when reading, the clinician may draw a bright red line down the left margin of the page. Also, family members may be taught to present information to the client in ways that enhance his or her understanding. Often, a clinician will combine the facilitation and compensation approaches in the treatment sessions, with more facilitation work being done in the early stages of treatment, which gradually transitions to more of a compensation emphasis in the later stages. [*The clinician expands the answer to give more treatment information relevant to the client's RHS disorder.*]

When do we start treatment? It is better to start treatment as soon as possible. The sooner we start, the better the outcome. [*The clinician gives additional information, depending on whether the client needs to be referred to other specialists before starting treatment; also, depending on the service setting, the clinician tells when and how the treatment might begin.*]

References

Adolfs, R., Damasio, H., & Tranel, D. (2002). Neural systems for recognition of emotional prosody: A 3-D lesion study. *Emotion, 2,* 23–51.

Ardila, A., & Rosselli, M. (1993). Spatial agraphia. *Brain and Cognition, 22,* 137–147.

Bihrle, A. M., Browell, H. H., Powelson, J. A., & Gardner, H. (1986). Comprehension of humorous and nonhumorous materials by left and right brain damaged patients. *Brain and Cognition, 5,* 399–411.

Blake, M., Duffy, J., Myers, P., & Tompkins, C. (2002). Prevalence and patterns of right hemisphere cognitive/communicative deficits: Retrospective data from an inpatient rehabilitation unit. *Aphasiology, 16,* 537–548.

Brookshire, R. (2007). *An introduction to neurogenic communication disorders* (7th ed.). St. Louis, MO: Mosby Year Book.

Bryan, K. L. (1988). Assessment of language disorders after right hemisphere damage. *British Journal of Disorders of Communication, 23,* 111–125.

Bryan, K. L. (1995). *The Right Hemisphere Language Battery* (2nd ed.). London, UK: Whurr.

Burns, M. (1997). *Burns Brief Inventory of Communication and Cognition.* San Antonio, TX: The Psychological Corporation.

Critchley, M., & Henson, R. A. (Eds.). (1977). *Music and the brain.* London, UK: Heinemann.

Foldi, N. F. (1987). Appreciation of pragmatic interpretations of indirect commands: Comparison of right and left brain-damaged patients. *Brain and Language, 31,* 88–108.

Halper, A. S., Cherney, L. R., & Burns, M. (1996). *Rehabilitation Institute of Chicago clinical management of right hemisphere dysfunction* (2nd ed.). Rockville, MD: Aspen.

Heilman, K. M., Bowers, D., Speedie, L., & Coslett, H. B. (1984). Comprehension of affective and nonaffective prosody. *Neurology, 34,* 917–921.

Horner, R. D., Swanson, J. W., Bosworth, H. B., & Matchar, D. B. (2003). Effects of race and poverty on the process and outcome of inpatient rehabilitation services among stroke patients. *Stroke, 43*(4), 1027–1038.

House, A., Rowe, D., & Standen, P. (1987). Affective prosody in the reading voice of stroke patients. *Journal of Neurology, Neurosurgery, and Psychiatry, 50*, 910–912.

Joanette, Y., Ska, B., & Côté, H. (2004). *Protocole Montréal d´évaluation de la communication (MEC).* Isbergues, France: Ortho-Edition.

Lehman-Blake, M. (2007). Perspectives on treatment for communication deficits associated with right hemisphere brain damage. *American Journal of Speech-Language Pathology, 16,* 331–342.

Myers, P. S. (1999). *Right Hemisphere Disorder.* San Diego, CA: Singular.

Myers, P. S., & Blake, M. L. (2008). Communication disorders associated with right hemisphere damage. In R. Chapey (Ed.), *Language intervention strategies in aphasia and related neurogenic communication disorders* (5th ed., pp. 963–987). Philadelphia, PA: Lippincott Williams and Wilkins.

Payne, J. C. (1997). *Adult neurogenic language disorders: Assessment and treatment.* San Diego, CA: Singular.

Pell, M. D. (1999). The temporal organization of affective and non-affective speech in patients with right-hemisphere infarcts. *Cortex, 35,* 455–477.

Pimental, P. A., & Knight, J. A. (2000). *The Mini Inventory of Right Brain Injury* (2nd ed.). Austin, TX: Pro-Ed.

Pimental, P. A., Knight, J. A., & Allen, E. A. (1999). The mini inventory of right brain injury-2 (MIRBI-2): Restandardization and statistical characteristics. *Archives of Clinical Neurology, 14*(8): 736–737.

Schmitt, J., Hartje, W., & Willmes, K. (1997). Hemispheric asymmetry in the recognition of emotional attitude conveyed by facial expression, prosody and prepositional speech. *Cortex, 33,* 65–81.

Stone, S. P., Halligan, P. W., & Greenwood, R. J. (1993). The incidence of neglect phenomena and related disorders in patients with an acute right or left hemisphere stroke. *Age and Ageing, 22,* 46–52.

Tompkins, C. A. (1995). *Right hemisphere communication disorders.* San Diego, CA: Singular.

Tompkins, C. A., Bloise, C. G., Timko, M. L., & Baumgaertner, A. (1994). Working memory and inference revision in brain-damaged and normally aging adults. *Journal of Speech and Hearing Research, 37,* 896–912.

Walker, J. P., Daigle, T., & Buzzard, M. (2002). Hemisphere specialization in processing prosodic structures: Revisited. *Aphasiology, 16,* 1155–1172.

Winner, E., & Gardner, H. (1977). The comprehension of metaphor in brain damaged patients. *Brain, 100,* 717–723.

Zanini, S., Bryan, K., De Luca, G., & Bava, A. (2005). Italian right hemisphere language battery: The normative study. *Neurological Sciences, 26,* 13–25.

CHAPTER 10

Assessment of Right Hemisphere Syndrome (RHS): Protocols

- Overview of RHS Protocols
- Assessment of RHS: Interview Protocol
- RHS Assessment Protocol 1: Visual Neglect and Visuospatial Skills
- RHS Assessment Protocol 2: Communication Skills
- RHS Assessment Protocol 3: Abstract Language

Overview of RHS Protocols

Assessment protocols provided in this chapter help assess RHS disorders in adults in an efficient manner. The protocols offer ready-made formats that clinicians can use in structuring their client and family interviews and assessing various parameters of RHS disorders.

The protocols offered in this chapter also are available on the accompanying CD. The clinician may print the needed protocols in evaluating his or her clients. The clinician may combine these protocols in suitable ways to facilitate the evaluation of an adult's RHS disorders.

In assessing adults with multiple disorders, the clinician may combine these protocols with protocols from other chapters. For example, the clinician may combine the RHS assessment protocols with dysarthria assessment protocols (Chapter 6) or aphasia assessment protocols (Chapter 8).

The protocols given in this chapter are specific to RHS disorders in adults. To complete the assessment on a given client, the clinician should combine these disorder-specific protocols with the common assessment protocols given in Chapter 2:

- The Adult Case History
- Orofacial Examination and Hearing Screening Protocol
- Diadochokinetic Assessment Protocol for Adults
- Adult Assessment Report Outline

Assessment of RHS: Interview Protocol

Name _____ DOB _____ Date _____ Clinician _____

Individualize this protocol on the CD and print it for your use. 💿

Preparation

- Review the guidelines given under *The Initial Clinical Interview* in Chapter 1.
- Arrange for comfortable seating and lighting.
- Record the interview on audio or video.
- Initially interview the client alone and then have the accompanying person join the interview.
- Review the case history ahead of time and take note of areas you want to explore during the interview.

Introduction

☐ Introduce yourself. Describe the assessment plan and tell the client the time it will take.

Example: "Hello Mr./Mrs. [*client's name*]. My name is [*your name*] I am the speech-language pathologist who will be assessing you today. I would like to start by reviewing the case history and asking you a few questions. After we finish talking, I will work with you. Today's assessment should take about [*estimate the amount of time you plan to spend*]."

Interview Questions

The questions are generally directed toward the adult client. When interviewing the client and the accompanying person together, it is essential to pose the same, but reworded, question to the accompanying person. A few examples are shown within the brackets; the clinician may use this strategy whenever necessary.

- What is your main concern following your illness? [What do you think is his (her) main problem?]
- How would you describe your (visual, speech, language, memory, attention) problem? [How would you describe her (his) problem?]
- When did you first notice that your (visual, speech, language, memory, attention) was different? [When did you notice that his (her) abilities are different?]
- Has your (visual, speech, language, memory, attention) changed over time? If so, how? [Have you noticed any changes in behavior or personality since the stroke?]

(continues)

Assessment of RHS: Interview Protocol (continued)

- What does your family doctor say about your (visual, speech, language, memory, attention) problem?

- Did your family doctor refer you to other specialists?

- What did the doctor(s) tell you?

- Have you seen a speech-language pathologist before? What was the advice?

- Did you follow the advice? Have you received speech therapy before?

- Besides a (visual, speech, language, memory, attention) problem, are you concerned with any other aspects of your speech, memory, or attention abilities?

- How would you describe these other problems? [How would you describe his (her) overall speech?]

- Are there times when your (vision, speech, language, memory, attention) is better or worse? For example, is it better in the morning than in the evening? [Do you also think her (his) (vision, speech, language, memory, attention) varies throughout the day?]

- Do you believe that your (visual, speech, language, memory, attention) problem is affecting your social interactions? Would you describe how?

- Do you think that your (visual, speech, language, memory, attention) problem is affecting your job performance? How is it affected?

- Do you have any other chronic health conditions or concerns?

- Are you currently on any medications?

- Is there anything you would like to add about your problem?

- It looks like I have most of the information I wanted from you. Do you have any questions for me at this point?

- Thank you for your information. It will be helpful in my assessment. I will now work with you to better understand your problem. When we are done, we will discuss our findings.

Review the case history again and ask additional questions if needed.

RHS Assessment Protocol 1:
Visual Neglect and Visuospatial Skills

Name _____ DOB _____ Date _____ Clinician _____

Individualize this protocol on the CD and print it for your use.

Line Cancellation

Instructions: Ask the client to draw a line through each line on this page.

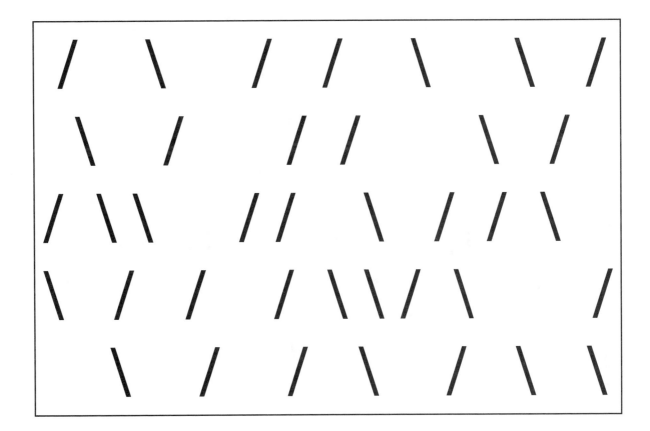

RHS Assessment Protocol 1:
Visual Neglect and Visuospatial Skills

Name _____ DOB _____ Date _____ Clinician _____

Individualize this protocol on the CD and print it for your use.

Letter Cancellation

Instructions: Ask the client to draw a line through each Q on this page.

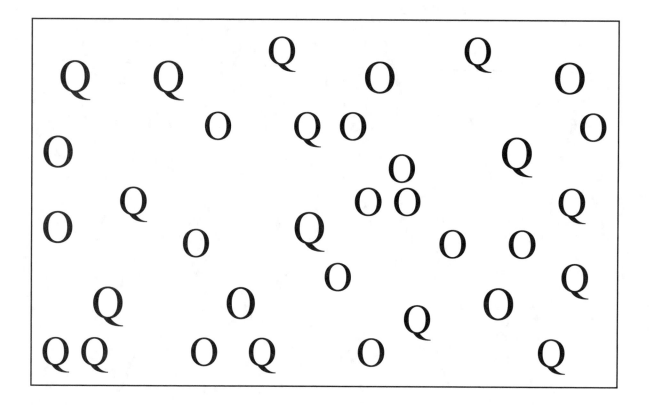

RHS Assessment Protocol 1:
Visual Neglect and Visuospatial Skills

Name _____ DOB _____ Date _____ Clinician _____

Individualize this protocol on the CD and print it for your use. 💿

Copy a Drawing

Ask the client to copy the following drawings.

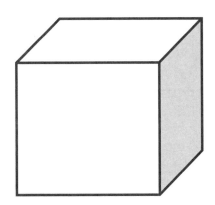

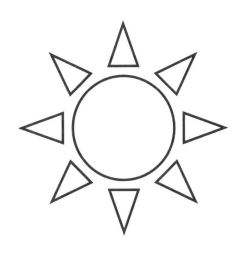

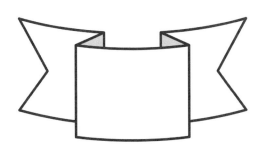

RHS Assessment Protocol 1:
Visual Neglect and Visuospatial Skills

Name _____ DOB _____ Date _____ Clinician _____

Individualize this protocol on the CD and print it for your use. 💿

Line Bisection

Instructions: Ask the client to draw a line through the middle of both lines on this page.

_____

_____

RHS Assessment Protocol 1:
Visual Neglect and Visuospatial Skills

Name _____ DOB _____ Date _____ Clinician _____

Individualize this protocol on the CD and print it for your use. 💿

Reading Multisyllabic Words

Instructions: Ask the client to read the following words aloud. Place a check mark in the left margin by each word read correctly. If the client does not begin reading a word with its first letters, place a check mark within the word where the client began reading.

Aggravation

Skillfulness

Information

Environmental

Impossibility

Eventuality

RHS Assessment Protocol 1:
Visual Neglect and Visuospatial Skills

Name _____ DOB _____ Date _____ Clinician _____

Individualize this protocol on the CD and print it for your use.

Reading Sentences

Instructions: Ask the client to read the following sentences aloud. Place a check mark in the left margin by each sentence read correctly. If the client does not begin reading a sentence with its first words, place a check mark within the sentence where the client began reading.

What is her name?

I liked him better than before.

Try to think of another word for it.

I was pretty tired, and I had to go home.

She turned on the computer yesterday.

Why is she always late for everything?

Please turn on the air conditioner because it is hot.

We left the water running all day.

I took a trip to Holland and France.

That school is one of the best in the city.

Clean the rug a little better next time you do it.

She is a good writer, and I got to meet her.

RHS Assessment Protocol 1:
Visual Neglect and Visuospatial Skills

Name _____ DOB _____ Date _____ Clinician _____

Individualize this protocol on the CD and print it for your use. ⊙

Reading a Paragraph

Instructions: Ask the client to read the following paragraph aloud. Place a check mark in the left margin by each line read correctly. If the client does not begin a line at the left margin, place a check mark within the sentence where the client began reading.

One cool October evening—it was the last day of the month, and unusually cool for the time of year—I made up my mind to go and spend an hour or two with my friend Robert. Robert was an artist (as well as a musical amateur and poet) and had a very delightful studio built onto his house, in which he liked to sit during the evenings. The studio had a cavernous fireplace, designed in imitation of the old-fashioned fireplaces of Elizabethan manor houses. In it, when the temperature outdoors warranted, he would build up a cheerful fire of dry logs. It would suit me particularly well, I thought, to go and have a quiet pipe and chat in front of that fire with my friend.

(Adapted from "Ken's Mystery" by Julian Hawthorne)

RHS Assessment Protocol 1:
Visual Neglect and Visuospatial Skills

Name _____ DOB _____ Date _____ Clinician _____

Individualize this protocol on the CD and print it for your use. 💿

Copying Sentences

Instructions: Give the client a blank, unlined piece of paper. Ask the client to copy the following sentences.

It tastes sweet.

I sat by him today.

What is wrong with the TV?

I do it by myself.

Marge is coming over later.

He cut the grass, and I pulled the weeds.

I bought a new one just the other day.

Do you really like it, or are you just saying so?

It was an old movie, but I liked it.

Open the door, and let the cat out.

That test was not so hard, but it took time.

Is that the right part for the car?

We can eat it now and then get another one.

Yes, he is kind of fun in a crazy sort of way.

RHS Assessment Protocol 2: Communication Skills

Name _____ DOB _____ Date _____ Clinician _____

Individualize this protocol on the CD and print it for your use. ⊙

Understanding a Narrative (Making Inferences)

Instructions: Ask the client to read the following paragraphs either silently or aloud. (If he or she cannot read it, the clinician may read it aloud.) Let the client choose the correct moral of the story from the choices listed.

1. By an unlucky chance, a fox fell into a deep well from which he could not get out. A goat passed by shortly afterward, and asked the fox what he was doing down there. "Oh, have you not heard?" said the fox, "There is going to be a great drought, so I jumped down here in order to be sure to have water by me. Why don't you come down, too?" The goat thought this was good advice, and jumped down into the well. But the Fox immediately jumped on her back, and managed to climb out of the well. "Goodbye, my friend," said the fox, "remember next time . . . "

   A. Never jump into a well when you cannot get out.

   B. That it always rains on a wet day.

   C. Never trust the advice of a person in trouble.

   D. That people often tell lies.

2. A singing bird was confined in a cage that hung outside a window and had a way of singing at night when all other birds were asleep. One night a bat came and asked the bird why she was silent by day and sang only at night. "I have a very good reason for doing so," said the bird. "It was when I was singing in the daytime that a fowler was attracted by my voice and set his nets and caught me. Since then I have never sung except by night." But the bat replied, "It is no use to do that now when you are a prisoner: If only you had done so before you were caught, you might still have been free."

   A. Never sing at night.

   B. Precautions are useless after the crisis.

   C. When caught, always keep your mouth shut.

   D. Bats are wiser than birds.

3. A wagoner was once driving a heavy load along a very muddy way. At last he came to a part of the road where the wheels sank halfway into the mire, and the more the horses pulled, the deeper sank the wheels. So the Wagoner threw down his whip, and knelt down and prayed to Hercules the Strong.

(continues)

Assessment of RHS: Communication Skills Protocol (continued)

"O Hercules, help me in this my hour of distress," cried the man. But Hercules appeared to him, and said: "Tut, man, stop kneeling. Get up and put your shoulder to the wheel."

A. The gods help those who help themselves.

B. The best way is the old-fashioned way.

C. Wagons always get stuck in the mud.

D. Slow and steady wins the race.

RHS Assessment Protocol 2: Communication Skills

Name _____ DOB _____ Date _____ Clinician _____

Individualize this protocol on the CD and print it for your use. 💿

Producing a Narrative

Instructions: Ask the client to "tell a story" about what is happening in the picture on the following page. If unable to proceed at any point, cue the client with general comments or questions such as, "Tell me what is happening here." or "What do you think this means?" Score the accuracy and clarity of the client's narrative according to the following qualities:

1. *Efficiently identifies the main concept of the illustration*

    ☐ Efficiently described the main concept of the illustration (a shipwreck).

    ☐ Has initial difficulty, but after cueing, efficiently described the main concept.

    ☐ Even with cueing, was unable to efficiently describe the main concept.

2. *Includes relevant information in the narrative*

    ☐ Only included relevant information in the narrative.

    ☐ A majority of the narrative contained relevant information, but some irrelevant details also were included.

    ☐ A majority of the narrative contained irrelevant details.

3. *Includes correct inferences in narrative*

    ☐ The client made correct inferences about the illustration (e.g., the rope means that someone is trying to rescue the survivor).

    ☐ The client made correct inferences about the illustration only after cueing.

    ☐ The client made no inferences about the illustration.

4. *Provides an organized, logical narrative of the illustration*

    ☐ The narrative was logically organized with little or no extraneous detail.

    ☐ The narrative contained some extraneous or illogical details that affected organization, yet the overall description was adequate.

    ☐ The narrative was not logically or efficiently organized because of excessive amounts of nonessential or illogical details.

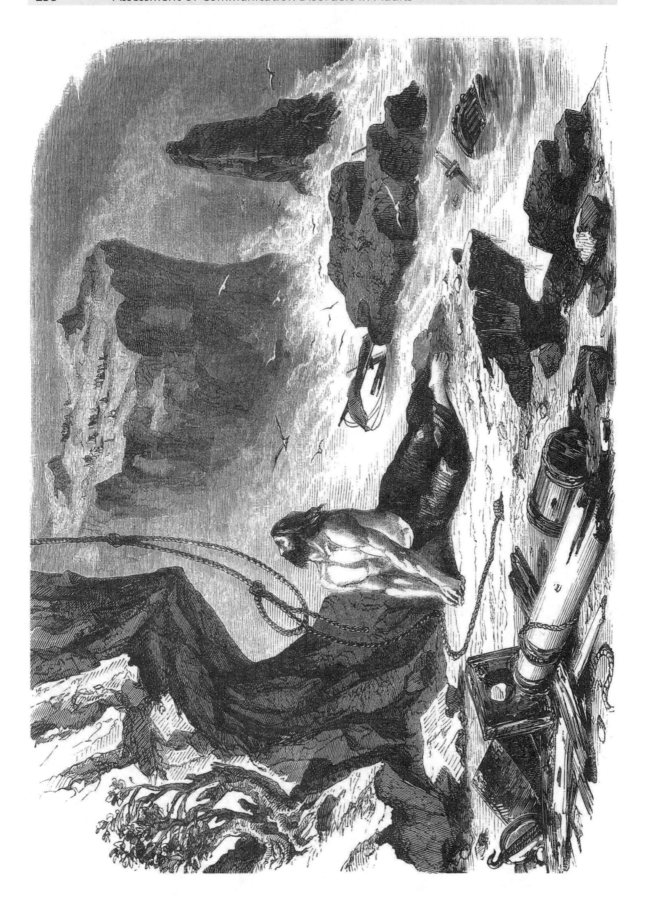

RHS Assessment Protocol 2: Communication Skills

Name _____ DOB _____ Date _____ Clinician _____

Individualize this protocol on the CD and print it for your use. 💿

Receptive Emotional Prosody

Instructions: Read the following sentences aloud to the client, using prosody that conveys the indicated emotional state. If cueing is needed, write the target emotions (happy, sad, mad, bossy, worried) on a piece of paper and allow the client to refer to it during the task.

Clinician's stimulus	Correct	Correct with Cues	Incorrect
I walked the dog this morning. (Bossy)			
She went to work at 10 o'clock. (Happy)			
We have two cars in the garage. (Worried)			
I read the magazine. (Mad)			
He was taking a nap. (Sad)			

Pragmatics and Expressive Linguistic Prosody

Instructions: Engage the client in a conversation for approximately 4 to 5 minutes. This can be initiated by asking for the client to describe his or her career, favorite vacations, hobbies, or similar topics. After 4 to 5 minutes have passed, end the conversation by indicating that there is more testing to do. Judge the client's pragmatic and expressive prosody on the following checkoff list.

Client's pragmatic and prosodic behaviors	Correct	Incorrect
Appropriate turn taking		
Appropriate eye contact		
Maintains the topic of conversation		
Demonstrates appropriate melody in connected speech		
Recognizes a conversational breakdown and tries to repair it		
Appropriate facial expressions for topic		
Appropriate body posture during conversation		
Uses hand gestures to emphasize points		

(continues)

RHS Assessment Protocol 2: Communication Skills (continued)

Client's pragmatic and prosodic behaviors	Correct	Incorrect
Modifies utterances for clarification when asked, "What?"		
Does not assume listener knows more about the topic than normal		
Uses intonation to indicate communicative intent (e.g., a question)		
Does not try to extend the conversation once it has ended		
Clinician summative statement:		

RHS Assessment Protocol 3: Abstract Language

Name _____ DOB _____ Date _____ Clinician _____

Individualize this protocol on the CD and print it for your use. 💿

Understanding Idioms

Instructions: "I am going to tell you a saying that means more than what it says. For example, "Save it for a rainy day" really means that people should save money for hard times. I want you to tell me the real meaning of these sayings." (Note: these are American idioms and should only be used with native English speakers.)

Idiom	Score 0 = Incorrect 1 = Correct
1. A piece of cake (Something that is easy)	0　1
2. To bend over backward (Very willing to help or satisfy)	0　1
3. Can't cut the mustard (Someone who is not good enough to do something)	0　1
4. To drive someone up the wall (Something that is very annoying or aggravating)	0　1
5. Go out on a limb (To take a risky chance to help someone or do something)	0　1
6. Spill the beans (To reveal a secret)	0　1
7. Know the ropes (To understand all the details of something)	0　1
8. Pulling your leg (Someone is joking)	0　1
9. To buy the farm (To die)	0　1
10. To hit the hay (To go to sleep)	0　1
Clinician's summative statement:	

(continues)

RHS Assessment Protocol 3: Abstract Language (continued)

Understanding Proverbs

Instructions: "I am going to tell you a number of sayings that have a wise lesson in them. For example, "Actions speak louder than words" really means that what a person does is more important than what he says. I want you to tell me the lessons from the following sayings." (Note: these are American proverbs and should only be used with native English speakers.)

Proverbs	Score 0 = Incorrect 1 = Correct	
1. An apple a day keeps the doctor away. (Leading a healthy lifestyle will keep you from needing a doctor frequently.)	0	1
2. Rome wasn't built in a day. (It takes time to create something great.)	0	1
3. Two heads are better than one. (It is better to have a number of people working on a problem or task.)	0	1
4. Don't put all your eggs in one basket. (Don't rely completely on just one person or event.)	0	1
5. A good example is the best sermon. (It is more convincing when someone does the right thing, rather than just talking about it.)	0	1
6. Haste makes waste. (Doing something too quickly will result in a poor result)	0	1
7. Don't cry over spilled milk. (It is useless to fret over something that has already happened.)	0	1
8. Birds of a feather flock together. (A person is attracted to similar people.)	0	1
9. All that glitters is not gold. (Worthless things can initially be attractive.)	0	1
10. A fool and his money are soon parted. (A person with poor judgment will quickly lose possessions of value.)	0	1
Clinician's summative statement:		

Detecting Verbal Absurdities

Instructions: "I am going to read to you a number of sentences that do not make sense . . . For example, "It was so hot today that I wore my heaviest coat," does not make sense because we don't wear coats on hot days. I want you to tell me why the following sentences do not make sense.

Verbal Absurdity	Score 0 = Incorrect 1 = Correct
1. Susan wasn't home when I went to her house, and I talked to her for an hour.	0 1
2. The window was so clean that I couldn't see out of it.	0 1
3. The chair cost 10 dollars, so I gave her a 5-dollar bill.	0 1
4. When the sun is up, we can see all the stars in the sky.	0 1
5. I was really sleepy, so I drove the car another 200 miles.	0 1
6. The food looked so good that I threw it all in the trash.	0 1
7. He ran the race in the fastest time and finished in last place.	0 1
8. The roses were just beautiful, so she pulled them all up.	0 1
9. I was so hungry that one bite of food really filled me up.	0 1
10. I didn't like the movie very much, so I saw it at least five times.	0 1
Clinician's summative statement:	

PART V

Assessment of
Dementia

CHAPTER 11

Assessment of Dementia: Resources

- Overview of Dementia
- Epidemiology of Dementia
- General Etiology and Pathology of Neurodegenerative Diseases
- Treatment of Irreversible and Reversible Dementia
- Dementia of the Alzheimer Type
- Other Forms of Dementia
- Overview of Dementia Assessment
- Screening and Diagnostic Tests for Dementia
- Assessment of Dementia in Ethnoculturally Diverse Adults
- Diagnostic Criteria and Differential Diagnosis
- Postassessment Counseling

Overview of Dementia

Dementia is a neurological disorder that causes progressive deterioration in intellectual skills and general behavior. Several better known forms of dementia are persistent and progressive, although some forms of dementia can be nonprogressive (transient). The progressive forms are irreversible, whereas the transient forms are reversible.

Definitions of dementia differ, but most emphasize intellectual and behavioral deterioration. The fourth edition of the *Diagnostic and Statistical Manual of Mental Diseases* (DSM-IV) (American Psychiatric Association, 1994) and its 2000 text revision (American Psychiatric Association, 2000) describes dementia as an impairment in memory plus at least *one* of the following: aphasia (language disturbances), apraxia, agnosia, or impaired executive functions (e.g., abstract thinking and planning). Others do not necessarily include memory impairment. For instance, Cummings and Benson (1992) define dementia as an "acquired persistent impairment of intellectual function with compromise in at least three of the following spheres of mental activity: language, memory, visuospatial skills, emotion or personality, and cognition (abstraction, calculation, judgment, executive function, and so forth)" (1992, pp. 1–2). These authors do not consider memory impairment as a necessary condition for diagnosing dementia because, in certain forms of dementia (e.g., dementia due to Pick's disease), memory may not be impaired in the early and middle stages of the disease.

The acquired nature of pathology that underlines dementia helps distinguish it from congenital intellectual disability. Also, dementia is a *deterioration* in normal intellectual functions whereas a lower intellectual level is relatively stable across the lifespan of individuals with intellectual disability. Furthermore, although the features of irreversible dementia persist and get worse, confusion due to acute cerebral trauma, metabolic disorders, and toxicity are transient. Confusion due to cerebral trauma is of more sudden onset than that due to dementia.

The pathology of aphasia and dementia may be distinguished by the more focal pathology in the former, and more diffuse pathology in the latter. In addition, the onset of dementia is gradual, whereas that of aphasia is typically more acute. Furthermore, intellectual deterioration is not a feature of aphasia. Most individuals with aphasia typically have normal cognitive abilities for tasks unrelated to language, such as reasoning, making judgments, goal setting, and orientation. Personality and behavior usually are unaffected by aphasia, but these can change significantly in persons with dementia.

Epidemiology of Dementia

Dementia primarily affects the elderly, and the consequences of having a dementing illness can be profound. Because of the slow progression of most types of dementia, affected individuals need the services of multidisciplinary teams that are able to provide long-term care. Treating individuals with dementia consumes much of the healthcare finances in the United States. It is estimated that that the annual cost of caring for these patients is more than $30 billion, a number that is certain to increase in the coming years.

As birth rates fall and the elderly live longer, the prevalence of dementia grows. Jorm, Korten, and Henderson (1987) stated that the number of individuals with dementia doubles every 5 years after the age of 65. In the United States, the number of individuals with dementia and related disorders may reach 15 million by 2030. In some parts of the world, estimating the prevalence of dementia can be difficult because early signs of dementia are often considered to be associated with normal aging. In fact, Payne (1997) found that it is not uncommon for many cases of dementia to go undetected in societies where the elderly receive nearly all their care in the family home. The following list provides additional information on the occurrence of dementia:

- A new patient is diagnosed with dementia somewhere in the world every 7 seconds.

- Dementia shortens life expectancy; the median survival rate of a person with dementia is 5 to 9.3 years.

- As the population ages, the prevalence of dementia increases. Found in 1% of people in their early 60s, it increases to 10% in those over 65. For individuals in their mid to late 80s, the prevalence may be as high as 30%. Some evidence suggests that the incidence of dementia declines slightly in people in their 90s.

- Dementia may affect as many as 20% of nursing home residents. It is the single most common illness in nursing homes.

- As healthcare improves around the world and people live longer, the incidence of dementia grows. In addition, dementia may be more common in urban areas of the world than in rural areas.

- Dementia does not affect all ethnocultural groups equally:
  - *Alzheimer's disease* may be more common in whites than in Asian Americans or African Americans.
  - *Vascular dementia* may be more common in Asian and African Americans than in whites or Hispanics. In Japan, vascular dementia is more common than other types of dementia.
  - *Lewy body dementia* may be more common in whites than in Asian Americans, African Americans, and Hispanics.
  - *Frontotemporal lobar degeneration* may be more common in whites, Asian Americans, and Pacific Islanders than in African Americans or Hispanics.
  - *Progressive supranuclear palsy* may be more common in Asian Americans and Pacific Islanders than in whites. It is equally common in African Americans and Hispanics.
  - *Late onset dementia* may be more common in African Americans than in other groups.
  - *The prevalence of dementia varies by geography.* Nigeria and India's Kashmir region report low numbers of individuals with dementia.

General Etiology and Pathology of Neurodegenerative Diseases

There are many general neuropathological factors linked to progressive dementia. Overall, these factors tend to affect the metabolic functions of neurons via abnormal growths, neuronal degeneration, or neurochemical disorders. Here is a listing of the pathological conditions associated with the more well-known types of dysarthria:

- *Neurofibrillary tangles*—abnormal, twisted formations inside the cytoplasm of neuron cell bodies, dendrites, and axons.

- *Neuritic plaques*—microscopic lesions in dendrites and at the ends of axons. They also are known as *senile plaques*.

- *Granulovacuolar degeneration*—a condition where cells develop microscopic spaces (vacuoles) filled with granulated protoplasm.

- *Reduced dendritic connections*—inhibit the transmission of neuron impulses.

- *Neurochemical disorders*—also inhibit the transmission of neuron impulses. Deficiencies of dopamine and cholinergic neurotransmitters are common to several types of dementia.

- *Neuron loss*—both gray and white matter is lost, particularly evident in the frontal and temporal lobes of the brain. As much as 10% of brain weight can be lost in some dementing conditions.

- *Enlarged ventricles and wider sulci*—occur as the neurons in the brain cells degenerate.

- *Reduced cerebral metabolism*—reflects the pathological conditions occurring at the neuronal level. As neurons in the brain develop neurofibrillary tangles, neuritic plaques, and other impairments, their metabolic function slows.

Treatment of Irreversible and Reversible Dementia

One way to categorize dementia is to divide it into those that can be treated successfully (reversible) and those that cannot (irreversible). The most well-known types of dementia are irreversible. These include Alzheimer's disease, Huntington's disease, Parkinson's disease, frontotemporal dementia, vascular dementia, and the infectious dementias such as Creutzfeldt-Jakob disease and AIDS dementia complex. In each of these conditions, the available medical treatments are limited, and nothing has been found to reverse the decline of cognitive abilities. Nevertheless, there are some medications that can improve the quality of life for many patients with irreversible dementia. For example, cholinesterase inhibitors have been shown to improve the cognitive abilities of patients with early Alzheimer's disease, at least temporarily. Other medications can ease the anxiety, sleeping disorders, and behavioral problems experienced by many individuals with irreversible dementia. Likewise, medical treatments for vascular dementia may greatly reduce the heart attacks, strokes, blood clots, and hypertension associated with this condition. Unfortunately, they cannot reverse the damage that has been done to the patient's brain and vascular system. Although these types of treatments may reduce a few of the patient's symptoms, most of the medical treatment for the irreversible dementia consists of palliative care, ensuring that the patient is as comfortable and healthy as possible.

The treatment options are different for the reversible dementias. This type of dementia usually appears as a secondary symptom of a primary disorder. For example, cognitive impairments can be a secondary symptom in some cases of nonconvulsive epilepsy. Other examples of reversible dementia may be found in these conditions:

- Normal pressure hydrocephalus
- Operable brain tumors
- Hypoglycemia
- Chronic drug intoxication
- Vitamin B12 deficiency and related metabolic disorders
- Hypothyroidism
- Depression
- Chronic subdural hematoma
- Cerebral vasculitis and related inflammatory conditions
- Tuberculosis and some types of fungal meningitis
- Heavy-metal intoxication

In each of these conditions, the co-occurring dementia will resolve once the primary disorder is treated successfully.

Although it is encouraging to know that some dementias can be reversed, the actual number of such cases may be quite low (Weytingh, Bossuyt, & van Crevel, 1995). Some estimates have found that less than 1% of all dementia cases are reversible (Geldmacher, 2004). For instance, Freter, Bergman, Gold, Chertkow, and Clarfield (1998) found that of 196 patients seen at a memory clinic, only 23% had potentially reversible dementias. Of those, only 3.6% (*n* = 7) actually showed improvement with treatment. The authors noted that improvements were seen only in those patients with early and mild cognitive impairments, suggesting that prompt and complete medical examinations are essential for a positive outcome.

Dementia of the Alzheimer Type

Alzheimer's disease (AD) is characterized by a progressive decline in memory, cognitive abilities, speech, and language. Changes in personality and behavior also are associated with this condition. AD is a degenerative neurological disorder that accounts for approximately 50% of dementias. The first description of this dementia was published in 1906 by Alois Alzheimer, who reported on a middle-aged patient's steady decline in intellectual and self-care abilities. Originally, the term *Alzheimer's disease* was used only in reference to relatively young individuals who demonstrated the behaviors described by Alzheimer. Currently, however, all individuals experiencing the cognitive decline associated with this condition can be diagnosed as having AD, regardless of age.

- **Epidemiology and Other Variables of AD**
  - Age of onset varies. Individuals in their 40s have been diagnosed with AD, but this is uncommon. Prevalence increases with age, with symptoms first appearing near the age of 65. As many as 3% of people 75 years old are estimated to have the disease. In the 75 to 84 age group, 6% are thought to be affected; and perhaps as many as 15% of 85-year-olds have AD.

- o Having Down syndrome is strongly associated with developing AD later in life. In fact, just having a family history of Down syndrome increases the risk factors for developing the condition.
- o Women develop AD about twice as frequently as men. This is partly due to women living longer than men, but there are gender-specific risk factors that increase the chances of women developing AD. There is no difference in the course of the disease in women or men.
- o The average duration of AD is 10 years.
- o The incidence of AD is increasing as the number of elderly people grows. About 2.3 million individuals had AD in the United States during the 1990s. It is estimated that this number will reach 8.64 million by 2047.
- o There seems to a familial link in the appearance of AD. First-degree relatives of a person with AD have a slightly increased chance of developing the condition.
- o AD may be more common among white individuals compared to African Americans, Hispanic Americans, and Asian Americans.
- o There have been cases where one identical twin acquired AD and the other did not, suggesting that environmental factors probably play a role in the development of AD.
- o Chromosomal abnormalities have been found in some clients with AD. A rare type of early-onset inherited AD is associated with mutations on chromosome 21. Abnormalities in chromosome 14 have been linked to another type of inherited AD.
- o Other factors that may increase the risk for developing AD include prior head injuries, lower levels of education, vascular diseases that reduce blood flow to the brain, and epilepsy (which can create neuritic plaques in the brain at a young age).

- **Onset of AD and Early Symptoms**
  - o AD begins with a subtle, gradual progression of symptoms.
  - o Memory lapses are the most commonly reported early symptom.
  - o Affected individuals have problems learning and remembering new tasks.
  - o Mild changes in behavior may be noted by family members, such as a lack of initiation, irritability, moodiness, and confusion in new situations or locations. As the disease progresses these behaviors intensify and may include suspiciousness, disorientation, and depression.
  - o Some affected individuals will not show awareness of their problems, although other individuals with early-stage AD will notice the changes in their cognitive abilities.
  - o Speech and language deficits may appear in the early stages of AD. For example, the individual may have difficulty giving instructions or telling a story. Frequently asking for clarification and drifting from the topic of conversation may be noted. Word-finding difficulties also begin to appear during this stage of AD. Word-fluency tasks ("Tell all the words you can

think of that start with the letter 'A'.") can be quite difficult for these individuals.

- o Problems with activities of daily living (ADLs) can appear. Bills may not be paid or perhaps be paid twice in the same month. Changes in self-care may become evident, with personal hygiene often being neglected.

- o There may be impairment in the ability to understand implied meanings in a conversation.

- o Visual-spatial deficits can appear in the early stages of AD. This may be noted in attempts to draw shapes or completing block design tasks. Forgetting where frequently used objects are kept will be noted.

- **Middle and Late Stage Symptoms of AD**
  - o The progression of early symptoms of AD continues, and they become more frequent and intensify in severity. Additional problems develop as the disease advances.

  - o Obvious memory difficulties appear for both recent and remote events.

  - o ADLs deteriorate significantly. Individuals are unable to take care of personal finances; maintenance of personal hygiene is difficult; and they cannot safely cook or travel independently.

  - o Aberrant behaviors can be noted. Apathy, paranoia, delusions, hoarding, inappropriate sexual behaviors, restlessness, and sleeping disturbances may appear in the middle and late stages of AD.

  - o In some cases, violence and emotional lability can be observed. These can be especially troublesome for family members.

  - o Speech and language difficulties increase in severity. Confusing use of pronouns and poor topic maintenance may be evident. The individual may repeat topics that were just discussed moments before. Word-finding problems intensify, while the person's vocabulary decreases. Comprehension of complex conversations is severely impaired. In the final stages of AD, individuals can demonstrate problems with eye contact, and their spoken utterances often are unintelligible. Palilialia or echolalia may be noted, or they may speak only in sentence fragments. They often are mute in the final stages of AD.

  - o The progression of visual-spatial deficits can make walking, dressing, and eating very difficult or impossible.

  - o Significant disorientation and wandering behaviors can be observed in the middle and late stages of AD. Affected persons may get lost in very familiar locations, and they eventually will become disoriented to person, place, and time.

  - o Motor deficits, such as muscular rigidity and tremor, may appear. Walking can be unsteady, often resembling the festinating gait of someone with Parkinson's disease. In fact, the early appearance of Parkinsonian-like movement difficulties may indicate an accelerated course of AD.

  - o Swallowing difficulties are common, often in association with repeated instances of aspiration pneumonia.

- **The Diagnosis of AD**

  Because AD is the most common form of dementia, medical professionals frequently are called upon to make the initial diagnosis or to document changes in cognitive ability as the disease progresses.

  - Currently, the only way to diagnose AD with certainty is through autopsy or brain biopsy (a procedure that is seldom, if ever, done for this condition). Consequently, medical doctors often will diagnose patients thought to have this disorder as having "dementia of the Alzheimer's type."

  - AD can be diagnosed with high levels of reliability via an examination that includes (a) a review of the patient's medical history and psychiatric background, (b) a full neurological examination, (c) detailed discussions about the patient with family members, (d) a mental status examination to assess cognitive abilities, and (e) laboratory testing to rule out medical conditions that can cause dementia-like behaviors (e.g., hypoglycemia).

  - By themselves, mental status examinations (also commonly known as memory screening tests) cannot diagnose AD. The results of such testing can only suggest that further evaluation is needed. Qualified professionals should conduct these mental status examinations, such as physicians, psychologists, nurse practitioners, social workers, or speech-language pathologists.

  - The results of mental status examinations need to be kept confidential. If further testing is recommended, a referral to a medical doctor specializing in dementia should be made.

  - Noninvasive neuroimaging procedures such as CAT scans or MRIs cannot provide sufficient information to confirm a diagnosis of AD, although they may provide a degree of corroborative evidence. Nevertheless, they rarely are performed in cases of suspected AD.

Other Forms of Dementia

Although Alzheimer's disease is the most well-known form of dementia, there are a significant number of other conditions that have irreversible dementia as a prominent symptom. They are a diverse collection of disorders with varied etiological factors. Some of these dementias are due to vascular disorders; a few are caused by abnormal chromosomes; most have unknown etiologies.

Huntington's disease is an inherited condition that causes the degeneration of neurons in the basal ganglia (which causes involuntary, hyperkinetic movements) and the cortex (which is associated with the dementia). It is an autosomal dominant disease, meaning that each child of a parent with the disease has a 50% chance of having the condition as well. The course of the disease is about 15 years, although cases lasting over 25 years have been documented. The first symptoms are subtle cognitive impairments that are evident only on neuropsychological tests. Months or years may pass until these deficits become directly observable, usually taking the form of impaired memory for both recent and remote events. A significant, generalized reduction in intellectual abilities becomes evident as the condition progresses.

The behavioral and psychiatric disturbances that eventually develop include irritability, emotional outbursts, and inattentiveness. In the more advanced stages of the disease, depression, delusions, suicidal thoughts, and paranoia often are present. As the basal ganglia neurons degenerate, Huntington patients demonstrate a hyperkinetic movement disorder known as *chorea*. These involuntary movements initially may appear as only a general restlessness. But over time, they develop into a complex collection of uncontrollable head, neck, limb, and torso movements that sometimes have a fluid, dance-like quality. The chorea significantly impairs the patient's ability to perform such voluntary movements as speaking, walking, and eating. Patients with Huntington's disease are mute and bedridden in the final stages of the disorder.

Parkinson's disease is a slowly progressive disorder primarily associated with disturbances in voluntary movement. This condition results from the degeneration of neurons in the substantia nigra, a small gray-matter collection of neuron cell bodies near the basal ganglia. Neuron degeneration also occurs in the brainstem as the condition progresses. In a normally functioning brain, neurons in substantia nigra neurons provide dopamine to large portions of the basal ganglia, a key part of the motor system for refining voluntary movements. The proper functioning of the basal ganglia is dependent on balanced amounts of an excitatory neurotransmitter (acetylcholine) and an inhibitory neurotransmitter (dopamine). In patients with Parkinson's disease, the neurons in the substantia nigra degenerate causing the dopamine levels in the basal ganglia to decline. This disrupts the balance of acetycholine and dopamine, leaving the basal ganglia in an overly excited state. As a result, the basal ganglia are unable to refine movements normally, leading to the well-known collection of motor deficits found in this disease:

- **Tremor** is one of the most common symptoms of Parkinson's disease, and it often is the first one noticed by patients with this condition. It is a resting tremor, meaning it is most evident while the body is at rest. When the body is in motion, the tremor will be greatly reduced, or it will disappear.

- **Bradykinesia** is the slowed and reduced range of movement seen in this disease. Voluntary movements can be labored, slow, and limited, such as in the shuffling walk demonstrated by many patients. Bradykinesia is caused by the neurochemical imbalance in the basal ganglia. It is not the result of muscle weakness, as might be assumed by watching someone with this condition struggle to complete simple tasks.

- **Muscle rigidity** is seen frequently in Parkinson's disease due to increased muscle tone, especially in the neck, torso, and limbs. When pulling an affected body part to full extension, constant resistance to the movement will be noted.

- **Akinesia** causes a delay in the initiation of a voluntary movement. Usually, the delay is only for a few seconds, but it may be significantly longer in more advanced cases. In the most severe instances of akinesia, patients may become "frozen" in position and are unable to move voluntarily.

- **Disturbed postural reflexes** are most evident when the affected individual is attempting to perform normal movements, such as walking, getting up from a chair, or even standing still. For example, if lightly pushed while standing, the patient may fall because of an inability to rapidly shift his or her center of balance.

Not all individuals with Parkinson's disease develop a dementia, and there is significant variability in the number of dementia cases reported in this disease—ranging from 8% to 50%, with 30% being an often cited percentage. Dementia is more common in individuals who develop Parkinson's disease after the age of 60. The process causing the dementia is unclear, but neurofibrillary tangles and neuritic plaques have been noted in the brains of parkinsonian patients with dementia. Impairments of memory, naming, word fluency, narrative comprehension, and visuospatial perception have all been noted in this type of dementia.

Frontotemporal dementia is an umbrella term for several dementing illnesses, all of which are linked to neural degeneration of the frontal lobe, temporal lobe, or both. This type of dementia may account for 12% of dementia cases in individuals who are under 65 years of age. It is one of the more common non-Alzheimer types of dementia. *Pick's disease* is the most well-known frontotemporal dementia. It is associated with two primary neuropathological conditions: Pick bodies and Pick cells. Pick bodies are intracellular growths in the neuronal cytoplasm, and Pick cells are enlarged, "ballooned" neurons. The posterior inferior frontal lobes and the anterior temporal lobes are affected most by Pick's disease. The cause of the condition is unknown.

A unique aspect of frontotemporal dementia is the early appearance of behavior and personality disorders, with memory remaining relatively intact, at least for a substantial period. Patients with neuron degeneration predominately in the right hemisphere tend to demonstrate more significant behavior problems than patients with degeneration occurring mostly in the left hemisphere. These behaviors include impulsive and inappropriate social comments, uncaring attitudes about loved ones, inappropriate sexual advances, moodiness, and even aggression in severe cases. The patient's conduct can be particularly distressing for family members who often comment on how out of character these actions are. Depression may alternate with euphoria, and persecution delusions may be observed in some individuals. Compulsive eating may be noted, even for nonedible materials. (One of the authors had a patient with this disease who regularly would attempt to eat bars of soap.) Ultimately, judgment and reasoning abilities also decline significantly. Patients with frontotemporal dementia show little insight into their condition.

Language deficits are noted in frontotemporal dementia that is primarily affecting the left hemisphere. Vocabulary decreases as word-finding difficulties increase. Indefinite pronouns, circumlocutions, and verbal paraphasias may be evident. The word-finding difficulties in this dementia seem to have a semantic basis, suggesting that the patient's knowledge of word meaning is being lost as the disease progresses. (This contrasts to word-finding problems in aphasia, which often, but not always, have a phonological basis—the aphasic patient knows what to say but cannot think of the word.) Word fluency performance is impaired, along with the ability to participate in a spontaneous conversation. In the later stages, a patient's speech may be restricted primarily to echolalia, palilalia, and stereotypic utterances.

Infectious dementia results from a communicable condition. A typical example of infectious dementia is that associated with acquired immune deficiency syndrome (AIDS). Many patients with AIDS develop a dementia, known variously as *AIDS dementia complex, HIV-1-associated dementia,* or *HIV encephalopathy.* This dementia is a result of the HIV infection directly affecting brain tissue, causing the degeneration of cortical neurons and subcortical white matter. The basal ganglia also can be affected. In some patients with AIDS, the dementia may be the first obvious indication of the disease. The early symptoms of AIDS dementia complex include forgetfulness, slowed thinking, apathy, and decreased ability to concentrate. Depression and mania, disorientation, delusions, and significantly reduced memory may appear late in the condition. Fortunately, medical treatment of AIDS has progressed considerably in recent years. Antiretroviral medications have reduced the occurrence of AIDS dementia complex by approximately 50%, as well as prolonged the life of affected patients.

Creutzfeldt-Jakob disease is another infectious dementia. It is a very rare condition and is associated with diffuse neuron loss following the transmission of protein particles known as prions into brain tissue. One well-documented method of prion transmission is the use of human growth hormone created from the cadaver of an individual who died from Creutzfeldt-Jakob disease. There are several subcategories of this disease including an inherited version, which accounts for about 10% of cases.

Creutzfeldt-Jakob disease progresses rapidly, especially compared to other types of dementing illnesses. Most patients die within one year, although in some variations of the disease the progression is slower. The first noted symptom is dementia, which initially reveals itself as forgetfulness and impaired concentration. Eventually this leads to significant memory loss and personality changes, as well as hallucinations, delusions, and depression. Motor problems also appear including ataxia, chorea, tremor, and rigidity. Seizures are common. Unfortunately, there is no cure or effective treatment for Creutzfeldt-Jakob disease.

Progressive supranuclear palsy typically first appears in late middle age, and causes neural degeneration in the basal ganglia, brainstem, and cerebellum, where neurofibrillary tangles, reduced dopamine, granulovacuolar degeneration, gliosis, and demyelination can be observed. It is rare and usually is fatal after only a few years. Several of the symptoms are similar to those seen in Parkinson's disease, such as hypokinetic dysarthria and reduced facial expressions. Restricted voluntary eye movement is another common characteristic of this disease, which makes it difficult for the affected individual to read or walk down stairs. Generalized muscular rigidity occurs in the later stages.

The dementia associated with progressive supranuclear palsy includes such symptoms as forgetfulness, a slowing of intellectual processes, apathy, and depression. Significant intellectual decline is not evident until the final stages. Dysarthria may be present, including hypokinetic, spastic, and mixed hypokinetic-spastic during the course of the disease (Duffy, 2005). Language disorders are not evident until late in the progression, eventually reaching the point where the patient is mute.

Vascular dementia is linked to a number of neuropathological conditions that are secondary to vascular disorders. It has long been known that dementia can result from cerebrovascular disease, but the concept of a "vascular dementia" has been the subject of debate. Questions about vascular dementia as a standalone diagnostic entity have centered on how to detect the lesions and the degree and location of damage. Despite the lack of agreement on the classification of this disorder, vascular dementia has been divided into three subcategories: (a) dementia due to multiple lesions, (b) dementia due to a specific single lesion, and (c) dementia due to widespread subcortical white matter lesions. *Binswanger's disease* is a good example of the third category. It is a vascular dementia associated with demyelination of subcortical white matter. A complicating factor in diagnosing vascular dementia is the finding that about 30% of patients with AD also have significant cerebrovascular disease, something that blurs the diagnostic boundary between these two conditions.

Additional dementia syndromes include the following disorders:

- *Multiple sclerosis* is caused by the demyelination of white matter in the central nervous system. A dementia may be present in the more advanced or severe cases of this disorder.

- *Lewy body dementia* is linked to the development of abnormal proteins in neuron cell bodies. These proteins (Lewy bodies) affect dopamine and acetylcholine production in the brain, resulting in motor deficits similar to that found in Parkinson's disease and a dementia similar to AD.

- *Traumatic brain injury* can be associated with dementia. External trauma to diffuse areas of the brain is the primary pathological factor. This damage can result in widespread axon and vascular injuries, which are often linked to the appearance of dementia later in life. Intracranial hematoma, infection, elevated intracranial pressure, and ischemia are additional brain injuries that have been associated with the development of dementia.

- *Wilson's disease* is a rare, inherited condition that prevents the body from metabolizing dietary copper. The copper accumulates in the cornea, liver, kidney, and brain. These deposits are toxic to the affected tissue, and in the brain, they are primarily found in the lenticular nuclei of the basal ganglia. As the disease progresses, dementia, dysarthria, hyperkinetic movements, depression, mania, and limb ataxia may be observed in untreated cases. Fortunately, Wilson's disease can be managed successfully if the treatment is started early in its development.

Overview of Dementia Assessment

The assessment of dementia frequently begins with an inquiry from worried family members who have noted cognitive changes in the patient. In most cases, the troublesome changes are related to a decline in memory. Forgetting newly learned information such as names and appointments often is what family members notice first. Although forgetting such information is not unusual, it is the increased frequency of these forgetful moments that catches the family's attention, especially if they are out of character for the person in question. Although memory difficulties are the most common first indication that dementia may be present, a variety of others also may be observed, including:

- **Word-finding difficulties** for common objects or tasks. For example, the individual may say, "Those things I use for starting the car" when the word *key* cannot be recalled.

- **Demonstrating poor judgment** in a way that is unusual for the individual. Someone who usually is careful with money may suddenly write checks to a questionable organization or buy objects for which he or she has no use.

- **Uncharacteristic moodiness** can be observed in early cases of dementia. An individual who normally is emotionally stable may show rapid changes in mood, such as suddenly showing anger for little or no reason.

- **Problems doing ordinary tasks** may include confusion when doing everyday chores, such as cooking food, paying bills, or using a TV remote control.

- **Losing objects around the house** may happen to anyone, but when the frequency of this behavior increases or objects are left in unusual places, it may indicate a developing cognitive problem.

- **Decreased initiative** can be seen when an individual begins to show signs of passivity or apathy, such as refusing to do normally enjoyable activities, choosing instead to sleep or watch television.

- **Disorientation in familiar places** might be observed when an individual gets lost while walking alone in a well-known neighborhood or shopping mall.

Screening Tests for Dementia

When one or more of these behaviors cause a family member to make a referral to a medical professional, the first assessment to be completed is usually a screening test of cognitive function. These tests are quick (usually taking no more than 10 minutes), and most of them examine four areas of intellectual ability: orientation, memory, praxis, and language. The orientation tasks typically ask about the current day, week, and location. The memory tasks often ask the patient to remember several words and then repeat them at the end of the test. The praxis portion may have the patient to draw geometric shapes or the face of a clock. The language task may ask the patient to name common items or answer questions about a story. *The Mini Mental State Examination* (MMSE Folstein, Folstein, & McHugh, 1975) is probably the best known dementia screening test. *The Saint Louis University Mental Status Examination (SLUMS)* is another. Both tests are described later in this chapter, and a copy of the SLUMS can be found in Chapter 12.

Diagnosing Dementia

Dementia screening tests never should be used to make the diagnosis of dementia. They are designed only to indicate whether further testing is needed. If a patient does not pass a test like the MMSE or SLUMS, it does not mean he or she has dementia. That must be determined by a much more detailed evaluation that can involve psychologists, physicians, social workers, nurses, and other related professionals. It is a team effort, as can be seen in the following description of a full diagnostic evaluation for dementia:

1. **An interview with the patient** is often the place to start the full diagnostic process. This interview examines the patient's perceptions of the deficits, behavior problems, onset of memory problems, safety concerns, and current level of ability. Note: All information obtained in this interview should be confirmed with family members.

2. **An interview with the family** (without the patient present) to explore their perceptions of the patient's abilities and the degree of caregiver strain that may be present.

3. **A review of past medical history** to look for risk factors (e.g., prior head injuries, level of education, presence of vascular disease).

4. **A geriatric review** that examines driving skills, continence, balance and mobility, and vision and hearing.

5. **Review of medications** to determine if the behaviors of concern may be caused or aggravated by current prescription or over-the-counter medications.

6. **Advance healthcare directives** to determine the patient's end-of-life wishes and to identify a surrogate to make medical decisions.

7. **A full medical evaluation** that includes both a physical examination (e.g., blood pressure, respiration) and a neurologic examination (e.g., reflexes, muscle tone, cranial nerve function).

8. **Functional status evaluation** to assess the patient's independence in self-care tasks and other activities of daily living.

9. **A cognitive mental status examination** that goes beyond the tasks found in the MMSE and other screening tests.

10. **Evaluate the patient for depression** or other reversible, treatable conditions that sometimes can be incorrectly diagnosed as dementia.

11. **Conduct laboratory tests** to evaluate glucose, serum electrolytes, and drug levels. This may determine whether the suspected dementia is reversible.

When these interviews, evaluations, and tests are complete and the results collected, the diagnosis of dementia can be made, usually by a physician or cognitive neuropsychologist specializing in dementia. Diagnostic evaluations such as this have been shown to be 90% accurate for identifying AD. After the dementia diagnosis is made, the patient and family can move into the management and family support phase of the process, which once again can involve numerous medical professionals working as a team.

Screening and Diagnostic Tests for Dementia

Given the large number of screening and diagnostic tests available for assessing dementia, it is not surprising to find different approaches to evaluating this disorder. Some tests are designed as research-based analytical tools, and others take a more patient-centered approach to evaluating the presence and severity of dementia. Mohs (1995) described the necessary characteristics of dementia tests when they are used during clinical trials of treating AD. Although treatment of dementia is beyond the scope of this book, Mohs criteria are useful for evaluating the appropriateness of performance-based cognitive tests for both screening and diagnosis:

- The test should provide consistent results even when conducted by different examiners (i.e., have high inter-rater reliability).

- The test should provide consistent results each time it is given to a particular patient (i.e., have high test-retest reliability). To facilitate repeated testing, dementia tests also should provide a number of different but equivalent forms. In clinical use, repeated testing might be necessary in situations where a patient's cognitive status needs to regularly monitored or where a cognitive decline must be documented.

- The test should be short enough to complete in one hour or less.

- The test should examine all of the clinically important symptoms that are relevant to dementia.

- The test should be able to assess patients with a range of dementia severity because not all individuals are referred during the early stages of the disorder.

- The test should be able to assess the changes in symptom severity that will occur as the dementia progress.

Screening Tests and Dementia Batteries

The following paragraphs briefly describe some of better known tests used to evaluate the cognitive abilities in patients suspected of having dementia (Mohs, 1995). Both screening tests and diagnostic batteries are examined. Although certainly not a complete listing, it is a representative sample of the types of instruments available. A listing of additional tests can be found in Table 11–1.

- *The Mini Mental State Exam (MMSE).* Before the copyright status of this test was enforced by its publisher, the MMSE was the most commonly used dementia screening instrument. The subsequent development of copyright-free alternative screening tests has reduced its usage in both clinical and research settings. Nevertheless, it remains a widely used screening tool. The MMSE contains 11 items that assess orientation, language, praxis, and memory. The total score ranges from 0 to 30. It is a quick assessment tool, and its extensive use for many years has provided much data for research. Mohs (1995) described several drawbacks of the MMSE, mentioning that it is not very sensitive because it is so brief and that alternative forms are not available.

- *The Saint Louis University Mental Status Examination (SLUMS).* The SLUMS was created by John Morley at Saint Louis University's division of geriatric medicine. It is one of the copyright-free screening alternatives to the MMSE. The SLUMS has many of the same advantages and drawbacks of the MMSE. It is brief, taking only about 7 minutes to administer. It contains 12 items; the total score ranges from 0 to 30. Its scoring is adjusted for the patient's educational level. Like the MMSE, there are no alternative forms for the SLUMS. It has been shown to be more sensitive at detecting mild dementia than the MMSE (Tariq, Tumosa, Chibnall, Perry, & Moore, 2006). The SLUMS is provided in the dementia protocols (Chapter 12).

- *The Informant Questionnaire on Cognitive Decline in the Elderly (IQCODE).* The IQCODE is a copyright-free screening test for dementia, originally developed by

Table 11–1. Selected Tests for Assessing Dementia

Test	Purpose
Activities of Daily Living Questionnaire (ADLQ) (M. Johnson, et al.)	A questionnaire-based assessment of activities of daily living.
Benton Revised Visual Retention Test (A. L. Benton)	A visual memory test.
The Blessed Dementia Scale (G. Blessed, et al.)	Information from family and friends is used to assess a patient's self-care abilities.
Brief Cognitive Rating Scale (B. Reisberg)	A rating scale to assess cognitive decline; can be used for conditions other than dementia.
Clinical Dementia Rating Scale (C. P. Hughes, et al.)	A 5-point rating scale to judge cognitive abilities.
Dementia Deficits Scale (DDS) (A. Snow, et al.)	An assessment of the patient's awareness of unsafe or dangerous behaviors.
Discourse Abilities Profile (B. Terrel & D. Ripich)	An assessment of the patient's conversational skills with family members and care givers.
Global Deterioration Scale (B. Reisberg, et al.)	A 7-point rating scale for assessing dementia.
Memory Assessment Scales (J. M. Williams)	A more detailed assessment of memory skills compared to the typical dementia scales.
The Progressive Deterioration Scale (PDS) (R. Dejong, et al.)	An assessment of declining cognitive abilities over time.
Wechsler Memory Scale—Revised (E. W. Russell)	A detailed test of many types of memory including visual and auditory tasks.

Jorm and Jacomb (1989). Unlike the other assessments discussed in this section, it is not a cognitive performance test. As its name indicates, it is a questionnaire to be completed by a family member, friend, or caregiver who has known the patient for at least 10 years. It is the most widely used informant questionnaire in the dementia literature (Jorm, 2004). The IQCODE has been shown to be a reliable measure of cognitive decline, and its administration time is brief. When screening patients for dementia, comparing scores from the IQCODE with those from a cognitive performance test (e.g., MMSE or SLUMS) can improve the accuracy of the assessment. A copy of the short version of the IQCODE is provided in the dementia protocols (Chapter 12).

- *Blessed Test of Information, Memory, and Concentration* (BMIC; Blessed, Tomlinson, & Roth, 1968). The BMIC is a brief screening tool that examines memory and orientation. A 27-item version of the test is commonly used in the United States. The total score ranges from 0 to 33. As with the MMSE, its wide use has provided a valuable collection of longitudinal data. The BMIC's primary drawbacks are that it does not assess all cognitive skills associated with dementia, and alternative forms are not available.

- *Syndrome Kurtztest* (SKT; Erzigkeit, 1989). The SKT is a brief screening test with nine subtests that assess visuospatial skills, naming, attention, and memory. Patients are given 1 minute to complete each subtest. A unique aspect of the SKT is its examination of attention. As with many of the dementia screening tests, its brevity makes it insensitive to some of the more subtle cognitive deficits seen in early dementia.

- *Alzheimer's Disease Assessment Scale* (ADAS; Rosen, Mohs, & Davis, 1984). This assessment examines many of the cognitive and psychiatric impairments associated with dementia. The cognitive subtests evaluate orientation, memory, praxis, and language; the psychiatric subtests address depression, anxiety, and psychosis. The cognitive scores range from 0 to 70. Its more detailed assessment of cognitive deficits makes it an attractive tool, although it can take nearly an hour to administer. This test does provide alternative forms to enhance test-retest reliability. The ADAS is widely used in clinical trials in the United States and Europe.

- *Mattis Dementia Rating Scale* (MDRS; Coblentz, Mattis, Zingesser, Kasoff, Wisniewski, & Katzman, 1973). The MDRS is a detailed test that examines memory, initiation, attention, visuospatial construction, and conceptualization. Total scores range from 0 to 144, with a score of 144 indicating severe impairment. The administration time varies because not all items in a subtest are administered if a patient fails the beginning items. A benefit of the MDRS is its wide-ranging assessment of cognitive skills. Mohs (1995) noted that the test's attention subtest is a major strength. It does not include alternative forms.

- *Neuropsychological Battery of the Consortium to Establish a Registry for Alzheimer's Disease* (CERAD; Heyman, Fillenbaum, & Mirra, 1991). The CERAD is an in-depth battery for assessing Alzheimer's disease. It includes seven subtests, some of which were adapted from other assessment tools, such as the ADAS. This test assesses memory, language, praxis, and orientation. Its detailed subtests allow for the evaluation of patients with varied levels of severity. The CERAD does not provide alternative forms.

- *Arizona Battery for Communication Disorders of Dementia* (ABCD; Bayles & Tomoeda, 1993). The ABCD standardized, norm-referenced test that examines the communication abilities of patients with AD. It does not assess all of the cognitive skills (e.g., praxis) usually found in dementia assessments, although orientation and memory tasks are included. It has 4 screening tasks and 14 subtests (e.g., story retelling, naming, object description, etc.). The administration time is between 45 and 90 minutes. Because of this, the test may be administered over several separate sessions.

- *Wechsler Adult Intelligence Scale* (WAIS; Wechsler, 1958). The WAIS is a widely used assessment of general intelligence. It has subtests that evaluate both verbal and nonverbal cognitive skills. However, it is not a recommended test for assessing dementia. It does not examine memory, nor is it appropriate for dementia patients of varied severity. The WAIS does not provide alternate forms.

Assessment of Dementia in Ethnoculturally Diverse Adults

When assessing ethnoculturally diverse patients, clinicians should consider how the patient and family view dementia. Understanding the patient's cultural and language background will help make the assessment valid. Here are some of the factors to consider when assessing individuals from diverse backgrounds:

- **Determine the patient's language**—This is the language the patient will be using during most of the interview and testing. The preferred language should be known to the examiner before the assessment begins. If the examiner is not proficient in the patient's preferred language, decide if an interpreter is going to be needed.

- **Address the patient correctly**—In general, the simple use of *Mister* or *Misses* is adequate for most individuals being assessed for dementia. The correct pronunciation and word order of the name should be determined early in the initial interview. It may be especially important to know if the patient prefers the use of professional titles, such as *Dr. Smith*, when he or she is being assessed for a disorder like dementia.

- **Level of education**—The education level of a patient should be determined before the assessment. It can have a significant effect on his or her ability to validly complete certain cognitive screening tests, such as the *Mini Mental State Examination*. Some tests, such as *The Saint Louis University Mental Status Examination*, modify cutoff scores for individuals with lower educational levels.

- **Determine the patient's English proficiency**—Patients may initially state that English is their preferred language, but occasionally they will overestimate their ability to speak English well enough to complete a cognitive assessment. Examiners must be aware of this possibility and modify or stop the assessment when it appears that the results will be invalid if the testing continues in English.

- **Religion**—It sometimes can be valuable to determine the patient's religion during dementia assessment. Knowing the religion can provide insight into how a patient and family may react to a diagnosis of dementia. It also can give guidance into how to conduct postassessment counseling.

- **Ethnic background**—This information can reveal the ways in which the patient interacts and communicates. It can give the examiner insight into language, values, history, and thoughts about illness. In other words, it gives a full view of the patient and family.

- **Country of birth**—This may provide information that can help determine the patient's cultural background.

- **Income**—Information about income is relevant to all patients seen for an assessment of any illness, including dementia. Knowing this information can guide the examiner during postassessment counseling in making recommendations for further assessment.

- **Family values and customs**—When decisions about illness and healthcare need to be made, families of different backgrounds may come to those decisions in a variety of ways. The decision may be based on the agreement of the whole immediate family, or it may be determined by only the eldest son. Understanding this gives the examiner valuable information for post-assessment counseling, such as ensuring that the person(s) making decisions are fully informed about the findings of the assessment.

- **Extended relationships**—It is valuable to know the kinds of extended relationships the patient has with family, friends, and religious leaders. Knowing their attitudes about caring for an infirm older person can guide recommendations for long-term care.

Choosing Assessment Tools for Patients from Diverse Backgrounds

Most cognitive assessments of dementia were created with the assumption that they would be administered to educated, English-speaking patients. A good example of this is the Mini Mental State Examination (MMSE). Originally created for an English-speaking population, the MMSE has been translated into scores of languages ranging from Afrikaans to Urdu. Unfortunately, there are certain words and concepts on the MMSE (and on similar tests) that do not translate well into other languages. Research has suggested that MMSE results are influenced by the patient's age, education, language, ethnicity, and socioeconomic background. For example, Storey, Rowland, Basic, and Conforti (2002) found that the frequently used clock drawing task was not a useful predictor of dementia in a multicultural, non-English-speaking-background population. Similarly, Escobar et al. (1986) reported that after culturally biased words were omitted from the MMSE, the number of multicultural patients scoring in the severe range dropped significantly. Findings of content bias in the MMSE were found by Scazufca, Almeida, Vallada, Tasse, and Menezes (2008), who reported that the test gave many false positive instances of dementia in illiterate Brazilian adults over the age of 65. Although they did find that the MMSE accurately screened those individuals with "minimal literacy" abilities, the authors recommended an MMSE cutoff score of 14 or 15 for individuals with no education and a cutoff score of 17 or 18 for those with less than a year of education.

Clinicians with concern about the possible cultural bias of dementia screening tools may want to consider using such tests as the *Mini-Cog* (Borson, et al., 2000) or the *Rowland Universal Dementia Assessment Scale* (RUDAS; Storey, Rowland, Basic, Conforti, & Dickson, 2004). Both of these screening tools seem to be more "culture neutral" than the MMSE. The RUDAS addresses similar cognitive domains as the MMSE and has been shown to be equally effective in screening for dementia (Rowland, Basic, Storey, & Conforti, 2006). It was designed specifically to be valid across cultures, gender, and educational levels. In addition, the words in the test were selected for their ease of accurate translation. The RUDAS can be downloaded for free from these websites: http://www.health.qld.gov.au/northside/documents/rudas2.pdf and http://www.alzheimers.org.au/content.cfm?infopageid=3955 .

Diagnostic Criteria and Differential Diagnosis

As mentioned at the beginning of this chapter, the *Diagnostic and Statistical Manual of Mental Diseases* (DSM-IV) (American Psychiatric Association, 1994) and its 2000 text revision (American Psychiatric Association, 2000) describes dementia as an impairment in memory plus at least *one* of the following: aphasia (language disturbances), apraxia, agnosia, or impaired executive functions (e.g., abstract thinking and planning). This criterion most easily fits the profile of patients with AD, and it may facilitate an accurate diagnosis of that condition. However, it often is not much help when attempting to diagnose other types of dementia because some dementing illnesses do not have prominent memory deficits as an early symptom. Moreover, this definition does little to help in the differential diagnosis between dementia and related cognitive disorders that share many symptoms with dementia. There are several reasons why an accurate and early differential diagnosis is so important:

- Pharmacological treatment of AD is most effective when it is started early in the progression of the disease and when the symptoms are mild.

- In vascular dementia, early treatment of the hypertension, strokes, and artery disease associated with this condition may affect its progression.

- Early identification and treatment of reversible dementia may facilitate a quicker recovery of intellectual abilities and minimize long-term complications.

- Treatments of nondementing cognitive and psychiatric conditions that share symptoms with dementia often are more effective when they are diagnosed early.

Because the differential diagnosis of dementia often is difficult, various agencies and publications have offered guidance for medical professionals in making a final diagnosis. Figure 11–1 is a diagnostic flow chart created by the Agency for Health Care Policy Research (Costa, Williams, Somerfeld, et al., 1996) to aid in the diagnosis of dementia and related conditions. It begins with a patient demonstrating symptoms that may indicate dementia. The second step is conducting a full clinical assessment, very much like that described earlier in this chapter. After the clinical assessment is complete, the decision process begins. To facilitate this decision-making process, Geldmacher (2004) described the distinguishing characteristics of disorders that are often confused with dementia, as well as for the best-known dementing illnesses:

- *Dementia vs. delirium*—Delirium nearly always has an acute onset, is reversible, and presents itself as a fluctuating mental status. Most instances of delirium are the result of two or more abnormal toxic-metabolic factors, such as acidosis, drug intoxication, or sepsis. Delirium may be confused with dementia because patients with dementia may have delirium as a secondary symptom.

- *Dementia vs. depression*—Depression can be distinguished from dementia in several ways. In depression, it usually is the patient who seeks treatment; in dementia, it usually is the family who first makes contact with medical professionals. Depression typically has a more sudden onset than in dementia. A prior history of depression enhances the likelihood of depression being responsible for any current cognitive difficulties, and first-time occurrences of unexplained depression over the age of 60 are rare. It is unusual for depression to cause focal deficits such as apraxia, which are not uncommon in dementia.

- *Dementia vs. thyroid dysfunction*—Severe hypothyroidism can result in lethargy, depression, and a generalized slowness, which are similar to symptoms in

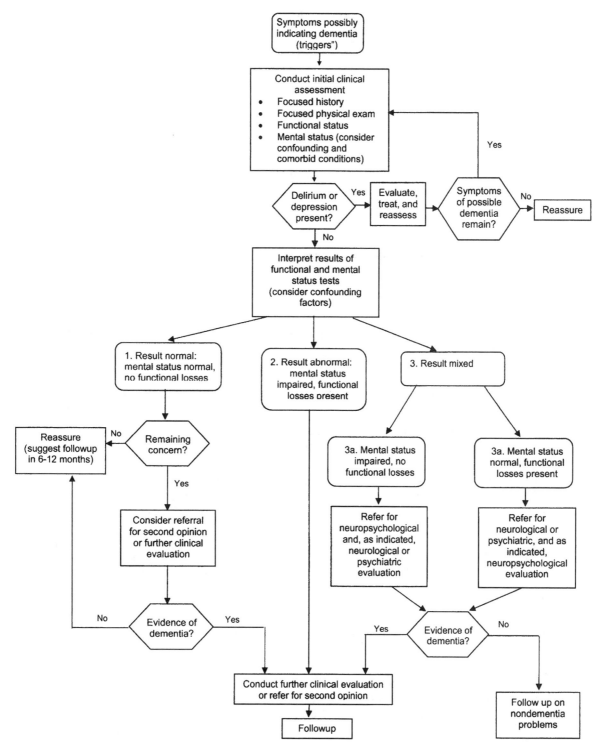

Figure 11–1. A diagnostic flow chart for the assessment of dementia created by the Agency for Health Care Policy Research (in the public domain).

dementia. However, the co-occurrence of the physical signs of hypothyroidism (fatigue, weight gain, dry hair, hair loss, weakness) typically ensures the correct diagnosis.

- *Dementia vs. alcohol abuse*—Memory deficits associated with Korsokoff's syndrome and Wenicke's encephalitis may superficially resemble the cognitive behaviors of some individuals with dementia. However, these alcohol-based problems are the result of nutritional deficiencies and are treatable though proper diet and supplements.

- *Dementia vs. B12 deficiency*—Significant deficiencies of this vitamin can cause a collection of symptoms similar to those in dementia, such as anxiety and forgetfulness. Psychosis has been reported in extreme cases. When cognitive or psychiatric features are present, concurrent neurologic complaints of tingling and numbness in the arms and legs almost always are present, which helps distinguish it from dementia.

- *Dementia vs. infection*—A number of infections of the brain may be confused with dementia. For example, the herpes simplex virus may damage areas of the brain linked to memory, but making the correct diagnosis usually is not a problem because co-occurring physical symptoms and the rapid, short-term progression of the condition easily distinguish it from dementia. Fungal and parasitic infections also may lead to dementia-like symptoms, but they usually can be recognized by CAT or MRI imaging.

- *Alzheimer's disease*—The central clinical aspects of mild AD that can help distinguish it from other dementing conditions include (a) insidious onset, (b) slowly progressive course, (c) compromised orientation, learning, and recent memory, (d) empty speech, word-finding difficulties, (e) apathy, (f) little self-awareness, and (g) emotional withdrawal.

- *Frontotemporal dementia*—The clinical characteristics of early frontotemporal dementia that can help distinguish it from other dementing conditions include (a) early appearance of behavioral changes and poor social judgment, (b) disordered executive function, (c) perseverative behaviors, (e) denial of illness, lack of awareness, (f) performance on cognitive screenings may be normal, and (g) periods of apathy are mixed with instances of disinhibited behavior.

- *Lewy body dementia*—Factors that can be distinguish mild Lewy body dementia from other dementias include (a) a progressive course with early appearance of sleep disturbances, (b) early development of visuospatial problems, (c) visual hallucinations, (d) impaired executive function, and (e) limb rigidity, masked faces, bradykinesia.

- *Vascular dementia*—This dementia can be differentiated from other types of dementia by (a) a gradual or abrupt onset, (b) variable progression that is often linked to episodes of vascular accidents, (c) presence of hypertension, heart disease, peripheral vascular disease, (d) specific cognitive impairments that often are associated with sites of vascular lesions, (e) awareness of deficits, (f) incontinence, (g) impaired executive function, and (h) focal neurological signs such as hemiparesis.

- *Creutzfeldt-Jakob disease*—The specific characteristics of this disease that distinguish it from other dementing conditions include (a) a rapid progression, changing weekly or monthly, (b) development of myoclonus, (c) distinctive electroencephalography patterns, (d) visual disturbances, blindness (e) decline in behavior and intellect is rapid, and (f) reduced affect.

Postassessment Counseling

The clinician concludes the assessment session with postassessment counseling, where the assessment results are shared with the patient, accompanying family members, and other caregivers. Subsequent to the postassessment counseling, the clinician makes an analysis of information obtained from the case history and interview, reports from other specialists, clinical assessment results, instrumental evaluations, and results of questionnaires or other tests. Integrating the information collected from all sources and means, the clinician writes a diagnostic report. See Chapter 1, "Assessment of Adults: An Overview," for details on the analysis and integration of assessment data and clinical report writing.

During the postassessment counseling of dementia screening, the clinician primarily offers recommendations. The clinician also takes time to answer questions from the client and the family members about the disorder and the recommendations.

Make Recommendations

The clinician cannot make a diagnosis of dementia from the assessment protocols offered in this book. The protocols are screening tools that only suggest whether further assessment is necessary. If the results of the screening indicate that further assessment is warranted, the clinician should carefully and sensitively describe the results of the test to the patient, stressing the preliminary nature of the findings. Because it would be inappropriate to make a prognosis or discuss treatment or long-term care, the remainder of the postassessment counseling session should be spent answering any general questions about dementia that the patient may have. A referral to a physician for a full assessment is the primary recommendation that should be made during this session.

If the screening does not indicate that additional testing is needed (i.e., the patient passes the test), the clinician will want to discuss the results with the patient and family with the same sensitivity as when the test is failed. Although the patient and family may be encouraged by this news, the behaviors that originally concerned them probably still will be an issue. The troubling episodes of forgetfulness or other actions will need to be explored and addressed. A passing score on the screening examination may nudge the family into reassessing the potential causes of these behaviors. Could depression, nutrition, illness, or other factors be the cause? Again, a recommendation to a physician for an evaluation of the patient's physical, neurological, or psychiatric status might be appropriate. Sometimes, when the screening results are negative and the patient and family feel that there is no need to see a physician, it might be appropriate to recommend readministering the screening test every six months to monitor the patient's cognitive abilities on a regular basis. If changes are noted during follow-up sessions, then the recommendation for a physician referral can be made again.

Finally, clinicians should remember that some individuals with frontotemporal dementia can pass or obtain a borderline score on a cognitive screening test during the early stages of their illness. If such a patient passes the screening but demonstrates the personality changes and uninhibited behaviors associated with this dementia, a referral to a physician should be the recommendation.

References

American Psychiatric Association. (2000). *Diagnostic and statistical manual of mental disorders-text revision* (4th ed.). Washington, DC: Author.

American Psychiatric Association. (1994). *Diagnostic and statistical manual of mental disorders* (4th ed.). Washington, DC: Author.

Bayles, K., & Tomoeda, C. (1993). Arizona Battery for Communication Disorders of Dementia. Austin, TX: Pro-Ed.

Blessed, G., Tomlinson, B. E., & Roth, M. (1968). The association between quantitative measures of dementia and of senile change in the cerebral grey matter of elderly subjects. *British Journal of Psychiatry, 114,* 797–811.

Borson, S., Scanlan, J., Brush, M., Vitaliano, P., & Dokmak, A. (2000). The Mini-Cog: A cognitive "vital signs" measure for dementia screening in multilingual elderly. *International Journal of Geriatric Psychiatry, 15*(11), 1021–1027.

Coblentz, J. M., Mattis, S., Zingesser, L.H., Kasoff, S. S., Wisniewski, H. M., & Katzman, R. (1973). Presenile dementia: clinical aspects and evaluation of cerebrospinal fluid dynamics. *Archives of Neurology, 29,* 299–308.

Costa, P. T., Williams, T. F., Somerfeld, M., et al. (1996). Early identification of Alzheimer's disease and related dementias. *Clinical practice guideline, quick reference guide for clinicians, no. 19.* Rockville, MD: U.S. Department of Health and Human Services, Public Health Service, Agency for Health Care Policy Research AHCPR Publication No. 97-0703.

Cummings, J., & Benson, F. (1992). *Dementia: A clinical approach.* Boston: Butterworth Heinemann.

Cummings, J. L., & Bensen, D. F. (1983). *Dementia: A clinical approach.* Boston, MA: Butterworth.

DeJong, R., Osterlund, O. W., & Roy, G. W. (1989). Measurement of quality-of-life changes in patients with Alzheimer's disease. *Clinical Therapeutics, 11,* 545–554.

Duffy, J. R. (2005). *Motor speech disorders: Substrates, differential diagnosis, and management* (2nd ed.). St. Louis, MO: Elsevier Mosby.

Erzigkeit, H. (1989). The SKT—a short cognitive performance test as an instrument for the assessment of clinical efficacy of cognitive enhancers. In W. Bergner, B. Reisberg (Eds.), *Diagnosis and treatment of senile dementia* (pp. 164–174). Heidelberg, Germany: Springer.

Escobar, J., Burnam, A., Karno, M., Forsythe, A., Landsverk, J., & Golding, J. M. (1986). Use of the Mini-Mental State Examination (MMSE) in a community population of mixed ethnicity: Cultural and linguistic artifacts. *Journal of Nervous and Mental Disease, 174,* 607–614.

Folstein, M. F., Folstein, S. E., & McHugh, P. R. (1975). "Mini-Mental-State." A practical method for grading the cognitive state of patients for the clinician. *Journal of Psychiatric Research, 12,* 189–198.

Freter, S., Bergman, H., Gold, S., Chertkow, H., & Clarfield, A. M. (1998). Prevalence of potentially reversible dementias and actual reversibility in a memory clinic cohort. *Canadian Medical Association Journal, 159*(6), 657–662.

Geldmacher, D. D. (2004). Differential diagnosis of dementia syndromes. *Clinical Geriatric Medicine, 20,* 27–43.

Heyman, A., Fillenbaum, G., & Mirra, S. S. (1991). CERAD: Clinical, neuropsychological, and neuropathological components. *Aging: Clinical and Experimental Research, 2,* 416–424.

Hughes, C. P., Berg, L., Danziger, W. L., Coben, L. A., & Martin, R. L. (1982). A new clinical scale for the staging of dementia. *British Journal of Psychiatry, 140,* 566–572.

Jorm, A. F. (2004). The Informant Questionnaire on Cognitive Decline in the Elderly (IQCODE): A review. *International Psychogeriatrics, 16*(3), 1–19.

Jorm, A. F., & Jacomb, P. A. (1989). The Informant Questionnaire on Cognitive Decline in the Elderly (IQCODE): Socio-demographic correlates, reliability, validity and some norms. *Psychological Medicine, 19,* 1015–1022.

Jorm, A. E., Korten, A. F., & Henderson, A. S. (1987).The prevalence of dementia: A quantitative integration of the literature. *Acta Psychiatrica Scandinavica, 76*(5), 465–479

Mohs, R. (1995). Neuropsychological assessment of patients with Alzheimer's disease. In F. E. Bloom & D. J. Kupfer (Eds.), *Psychopharmacology—4th Generation of Progress* (pp. 234–276). New York, NY: Raven Press.

Payne, J. C. (1997). *Adult neurogenic language disorders: Assessment and treatment.* San Diego, CA: Singular.

Reisberg, B., Ferris, S., De Leon, M., & Crook, T. (1982). The Global Deterioration Scale for assessment of primary degenerative dementia. *American Journal of Psychiatry, 139,* 1136–1139.

Rosen, W. G., Mohs, R. C., & Davis, K. L. (1984). A new rating scale for Alzheimer's disease. *American Journal of Psychiatry, 141,* 1356–1364.

Rowland, J. T. J., Basic, D., Storey, J. E., & Conforti, D. A. (2006). The Rowland Universal Dementia Assessment Scale (RUDAS) and the Folstein MMSE in a multicultural cohort of elderly persons. *International Psychogeriatrics, 18,* 111–120.

Russell, E. W. (1975). A multiple scoring method for assessment of complex memory functions. *Journal of Consulting and Clinical Psychology, 43,* 800–809.

Scazufca, M., Almeida, O. P., Vallada, H. P., Tasse, W. A., & Menezes, P. R. (2009). Limitations of the Mini-Mental State Examination for screening dementia in a community with low socioeconomic status. *European Archives of Psychiatry and Clinical Neuroscience, 259,* 8–15.

Snow, A., Norris, M., Doody, R., Molinari, V., Orengo, C., & Kunik, M. (2004). Dementia Deficits Scale: Rating self-awareness of deficits. *Alzheimer Disease and Associated Disorders, 18*(1), 22–31.

Storey, J. E., Rowland, J. T. J., Basic, D., & Conforti, D. A. (2002). Accuracy of the clock drawing test for detecting dementia in a multicultural sample of elderly Australian patients. *International Psychogeriatrics, 14*(3), 259–271.

Storey, J. E., Rowland, J. T. J., Basic, D., Conforti, D. A., & Dickson, H. G. (2004). The Rowland Universal Dementia Assessment Scale (RUDAS): a multicultural cognitive assessment scale. *International Psychogeriatrics, 16,* 13–31.

Tariq, S. H., Tumosa, N., Chibnall, J. T., Perry, M. H., & Morley, J. E. (2006). Comparison of the Saint Louis University mental status examination and the mini-mental state examination for detecting dementia and mild neurocognitive disorder–a pilot study. *American Journal of Geriatric Psychiatry, 14*(11), 897–899.

Terrell, B. & Ripich, D. (1989). Discourse competence as a variable in intervention. In J. Wilcox (Ed.) *Seminars in Speech and Language: Aphasia, 10*(4), 282–297.

Wechsler, D. (1958). *The measurement and appraisal of adult intelligence* (4th ed.). Baltimore, MD: Williams & Wilkins.

Weytingh, M. D., Bossuyt, P. M., & van Crevel, H. (1995). Reversible dementia: More than 10% or less than 1%? A qualitative review. *Journal of Neurology, 242*(7), 466–471.

Williams, J. M. (1991). *Memory assessment scales.* Odessa, FL: Psychological Assessment Resources.

CHAPTER 12

Assessment of Dementia: Protocols

- Overview of Dementia Protocols
- Assessment of Dementia: Interview Protocol
- Dementia Screening Protocol 1
- Dementia Screening Protocol 2
- Dementia Assessment Protocol 1: Mental Status and Intellectual Functioning
- Dementia Assessment Protocol 2: Communication Abilities
- Dementia Assessment Protocol 3: General Behavioral Evaluation

Overview of Dementia Protocols

Assessment protocols provided in this chapter help assess dementia in adults in an efficient manner. The protocols offer ready-made formats that clinicians can use in structuring their client and family interviews and assessing various parameters of dementia and its disorders.

The protocols offered in this chapter also are available on the accompanying CD. The clinician may print the needed protocols in evaluating his or her clients. The clinician may combine these protocols in suitable ways to facilitate the evaluation of adults with dementia.

In assessing adults with multiple disorders, the clinician may combine these protocols with protocols from other chapters. For example, the clinician may combine the dementia assessment protocols with dysarthria assessment protocols (Chapter 6) or aphasia assessment protocols (Chapter 8).

The protocols given in this chapter are specific to dementia in adults. To complete the assessment on a given client, the clinician should combine these disorder-specific protocols with the common assessment protocols given in Chapter 2:

- The Adult Case History
- Orofacial Examination and Hearing Screening Protocol
- Diadochokinetic Assessment Protocol for Adults
- Adult Assessment Report Outline

Assessment of Dementia: Interview Protocol

Name _____ DOB _____ Date _____ Clinician _____

Individualize this protocol on the CD and print it for your use. 💿

Preparation

- Review the guidelines given under The Initial Clinical Interview in Chapter 1.
- Arrange for comfortable seating and lighting.
- Record the interview on audio or video.
- Initially interview the client alone and then have the accompanying person join the interview.
- Review the case history ahead of time and take note of areas you want to explore during the interview.

Introduction

☐ Introduce yourself. Describe the assessment plan and tell the client the time it will take.

Example: "Hello Mr./Mrs. [*client's name*]. My name is [*your name*] I am the speech-language pathologist who will be assessing you today. I would like to start by reviewing the case history and asking you a few questions. After we finish talking, I will work with you. Today's assessment should take about [*estimate the amount of time you plan to spend*]."

Interview Questions

The questions are generally directed toward the adult client with suspected dementia. When interviewing the client and the accompanying person together, it is essential to pose the same, but reworded, question to the accompanying person. A few examples are shown within the brackets; the clinician may use this strategy whenever necessary.

- What is your main concern regarding your memory? [What do you think is his (her) main problem?]
- How would you describe your memory problem? [How would you describe her (his) memory problem?]
- When did you first notice that your memory was different? [When did you notice that his (her) memory was different?]
- Has your memory changed over time? If so, how?
- Have you seen your family doctor about your memory?

(continues)

Assessment of Dementia: Interview Protocol (continued)

- Did your family doctor refer you to a specialist?

- What did the doctor(s) tell you?

- Besides a memory problem, are you concerned with any aspects of your speech? [Have you noticed any changes in behavior or personality recently?]

- How would you describe these speech problems? [How would you describe his (her) overall speech?]

- Are there times when your memory is better or worse? For example, is it better in the morning than in the evening? [Do you also think her (his) memory varies throughout the day?]

- Do you believe that your memory problem is affecting your social interactions? Would you describe how?

- Do you think that your memory problem is affecting your job performance? How is it affected?

- Has anyone else in your family ever experienced memory problems?

- Do you have any other chronic health conditions or concerns?

- Are you currently on any medications?

- It looks like I have most of the information I wanted from you. Do you have any questions for me at this point?

- Thank you for your information. It will be helpful in my assessment. I will now work with you to better understand your memory problem. When we are done, we will discuss our findings.

Review the case history again and ask additional questions if needed.

Dementia Screening Protocol 1: Saint Louis University Mental Status (SLUMS) Examination

Name _____ DOB _____ Date _____ Clinician _____

Individualize this protocol on the CD and print it for your use. 💿

This mental status screening examination was created by John Morley at Saint Louis University School of Medicine. It has been shown to be more sensitive than the Mini Mental Status Examination in detecting mild cognitive impairments (Tariq, Tumosa, Chibnail, Perry, & Morley, 2006). It is a copyright-free assessment tool.

1. What day of the week is it? (1 point for the right answer)

2. What is the year? (1 point)

3. What state are we in? (1 point)

4. Please remember these five objects. I will ask you what they are later: apple, pen, tie, house, car. (No points yet)

5. You have $100 and you go to the store and buy a dozen apples for $3 and a tricycle for $20.
   ○ How much did you spend? (1 point)

   ○ How much do you have left? (2 points)

6. Please name as many animals as you can in one minute. (No point for naming 0–4; 1 point for naming 5–9; 2 points for naming 10–14; and 3 points for naming 15 or more.)

7. What were the five objects I asked you to remember? (1 point for each object remembered.)

(continues)

Dementia Screening Protocol 1: SLUMS Examination (continued)

8. I am going to say a series of numbers and I would like you to give them to me backwards. For example, if I say 42, you would say 24.

   o   87 (0 points)

   o   649 (1 point)

   o   8537 (1 point)

9. (Draw circle.) This circle represents a clock face. Please put in the hour markers and the time at ten minutes to eleven o'clock.

   o   (2 points for hour markers labeled correctly)

   o   (2 points for correct time)

10. (Show a triangle, a square, and a rectangle.) Please place an X in the triangle. (1 point)

11. (Show a triangle, a square, and a rectangle.) Which of those objects is the largest? (1 point)

12. I am going to tell you a story. Please listen carefully because afterward I'm going to ask you some questions about it.

    Jill was a very successful stockbroker. She made a lot of money in the stock market. She then met Jack, a devastatingly handsome man. She married him and had three children. They lived in Chicago. She then stopped working and stayed at home to bring up her children. When they were teenagers, she went back to work. She and Jack lived happily ever after.

o   What was the female's name? (2 points)

o   When did she go back to work? (2 points)

o   What work did she do? (2 points)

o   What state did she live in? (2 points)

SCORING: *High school education*: Normal: 27–30; Mild neurocognitive disorder: 21–26; Dementia: 1–20. *Less than high school education*: Normal: 25–30; Mild neurocognitive disorder: 20–24; Dementia: 1–19.

Dementia Screening Protocol 2: Short Form of the Informant Questionnaire on Cognitive Decline in the Elderly (Short IQCODE)

Name _____ DOB _____ Date _____ Clinician _____

Individualize this protocol on the CD and print it for your use.

IQCODE was developed by Jorm and Jacomb (1989) to measure cognitive decline via a respondent questionnaire. It evolved through a number of versions since its first publication, but the administration procedure has remained essentially the same. A relative or close friend is asked to answer a series of questions about the client's cognitive abilities over a 10-year period. Presented here is the short version of the IQCODE, which has been shown to be as accurate as the long version of the test for most clients (Jorm, 2004). The IQCODE is copyright free.

Instructions

Now we want you to remember what your friend or relative was like 10 years ago and to compare it with what he or she is like now. Ten years ago was in 20__. Below are situations where this person has to use his or her memory or intelligence, and we want you to indicate whether this has improved, stayed the same, or become worse in that situation over the past 10 years. Note the importance of comparing his or her present performance *with 10 years ago*. So, if 10 years ago this person always forgot where he or she had left things, and he or she still does, then this would be considered "Hasn't changed much." Please indicate the changes you have observed by *circling the appropriate answer*.

Compared with 10 years ago how is this person at:

		1	2	3	4	5
1.	Remembering things about family and friends, e.g., occupations, birthdays, addresses	Much improved	A bit improved	Not much change	A bit worse	Much worse
2.	Remembering things that have happened recently	Much improved	A bit improved	Not much change	A bit worse	Much worse
3.	Recalling conversations a few days later	Much improved	A bit improved	Not much change	A bit worse	Much worse
4.	Remembering his/her address and telephone number	Much improved	A bit improved	Not much change	A bit worse	Much worse

		1	2	3	4	5
5.	Remembering what day and month it is	Much improved	A bit improved	Not much change	A bit worse	Much worse
6.	Remembering where things are usually kept	Much improved	A bit improved	Not much change	A bit worse	Much worse
7.	Remembering where to find things which have been put in a different place from usual	Much improved	A bit improved	Not much change	A bit worse	Much worse
8.	Knowing how to work familiar machines around the house	Much improved	A bit improved	Not much change	A bit worse	Much worse
9.	Learning to use a new gadget or machine around the house	Much improved	A bit improved	Not much change	A bit worse	Much worse
10.	Learning new things in general	Much improved	A bit improved	Not much change	A bit worse	Much worse
11.	Following a story in a book or on TV	Much improved	A bit improved	Not much change	A bit worse	Much worse
12.	Making decisions on everyday matters	Much improved	A bit improved	Not much change	A bit worse	Much worse
13.	Handling money for shopping	Much improved	A bit improved	Not much change	A bit worse	Much worse
14.	Handling financial matters, e.g., the pension, dealing with the bank	Much improved	A bit improved	Not much change	A bit worse	Much worse
15.	Handling other everyday arithmetic problems, e.g., knowing how much food to buy, knowing how long between visits from family or friends	Much improved	A bit improved	Not much change	A bit worse	Much worse
16.	Using his/her intelligence to understand what's going on and to reason things through	Much improved	A bit improved	Not much change	A bit worse	Much worse

(continues)

Dementia Screening Protocol 2: Short IQCODE (continued)

Scoring the Short IQCODE

Score the Short IQCODE by finding the average response score. This is done by adding the circled number scores in all the columns together and dividing that number by the number of items on the test (16). For example, if the caregiver circled 15 items in column number 3 and one in column 4, compute the final score like this: ($15 \times 3 + 4 = 49$), then divide by 16 ($49 / 16 = 3.06$ final score). Final scores can range from 1 to 5, although a significant majority of clients will be grouped somewhere near the middle of this range. For the Short IQCODE, a final score of 3.44 or higher suggests that dementia may be present and a referral for more testing is warranted (Jorm, 2004).

Dementia Assessment Protocol 1:
Mental Status and Intellectual Functioning

Name _____ DOB _____ Date _____ Clinician _____

Individualize this protocol on the CD and print it for your use. ☺

The following three dementia assessment protocols (Mental Status and Intellectual Functioning, Communication Evaluation, and General Behavioral Evaluation) are recommended when additional testing beyond the SLUMS and Short IQCODE is needed.

Ask the client each of the following questions. Score the responses as:

0 = *Incorrect*   1 = *Partially Correct*   2 = *Correct*

Discontinue the questioning in any section if the client appears to be anxious or frustrated with his or her performance. Describe the discontinuation in the "Clinician's summative statement" section at the end of protocol.

Orientation	Scoring
How old are you?	0 1 2
What year is this?	0 1 2
What month is this?	0 1 2
What day of the month is this?	0 1 2
What day of the week is this?	0 1 2
What is your birthday?	0 1 2
What city are we in right now?	0 1 2
What building are we in right now?	0 1 2
What time of day is it right now?	0 1 2
Short-Term Memory	
Repeat these numbers back to me: 7-2-9	0 1 2
Repeat these numbers back to me: 5-1-8-6	0 1 2
Repeat these numbers back to me: 4-9-2-6-8-3	0 1 2
Recent Memory	
What is my name?	0 1 2
What did you have for breakfast this morning?	0 1 2
Who is the president of the United States?	0 1 2

(continues)

Dementia Assessment Protocol 1: Mental Status and Intellectual Functioning (continued)

Recent Memory	Scoring
Who is the governor of this state?	0 1 2
What kind of shirt (blouse) did you wear yesterday?	0 1 2
Remote Memory	
Where did you go to high school?	0 1 2
What was the name of your high school?	0 1 2
Do you have brothers or sisters? What are their names?	0 1 2
What was the first car you owned?	0 1 2
How did you meet your wife (husband)?	0 1 2
Judgment	
What would you do if you found a lady's purse on the sidewalk?	0 1 2
What would you do if you had a flat tire while driving on a freeway?	0 1 2
What would you do if a fire alarm went off in your house late at night?	0 1 2
What would you do if a Girl Scout asked you to buy some cookies?	0 1 2
Attention	
I'm going to say a list of words. I want you to tap your hand on the table each time you hear the word "green."	
Water, sleep, many, green, look, raise	0 1 2
Open, market, baseball, face, candy, green	0 1 2
Fall, story, blue, point, green, snow	0 1 2
Rug, grass, record, purple, green, paper	0 1 2
Clinician's summative statement:	

Dementia Assessment Protocol 2: Communication Abilities

Client's Name _____ Age _____ DOB _____

Clinician _____ Date _____ Diagnosis _____

Assess Confrontation Naming

Ask questions after presenting a picture. Write down the incorrect responses; take note of the missing article. Score the self-corrections as:

No = *No attempt*   S = *Successful*   UnS = *Unsuccessful*

Clinician's questions	Correct Response	Incorrect	Self-Corrections
What is this?	"A dog"		No S UnS
What is this?	"A book"		
What is this?	"A pen"		
What is this?	"A house"		
What is this?	"A spoon"		
What is this?	"A tree"		
What is this?	"A glass"		

Assess Responsive Naming

Ask questions with no physical stimulus presentation. Write down the incorrect responses.

Clinician's questions	Correct Response	Incorrect Response
What do people wear to see better?	"Glasses"	
What is that you are sitting on?	"Chair"	
What do you use to unlock a door?	"Key"	
What do you use to cut vegetables?	"Knife"	
What do you do when you are sleepy?	"Sleep"	
What do you use to write?	"Pen"	
What do you want when you are thirsty?	"Water"	
What do you want when you are hungry?	"Food"	

(continues)

Dementia Assessment Protocol 2: Communication Abilities (continued)

Defining Words

Ask the client to define or describe the following words. Correct responses must contain complete sentences and include the underlined word or words in the correct response column. If a response is incorrect, write it in the incorrect response column.

Clinician's questions	Correct Response	Incorrect Response
What is a pencil?	"It's something to <u>write</u> with."	
What is a telephone?	"You <u>talk</u> to people on it."	
What is a key?	"It's used to <u>open</u> (or <u>unlock</u>) a door."	
What is a camera?	"You use it to <u>take pictures</u>."	
What is a cello?	"It's used to make <u>music</u>" or "It's a musical <u>instrument</u>."	
What is a sailboat?	"It's a boat that uses the <u>wind</u> to go."	
What is an umbrella?	"It's something to keep <u>rain</u> (or <u>water</u>) off of you."	
What is a triangle?	"It's a shape with <u>three sides</u> (or <u>three lines</u>)."	

Assess Categorical Naming (Word Fluency Test)

Give 1 minute for each category. Write down the responses or the number of responses given. Normative studies have shown that non-brain-damaged individuals generate an average of 17 animals in 1 minute. For words beginning with F, A, and S, they average approximately 37 total items (FAS scores combined) (Tombaugh, Kozak, & Rees, 1999).

Clinician's questions	Client's responses
"Tell me the names of all the animals you can think of."	
"I will say a letter of the alphabet. I want you to tell me all the words you can think of that start with that letter. Ready? Let's start with the letter 'F.'"	
"Now the letter 'A.'"	
"The last one is letter 'S.'"	

Reading for Comprehension (Single Sentences)

The clinician shows the client a sentence with the final word omitted; the client reads the sentence and chooses the correct final word in a field of three.

Sentences	A	B	C
Put the key in the _____.	cover	candy	door
I enjoyed reading the _____.	book	shoes	cotton
He plays music on his _____.	tooth	guitar	lamp
While sleeping, he often will _____.	run	snore	flower
The boy missed school because he was _____.	cable	picture	sick
The old movie was in black and _____.	purple	red	white
My doctor is a general _____.	practitioner	contractor	military
Why save money for a rainy _____?	morning	night	day
It is hard to learn a new _____.	language	day	friend
When I was gone, she cleaned the _____.	bathroom	event	better

Reading for Comprehension (Paragraph)

The client reads the following paragraph and then answers multiple choice questions about it. The client can respond either by verbally producing the answer or by pointing to it. Do not let the client see the paragraph while answering the questions.

A fox was taking her babies out for a walk one beautiful morning. As she came to a stream, the fox encountered a lioness with her cub. "Why such airs over one solitary cub?" sneered the fox, "Look at my healthy and numerous litter of five, and imagine, if you are able, how a proud mother should feel." The lioness gave her a squelching look, and lifting up her nose, walked away, saying calmly, "Yes, just look at that wonderful collection. What are they? Foxes! I've only one, but remember that one is a lion." Quality is better than quantity.

Clinician's questions	Choice A	Choice B	Choice C
What time of day were they out walking?	morning	afternoon	evening
Which animal had only one baby?	fox	lion	rabbit
The fox had how many babies?	three	four	five
What was the weather like in the story?	hot	cold	nice
Where did the fox encounter the lion?	on the grass	near the hill	at the stream

(continues)

Dementia Assessment Protocol 2: Communication Abilities (continued)

Writing the Names of Pictured Items

The clinician presents pictures of single objects or actions and asks the client to write the name of the pictured item. Use color photographs of common objects or activities as the stimuli.

Pictured Items	Correct	Incorrect
book		
bed		
shirt		
sleeping		
clock		
running		
lighthouse		
ironing board		
traffic sign		
watermelon		

Writing Sentences

The clinician asks the client to watch carefully as he or she performs an action. The client is asked to write a complete sentence that describes the action. A correct response contains correct spelling for all words and is a complete sentence (e.g., You snapped your fingers.).

Clinician's actions	Correct	Incorrect
Snap your fingers.		
Rub your chin.		
Knock once on the table.		
Clear your throat.		
Rub your hands together as if you were cold.		
Stretch your arms and yawn.		
Write something on a piece of paper.		
Stand up and sit down.		

Dementia Assessment Protocol 3: General Behavioral Evaluation

Name _____ DOB _____ Date _____ Clinician _____

Individualize this protocol on the CD and print it for your use. ⊙

Instructions: Please rate each item according to the rating scale specified. Please write any comments you may have about the amount or the frequency of actions you rate. Let me know if you need an explanation of an action.

Rating: 0 = never   1 = occasionally   2 = frequently   3 = always

Rating	Observed Behaviors	Your comments
	Problems remembering new information	
	Problems finding information in the phonebook	
	Forgets appointments	
	Changes in personal hygiene	
	Demonstrates sleeping problems or restlessness	
	Problems in getting dressed	
	Memory problems that affect job performance	
	More easily frustrated than in prior years	
	Problems with finding the correct words	
	Loses train of thought while talking	
	Has difficulty following long conversations	
	May wander from topic during a conversation	
	Misplaces objects; cannot find lost items	
	Consistent problems in keeping a checkbook	
	Confusion about time and place	
	Confusion about names of friends and relatives	
	Problems with fixing meals	
	Problems with paying bills	

(continues)

Dementia Assessment Protocol 3: General Behavioral Evaluation (continued)

Rating	Observed Behaviors	Your comments
	Rapid changes in mood without reason	
	Changes in personality	
	Increased apathy and passivity	
	Decreased participation in enjoyable activities	
	Lapses in personal or financial judgments	
	Uses vague, indefinite words in conversations	
	Confusion about location in familiar places	
	Frequently dwells on past events	
	Has difficulty maintaining attention	
	Has difficulty traveling to familiar places	
	Inappropriate laughing or crying	
	Less emotionally responsive than in prior years	
	Is more anxious or depressed than in prior years	
	Delusions about people or events	
Clinician's summative statement:		

References

Jorm, A. F. (2004). The Informant Questionnaire on Cognitive Decline in the Elderly (IQCODE): A review. *International Psychogeriatrics, 16*(3), 1–19.

Jorm, A. F., & Jacomb, P. A. (1989). The Informant Questionnaire on Cognitive Decline in the Elderly (IQCODE): Socio-demographic correlates, reliability, validity, and some norms. *Psychological Medicine, 19,* 1015–1022.

Tariq, S. H., Tumosa, N., Chibnall, J. T., Perry, M. H., & Morley, J. E. (2006). Comparison of the Saint Louis University mental status examination and the mini-mental state examination for detecting dementia and mild neurocognitive disorder—a pilot study. *American Journal of Geriatric Psychiatry, 14*(11), 897–899.

Tombaugh, T. N., Kozak, J., & Rees, L. (1999). Normative data stratified by age and education for two measures of verbal fluency: FAS and animal naming. *Archives of Clinical Neuropsychology, 14,* 167–177.

PART VI

Assessment of Traumatic Brain Injury

CHAPTER 13

Assessment of Traumatic Brain Injury (TBI): Resources

- Epidemiology of TBI
- Etiology of TBI
- Penetrating Brain Injuries
- Nonpenetrating Brain Injuries
- Primary and Secondary Effects of TBI
- Recovery from TBI
- Neurobehavioral Effects of TBI
- Communicative Disorders Associated with TBI
- Assessment of TBI
- Overview of Assessment
- Screening for TBI
- Diagnostic Assessment
- Assessment of Consciousness and Responsiveness
- Assessment of Memory and Reasoning Skills
- Assessment of Communicative Deficits Associated with TBI
- Postassessment Counseling

Speech-language pathologists assess traumatic brain injury (TBI) because of various communication deficits associated with this medical emergency. Also known as *cranio-cerebral trauma*, TBI is more common among children and adolescents and among those 65 years old or older. Throughout the world, TBI is a common cause of death and disability. Because of its potential long-standing effects, TBI is one of the most expensive medical disabilities (Adamovich, 1997; Bigler, 1990).

Speech-language pathologists, as members of an interdisciplinary team, help assess the multitudes of negative effects that follow TBI. The team is initially concerned with the medical emergency, and subsequently, with the overall rehabilitation of the individual. Eventual community reentry is the final goal of rehabilitation.

Brain injury associated with a variety of other conditions should be distinguished from TBI. For instance, brain injury associated with strokes, tumors, infection, progressive neurological diseases, metabolic disturbances, toxic agents, and inherited or congenital conditions are not classified as TBI. To be classified as **traumatic brain injury**, it should be caused by physical trauma or external force.

Head trauma, though always a part of brain injury, may or may not cause brain injury. In some cases head trauma may cause injury to facial structures, including the skull, but the brain may escape injury. Long-term rehabilitation needs and potential effects on communication and intellectual functions arise only when the brain is injured.

Epidemiology of TBI

Estimates of the prevalence of TBI vary across studies. This is because of methodological differences across studies. Some studies do not count head injury without brain injury, but others count them. The Center for Disease Control and Prevention (http://www.cdc.gov/traumaticbraininjury), which collects epidemiological data on diseases and medical conditions, reports that annually in the United States:

- Approximately 1.7 million people sustain a TBI; of these, about 52,000 individuals die.

- 275,000 persons are hospitalized due to injuries and complications related to TBI.

- 1.365 million, nearly 80% of those who sustain TBI, receive emergency room treatment.

- TBI is involved in 30.5% of all injury-related deaths.

- Direct medical costs and indirect costs due to lost productivity may be as high as $60 billion.

- The highest incidence of TBI is found in children aged 0 to 4 years, adolescents aged 15 to 19 years, and adults aged 65 years and older.

- Annually, nearly half a million (473,947) children aged 0 to 14 years make emergency department visits for TBI-related problems.

- Adults aged 75 years and older face the highest risk of TBI-related hospitalization and death rate.

- In all age groups, more males than females sustain TBI.

- TBI is believed to be more common among African Americans than in whites. Minorities living in poor and violence-prone neighborhoods may sustain more TBIs than those living in affluent neighborhoods.

Etiology of TBI

TBI has multiple causes, but a few causes are more common than others. The dominant causes in different age groups vary. For instance:

- **Falls are the leading cause of TBI.** A little over 35% of TBI is due to falls. Children aged 0 to 4 years and adults aged 75 years and older experience the highest incidence of TBI due to falls. Falls cause 50.2% of the TBIs among children aged 0 to 14 years and 60.7% among adults aged 65 years and older. The greatest number of emergency treatment for TBI is due to falls. Annually, more than half a million hospital visits (523,043) and hospitalizations (62,334) are caused by falls and the resulting TBI. From 2002–2006, there has been a significant increase in TBI caused by falls and the resulting hospitalization and death rate.

- **Motor vehicle–traffic injury is the second most frequent cause of TBI.** Traffic accidents cause 17.3% of all TBI in all age groups, although the death rates are the highest for adults aged 20 to 24 years. About 32% of TBI-related deaths are caused by traffic accidents. Nearly a third of TBIs sustained in traffic accidents may be due to drunk driving. Death rates in motorcycle riders due to accidents and TBI are about 15% higher than that found in the occupants of passenger cars. A significant number of pedestrians, especially children, and bicycle riders of all age group sustain TBI.

- **Struck-by and struck-against events are the third most frequent causes of TBI.** In about 16.5% of cases, TBI is caused by the head being struck by moving objects or struck against stationary objects.

- **Assaults and interpersonal violence cause about 10% of TBI.** The rate may be as high as 40% in large inner-city areas. The incidence of gunshot head injury is the highest among adolescents and young adults.

- **No precise data exist on several other causes.** Sports and recreational activities cause a certain number of TBI in all age groups, perhaps more in children. Drug abuse, learning disabilities, intellectual disabilities, and psychiatric disorders are thought to be related to TBI (Kraus & McArthur, 2000).

There are some seasonal variations in the incidence of TBI. More people sustain TBI in May through October. It is thought that increased outdoor activities during the warmer months account for this high rate of TBI in those months.

Brain injuries are classified as either *penetrating* or *nonpenetrating.* Penetrating TBIs are more prone to produce transitory effects than the nonpenetrating TBIs, which produce more lasting effects.

Penetrating Brain Injuries

Piercing objects or crushing forces produce **penetrating brain injuries**. Also known as *open head injuries*, penetrating objects or forces may fracture or perforate the skull, tear brain coverings (meninges), and damage the brain tissue. A variety of objects, including bullets, nail guns, lawn darts, knives, and crossbows may travel through the air and strike the skull. For this reason, such objects that cause penetrating TBIs are known as missiles. Some piercing objects may enter and exit the skull.

Depending on the speed with which they travel, penetrating objects may produce either **low-velocity impacts** (injuries) or **high-velocity impacts** (injuries). An arrow, nail gun, knife, civilian handguns, blows to the head, and automobile accidents tend to produce low-velocity injuries. A majority of low-velocity penetrating injuries are caused by bullets shot from handguns in the United States. Such injuries cause a mortality rate of up to 60% (Harrington & Apostolides, 2000). Often found in military personnel, **high-velocity injuries** are caused by weapons, rifles, and other automatic assault weapons.

The overall effects of penetrating brain injuries depend mostly on the size and velocity of the projectile and the course it takes after entering the skull. Generally, the higher the velocity (speed) of the projectile entrance, the greater the extent of injury. As can be expected, larger objects cause greater injury than smaller objects. The projectile that passes through the brain in a straight line will produce less severe injuries than the one that moves in a zigzag path. Such changes in the course of movement are called a projectile's *yaw*. Additional factors that affect the extent of brain injury include the amount of missile fragmentation and the number of wounds. Severe brain injuries are associated with missiles that shatter within the brain and those that cause multiple wounds (Harrington & Apostolides, 2000).

Penetrating brain injuries may be fatal. About 75% of those who receive gunshot wounds die immediately or soon thereafter. The mortality rate for low-velocity injuries is generally lower than that for high-velocity injuries. Those who survive penetrating brain injuries experience several consequences, including:

- **Increased intracranial pressure.** In less than 5 minutes of the impact to the head, the pressure within the skull increases and waves of pressure spread throughout the brain and the spinal cord. After some time, there may be another increase in intracranial pressure.

- **Varying blood pressure.** Soon after the impact, blood pressure drops, but it rises to abnormal levels and drops again.

- **Reduced blood flow and metabolic changes.** Blood flow to the brain tends to decrease, mostly because of lower cerebral metabolic rate and oxygen consumption.

- **Death of brain tissue.** More marked on the projectile tract, the extent of brain tissue death will depend on such variables as the velocity and size of the missile.

- **Bleeding, infection, swelling, and hydrocephalus.** These effects may cause destruction of additional brain tissue.

More long-term effects include physical, cognitive, and communication deficits. Assessment of these effects, especially those on speech and language will be the primary responsibility of speech-language pathologists.

Nonpenetrating Brain Injuries

The skull may or may not be fractured in nonpenetrating brain injuries. **Nonpenetrating brain injury** is caused by indirect force acting upon the head. There is no entry of a foreign substance into the brain and the meninges are intact. Complex and long-lasting symptoms follow nonpenetrating injuries, requiring extensive rehabilitation programs.

Nonpenetrating brain injuries may be caused by (a) an external object striking a stationary head or the head striking a stationary object, and (b) the head moving back and forth because of a force acting on it or elsewhere on the body. A blunt blow to the head or the collapse of an automobile onto the head of a mechanic working under it illustrates the impact of a force on a stationary head. Falls exemplify the head striking a stationary object, such as when the head hits the floor or a piece of furniture.

Automobile accidents typically cause injuries resulting from a rapidly moving head. A force may be applied directly to the head, which then moves violently and results in brain injury. On the other hand, a force applied elsewhere on the body (e.g., whiplash) also may set the head into back-and-forth movement, causing injury to the brain. The shaken-baby syndrome also illustrates moving forces applied to the head, causing intracranial, intraocular, and cervical spinal injuries and death in 19% of children who are subjected to this condition (King, McKay, & Sirnick, 2003).

Two kinds of injuries result from nonpenetrating forces that act upon the head: acceleration/deceleration injuries and nonacceleration injuries. Different biomechanics are involved in producing such differential injuries.

- **Some injuries are due to acceleration/deceleration of the brain.** When a force acts on the head, it accelerates first, and then decelerates, causing **acceleration/deceleration injuries** to the brain. The head also may accelerate and decelerate when a force is applied to another part of the body (e.g., the head movement due to an impact to the chest). An accelerating head may strike something (e.g., the automobile dashboard during an accident) and sustain additional injury, but mere acceleration/deceleration is sufficient to cause injury because the brain inside the skull moves back and forth.

- **Acceleration may be linear or angular.** The head and the brain inside may experience either a linear acceleration or an angular acceleration depending on the locus of the impact. The head moving back in a straight line because force is applied to its midline illustrates linear acceleration. Angular (nonlinear), rotation-like movements of the head are caused by forces that hit the head off-center. Angular acceleration, because it twists and rotates the tissue, produces a severe form of damage called *diffuse axonal injury* to the brain. In either case, the brain inside the skull initially does not move because of inertia; but soon it begins to move inside the skull, sustaining tissue damage. The bony protrusions at the bottom of the skull will cause additional tissue damage. When the head eventually stops moving, the brain inside the skull keeps moving for a few seconds, increasing the rate of tissue damage.

- **Coup and contrecoup injuries.** Brain injury at the point of impact trauma due to the skull compression is called *coup injury*. Injury that results on the opposite side of the impact because the moving brain hits the inside portion of the slowing or stationary skull is called *contrecoup injury*. These two types of injuries tend to damage meninges, cortex, and subcortical structures.

- **Blows to restrained heads cause nonacceleration injuries.** A moving object hitting and delivering a crushing blow to a restrained head can cause *nonacceleration injuries*. A force striking the head of a person standing against a wall, lying on a firm surface (as the auto mechanic under a car), or sitting with a rigid head support sustains nonacceleration injuries. Lack of acceleration also means an absence of deceleration.

Nonacceleration injuries are less frequent than acceleration/deceleration injuries. Compared to those with acceleration/deceleration injuries, neurological symptoms tend to be less severe and more transitory in patients who have sustained nonacceleration injuries. Skull fracture is the major concern in nonacceleration injuries.

Primary and Secondary Effects of TBI

TBI tends to produce a variety of negative neurological and other physical effects. Of these, some are described as primary and the others as secondary. In a later section, we will describe the neurobehavioral effects of TBI that the management team (including speech-language pathologists) will help assess.

- **Primary effects are more immediate than secondary effects.** A primary effect is the *laceration*, which is a torn or jagged wound on the skin surface. *Fracture of the skull,* another primary effect, is more serious than a laceration, and occurs in 80% of fatal cases. As noted previously, *diffuse axonal injury* (torn nerve fibers) is another primary effect of nonlinear (angular) acceleration/deceleration forces and may include focal lesions, especially in the corpus callosum and parts of the brainstem (Graham & Gennarelli, 2000). Diffuse axonal injury is often associated with severe long-term disability and the vegetative state. Other primary effects of TBI include brain stem injury, diffuse vascular injury, focal lesions, previously mentioned coup and contrecoup injuries, damage to cranial nerves, and abrading injuries. Brain stem injuries cause coma. Cerebral hemorrhage will follow vascular injury. Linear acceleration often results in focal injuries. Damage to cranial nerves V, VIII, X, and XII will affect speech production. Abrading injuries are due to acceleration and deceleration of the brain against the rough surfaces or projections of the skull. (Graham & Gennarelli, 2000).

- **Secondary effects are the consequences of primary effects.** They tend to occur sometime after the initial trauma to the brain. Three types of intracranial hematoma (i.e., the accumulation of blood due to hemorrhage) are among the serious secondary effects because they can cause death. In the *epidural (extradural) hematoma*, blood accumulates between the dura mater and the skull, and it may be cleared surgically. In the *subdural hematoma*, blood accumulates between the dura and the arachnoid and is associated with up to 60% mortality rate. In the intracerebral hematoma, blood accumulates within the brain itself, and it is often associated with diffuse axonal injury due to linear acceleration. Intracerebral hematoma is a frequent cause of coma and death (Graham & Gennarelli, 2000). Other secondary effects include increased intracranial pressure due to accumulation of blood and other fluids, ischemic brain damage due to oxygen deficiency, breathing difficulties, hypotension (reduced blood pressure), seizures, and increased chances of such secondary infections as meningitis (Gillis, 1996; Tien & Chesnut, 2000).

Prompt and competent intervention helps minimize the effects of TBI. Timely treatment to prevent or reduce the secondary effects will help stabilize the patient's physical condition and minimize more debilitating long-term effects.

Recovery from TBI

The course of recovery from the consequences of TBI varies across patients. Multiple variables influence the extent and rates of recovery. Although improvements in emergency treatment for patients with TBI have cut the death rate in recent years, nearly 50% of patients with severe forms of brain injury may die. Those who survive severe forms of TBI are likely to experience lasting effects that include memory deficits, intellectual disabilities, and more or less subtle communication problems (Andrews, 2000).

As can be expected, the lesser the severity of the injury, the greater the chances of recovery. Generally, those who recover from TBI do so within the first six months of injury. Chances of recovery for those in vegetative states are 50% for adults and 60% for children (Andrews, 2000). Chances of recovery are very low after the first year and any recovery is likely to be associated with permanent disabilities. Of the several factors that affect the pattern and rate of recovery from TBI, the following are among the most important:

- **Type of injury and secondary effects are critical variables.** Diffuse axonal injuries and multiple secondary effects are associated with slower or more partial recovery rates. Patients with subarachnoid hemorrhage, brainstem injuries, intracranial hematoma, and increased intracranial pressure have a relatively poor prognosis for recovery. Patients who experience such multiple secondary effects also may have a poor prognosis for fully recovered functions (Jeremitsky, Omert, Dunham, Protetch, & Rodriguez, 2003).

- **Level of consciousness and coma affect recovery.** Patients with higher levels of consciousness following TBI recover faster than those with lower levels. Patients with longer durations of coma recover less than those with shorter durations. Patients with reactive pupils have a 50% chance of good recovery or only a moderate disability.

- **Age is an important variable.** Generally, children with TBI, even those with diffuse axonal injury, may recover better than most older patients. Younger patients survive TBI better than older patients.

- **Drug abuse and alcoholism complicate recovery.** Consumption of alcohol and drug use before the injury negatively affects recovery. This is partly due to increased secondary effects, including edema, cerebral hypoxia, and hemorrhage.

Race and gender of the patient do not seem to affect the rate of recovery. Generally, it is difficult to predict recovery in individual cases with a mild to moderate degree of TBI. The overall symptom complex tends to vary across individuals with similar kinds of injuries.

Neurobehavioral Effects of TBI

Both short- and long-term neurological and behavioral changes follow TBI. Depending on the severity of the injuries, patients with TBI may exhibit some or most of the following:

- **Neurological symptoms may be initially more prominent.** *Altered consciousness*, which may vary from a dazed state to coma, may be among the more immediate neurological effects of TBI. A *dazed* patient is conscious and responsive to strong stimulation. A patient in a state of *stupor* is unresponsive except for pain stimuli. A patient lapsing into *coma* is unconscious, unresponsive to most or all external stimulation, and may die without recovering from it. Others who are comatose may survive in a *vegetative state* with intact sleep-wake cycle and reflexes and brief periods of alertness and intact reflexes. Those who do not recover from coma within 30 days of injury are said to be in a *persistent vegetative state*. Other symptoms include headache, dizziness, blurred vision, fatigue, lethargy, seizures, restlessness, agitation, and lack of motor coordination.

- **Behavioral symptoms may be just as prominent.** Initially, most patients who sustain TBI are *confused* and *disoriented*. *Confusion* and *disorientation* may be evident in patients who have just recovered from coma. *Lack of concentration*, *impaired thinking* and *judgment*, and *memory problems* are common in patients with TBI. Memory is typically impaired for events preceding and following the trauma. Reduced levels of consciousness and a state of excessive arousal (delirium) are associated with memory problems in patients with TBI. As described in the next section of this chapter, communication difficulties, especially speech disorders, may be prominent in patients with TBI.

- **Dysphagia may be present in 25% to 75% of patients.** Difficulty swallowing may be one of the initial problems. Intracranial bleeding and brainstem injury tend to increase the chances of dysphagia. Some children with TBI refuse to eat.

- **Psychiatric changes may be evident in some patients.** Some psychiatric symptoms appear soon after the trauma and diminish over time. Others may persist. During the period of recovery, some patients my experience auditory hallucinations, confabulations, and delusions. Some patients may be depressed and others may show apathy. Poor emotional control, social withdrawal, irritability, childishness, and unreasonable behavior may persist in some patients.

Communicative Disorders Associated with TBI

Minimal TBI may not produce significant communication problems except for a delayed response and an occasional irrelevant response. A slight disorientation to time (but not necessarily to place) may be present as well.

Communication problems emerge in patients with moderate to severe TBI. In most cases, effective communication, not grammar, tends to be impaired. If cerebellum, brainstem, or peripheral nerves are damaged, dysarthria may be present. In patients with severe TBI, subtle language deficits may be a lasting effect.

Language Problems of Patients with TBI

In the acute stage of TBI, some patients may not talk at all (*mutism*). Most patients, however, recover from their mutism. These and other patients who have not had an initial mutism tend to speak grammatically correctly. Their syntactic structures and morphologic features may be intact. Nonetheless, their communication may be less effective, mostly because of their impaired social interactions.

- **Language may be confused.** This may be a feature of most patients in their initial stage of TBI. Their responses to questions may be irrelevant, circumlocutory, incoherent, and confabulatory.

- **Naming difficulties may not be as severe as they are in aphasia.** Confrontation naming, or naming objects when shown and asked "What is this?" may be difficult for patients with TBI. This verbal task may be especially difficult possibly because of inattentiveness or impulsive and hasty responding when asked to name something.

- **Verbal responses tend to perseverate.** The patient may repeat the same response multiple times.

- **Word fluency is often impaired.** When asked to recall as many words as possible within a category (e.g., names of flowers or furniture items), patients with TBI may give an extremely limited number of responses. Naming difficulties and their general inattention may partly be responsible for this difficulty.

- **Conversational skills deficiencies are prominent.** Difficulty in producing and maintaining appropriate and spontaneous conversational speech is probably the most significant language deficiency seen in patients with TBI. These deficiencies include *difficulty in spontaneously initiating conversation*, problems in taking appropriate *conversational turns*, impaired *conversational topic selection*, lack of *topic maintenance*, absence of narrative cohesion, and production of *vague* and *imprecise words*.

- **Nonverbal communication also may be impaired.** Gestures, facial expression, and other nonverbal means of communication may not accompany verbal expression as they normally do. Patients with TBI may fail to understand facial expressions and gestures of speakers.

- **Auditory comprehension problems may be evident.** Patients with TBI may fail to give appropriate responses to speech stimuli, suggesting problems in understanding what they hear. Responding appropriately to metaphoric and ironic speech may be especially impaired.

- **Reading and writing may be impaired.** Understanding what they read, especially extended texts, may be impaired. In the absence of motor difficulties, printing words and a few sentences may or may not be impaired. Nonetheless, writing extended paragraphs may be incoherent and full of errors.

Speech Problems of Patients with TBI

Depending on the extent and the nature of brain injury, speech problems may be more dominant than language difficulties in patients with TBI. Approximately 30% to 35% of patients with TBI exhibit speech disorders. In acute rehabilitation settings, speech disorders may be found in 65% of patients (Beukelman, Burke, & Yorkston, 2002.

Speech disorders found in persons with TBI are called **dysarthria**, a group of motor speech disorders associated with impaired muscular control of the speech mechanism. Neuropathology that causes dysarthria may be central, peripheral, or both. Neuromotor control problems that result from TBI affect all aspects of speech production, including respiratory support for speech, articulation of speech sounds, speech prosody, resonance, voice quality, vocal pitch and loudness, and the rate of speech (Duffy, 2005; Freed, 2000). See Chapter 5 for more information on dysarthria and its types.

There are different types of dysarthria, although spastic dysarthria is probably more common in patients with TBI. Frontal lobe damage, frequent in patients with TBI, accounts for their spastic dysarthria, which is characterized by abnormal stress patterns, slow rate of speech, and imprecise production of consonants and vowels. Phonatory problems, typically not prominent in dysarthria associated with TBI may be found in some patients with spastic dysarthria (Murdoch & Theodoros, 2000). TBI may be associated with any type of dysarthria.

Patients with TBI are likely to produce the following dysarthric speech characteristics (Murdoch & Theodoros, 2000):

- **Hypernasality is typical.** A mild to moderate degree of hypernasal speech is found in up to 98% of the patients who have dysarthria associated with their TBI.

- **The rate of speech may be slower than normal.** Impaired speech rate, mostly a slower rate, is found in up to 95% of the patients with dysarthria due to TBI.

- **Production of consonants may be imprecise.** Precise production of consonants may be negatively affected in about 91% of the patients with dysarthria and TBI. Consequently, speech intelligibility may be impaired to varying degrees.

- **Breath support for speech tends to be reduced.** Breath support for speech may be reduced in about 88% of patients with dysarthria following a TBI.

- **Voice problems may be present.** Up to 88% of the patients with dysarthria may exhibit limited pitch variations. Loudness of voice may be limited in about 79% of patients with dysarthria due to TBI. Vocal quality deviations, often found in dysarthria associated with various neuropathologies, are not typical of TBI-associated dysarthria. Nonetheless, in about a third of patients with dysarthria due to TBI voice quality may be harsh, hoarse, and strained-strangled. Another voice problem can be glottal fry. (Murdoch & Theodoros, 2000).

- **Speech fluency may be reduced.** Fluency may be reduced because of increased speech dysfluencies. A slower rate of speech, frequent pauses or silent intervals, and short phrases also contribute to a judgment of reduced fluency.

- **Prosodic features of speech may be impaired.** The prosodic features, which include normal pitch variations, appropriate pausing, a speech rate within normal limits, typical stress patterns, and so forth, may be impaired. For instance, up to 86% of the patients with dysarthria due to TBI tend to speak with excess stress on unstressed syllables. Speech may be characterized by short phrases in about 84% of the patients. Silent intervals in speech may be prolonged in about 79% of the patients with dysarthria.

Thinking and Reasoning Skill

Often described as *cognitive deficits*, impairments in thinking and reasoning are a part of the TBI symptom complex. These difficulties affect the overall communication effectiveness of patients with TBI. Speech-language pathologists need to assess them to design effective treatment plans.

Some of the commonly found deficits in thinking, reasoning, and planning skills include the following:

- **Difficulty with abstract language may be the central problem.** Therefore, verbal behavior is still the main means of assessing problems in logical reasoning and planning sequenced activities. Patients with TBI find more abstract reasoning and planning tasks harder than less abstract (more concrete) tasks. The more severe is the brain injury, the greater is the difficulty with abstraction. Thinking and responses to complex verbal stimuli tend to be more concrete in patients with TBI.

- **Difficulty understanding proverbs, similes, and metaphors may be common.** Patients may concretely interpret proverbs, similes, and metaphors or may fail to respond when exemplars are provided. For example, a patient may either fail to interpret the meaning of *all that glitters is not gold*, or may interpret literally, by pointing to something that is shining, but not gold.

- **Similarities and differences may be a difficult discrimination.** The patient may not be able to tell how a *jasmine* and a *petunia* are similar or how a *table* and a *chair* are different.

- **Matching geometric forms may be difficult.** The patient may be unable to match (re-create) geometric forms presented visually. He or she may make errors in completing incomplete patterns. In addition, sorting objects based on shape, color, or other characteristics may be difficult as well.

- **Reasoned verbal answers or solutions may be difficult for them.** For example, the patient may not answer correctly when asked such questions as "What would you do if you found someone's car keys on the floor of a store?"

- **Logical inconsistencies may be difficult for the patient to specify.** For instance, the patient may give vague or incorrect answers when asked to specify what is wrong with such statements as, *he was very tired, so he easily walked seven miles.*

- **The patient may make errors in sequentially arranging story-telling pictures.** When the clinician randomly presents a set of story-telling pictures, persons with TBI may fail to correctly and sequentially arrange them to tell the story.

- **The patient may fail to tell why some pictures are absurd.** For example, when a picture shows a deer chasing a tiger, the patient may not say that it is usually the other way around.

- **The patient may not correctly describe the missing elements in drawings.** For example, the patient, looking at a picture of a man with no eyes may not say that the eyes are missing, or when the tail of a cat is missing, may not say the tail is missing.

- **Planning daily activities may be impaired.** When asked to describe how he or she would plan for a birthday party, book a hotel room, or prepare a sandwich for lunch, the patient may give partial or confused answers.

Assessment of TBI

Assessment of patients with TBI is a team effort. The typical team includes the emergency care physician, neurologist, radiologist, primary care physician, speech-language pathologist, clinical psychologist, physical therapist, nurse, social worker, and other professionals depending on the complexity of the patient's injury. A neurosurgeon's help, for example, may be requested if emergency brain surgery is needed. The team's initial concern is the patient's general health, levels of consciousness and awareness, and immediate medical or surgical intervention needed to save the life, stabilize the patient, and prevent infections and other complications that will worsen brain function.

Assessment of patients with TBI is a recurring activity. The patient's physical and behavioral status may continuously change for better or worse. To track these changes, a reliable assessment of the initial status of the patient would be essential. A brief initial assessment (or even results of observations) may be made at the time of emergency room admission. A more detailed examination, still initial, may be made soon after the patient is admitted to the hospital, if that is done. Subsequently, a more detailed assessment may be made when the client's physical and behavioral status improves to make it practical. As the patient improves over time, with or without treatment, and whether as inpatient or outpatient, assessment may be repeated at intervals considered appropriate. Assessment done over time may use different methods and tools and may target different skills. Assessment goals also may change over time. For instance, the initial goal may be to find ways to stabilize the patient. Subsequent assessment goals may be to identify short-term treatment goals. Later goals may be to design long-term rehabilitation goals. Such repeated and dynamic assessments help design flexible and effective rehabilitation programs.

A clear understanding of what each of the other specialists on the team does to help the patient with TBI is essential for speech-language pathologists to do their jobs effectively. Assessment and treatment of patients' communication skills and dysphagia are the main responsibilities of patients with TBI.

Overview of Assessment

All specialists in the team contribute to the initial assessment of patients. The team needs information on the patient and the family. As with any patient, the assessment begins with a quick evaluation of the patient's status and detailed information about the patient, the circumstances of injury, the family, and so forth.

- **A case history is completed.** A standard case history form may be completed by all patients or their informants. The case history may seek specific information on the events preceding the brain injury.

- **Family members or other informants are interviewed.** A family member, friend, colleague, or someone who is close to the patient should be interviewed to understand the premorbid status of the client. It is essential to know the patient's education and verbal (language) skills, social and occupational skills, and interests and hobbies. Such knowledge will help distinguish limitations in premorbid skills from the negative effects of brain injury. The clinician should explore any evidence of substance abuse and alcoholism that may have contributed to the accident that caused the brain injury. Anyone familiar with the accident or trauma scene will be especially helpful in providing information on the condition of the patient at the onset of TBI.

- **The current medical condition is evaluated.** An initial evaluation of the patient's current physical condition, organ injuries, medications, alertness, and responsiveness begins when the paramedical staff comes in contact with the patient. This evaluation continues upon admission to the emergency room.

- **Medical tests are ordered.** Laboratory and other tests, including radiological, blood, and scanning tests may be ordered as soon as possible. These tests and the physical examinations may help assess the extent of skull and brain injury.

- **Effects of the current medication are taken into consideration.** Drugs prescribed to the patient may influence general behavior, including communication. For instance, drugs prescribed to control thought disorders or anxiety may decrease attention by sedating the patient. Some drugs may have the effects of slurring the speech. It is important to distinguish the effects of drugs from those of TBI.

- **Patient's general behaviors are assessed.** A patient's behaviors and physical symptoms are likely to change, often quite rapidly. To assess such changes over time, it is essential to establish a base rate of behaviors and symptoms as soon as the patient's condition will allow. Therefore, as soon as practical, the patient's general and verbal behaviors should be assessed to establish initial levels to be compared against later levels.

- **Consciousness and responsiveness are initially assessed.** Whether the patient is conscious and responsive to environmental stimuli are assessed as soon as possible. The team may use standardized scales and make systematic observations of the patient to determine the degree of consciousness and responsiveness.

- **Memory and reasoning skills are assessed in due course.** As soon as it is practical, speech-language pathologists and psychologists evaluate memory, thinking, reasoning, and planning skills of the patient.

- **Speech-language pathologists assess communication skills.** This evaluation may include standardized and client-specific procedures and general observations of communication in the hospital or clinic settings. The clinician will be especially interested in assessing functional communication skills of the patient.

- **Any evidence of swallowing problems will trigger a special assessment.** Speech-language pathologists are typically in charge of this assessment.

- **Postassessment counseling summarizes the findings for the patient, caregivers, or both.** At the end of the initial or repeated assessment, the clinician counsels the family or other caregivers.

- **The assessment team will integrate the information.** The team of specialists who evaluated the patient may collectively or individually analyze their data and observations. They may prepare a summary of initial findings and impressions.

- **The team or individual professionals will write the report.** In most cases, individual professionals will write their separate reports. There may be a collective recommendation, however.

Depending on the physical condition of the patient, the initial assessment may be more or less comprehensive. Soon after the trauma, or soon after regaining consciousness, patients may be inconsistent, disorganized, confused, restless, irritated, and disoriented to time and place. A brief bedside evaluation is usually done to make a quick assessment of the patient's condition.

Screening for TBI

The assessment team or a specific professional on the team makes an initial screening of the patient's status as soon as it is practical. Clinicians may use a published screening protocol to gain an initial impression of the patient's level of consciousness, responsiveness to environmental stimuli, and status of general behavioral, including verbal behavior.

A published screening tool is the *Brief Test of Head Injury* (BTHI; Helm-Estabrooks & Hotz, 1991). It allows for a brief and quick assessment of orientation, following verbal commands, linguistic organization, naming, memory, visual-spatial skills, and reading comprehension. It may be administered to patients in the age range of 10–59+ years who have sustained brain injury. It helps establish a baseline of skills against which improvement may be monitored in subsequent assessments.

Other screening tests include the *Mini Mental Status Examination* (MMSE; Folstein, Folstein, & McHugh, 1975) and the *Galveston Orientation and Amnesia Test* (GOAT; Levin, O'Donnell, & Grossman, 1979). The MMSE helps screen orientation, attention, calculation, recall of previously tested names, pointing to selected objects, repeating phrases, following commands, and so forth. The GOAT is designed to screen orientation (to time, place, and person) and memory for events preceding and succeeding the brain injury.

All screening test results may be supplemented by systematic observations and clinician-prepared rating scales. Information made available from other professionals, medical charts, and medial test results also will help support a tentative status evaluation of the patient.

Diagnostic Assessment

A more complete diagnostic assessment than screening typically begins with an assessment of the patient's level of consciousness and responses to environmental stimuli. As the patient's physical condition is stabilized, additional assessment goals may be considered. Assessment of memory and reasoning skills, along with communication skills, will be the additional goals.

A detailed assessment of communication skills may be specifically targeted when judged appropriate. Nonetheless, the clinician gains some understanding of the patient's verbal behavior, including responses to speech directed to him or her (comprehension) while conducting other kinds of assessments. For instance, appropriate and timely response to speech is one of the elements of testing the level of consciousness. Assessment of memory and reasoning skills also involve verbal stimuli.

Assessment of Consciousness and Responsiveness

Even if the patient is not in coma or is not recovering from it, the level of consciousness and responsiveness to stimuli may have been affected. Even if fully conscious, the patient may be confused, disoriented, sleepy or agitated, inattentive, and irrelevant in speech. Those who are recovering from coma may go through various levels of consciousness and responsiveness. Therefore, an initial assessment targets the patient's *responsiveness to external stimuli*, which is the key element in assessing levels of consciousness and alertness. In addition, the clinician also targets orientation to time, space, and persons, including orientation to self for an initial assessment. An in-depth assessment of memory skills may be postponed to a later time, but a few questions about the events preceding and succeeding the trauma may be asked to get an initial impression of the effects the trauma had on the patient's memory.

Several standardized or semistandardized methods are available to make the initial as well as subsequent assessment. Some of them may be administered repeatedly to the same patient to make a continuous assessment of recovery—whether spontaneous or associated with rehabilitation.

Several specific tasks help assess responsiveness to stimuli as a clue to the levels of consciousness. Standardized tests or clinician-devised assessment protocols usually involve presentations of several specific verbal and nonverbal stimuli to assess the level of consciousness, orientation and attention, confusion or alertness, agitation or depression, memory and reasoning difficulties, verbal behavior including speech disorders, and swallowing problems. Several commonly targeted responses help assess patients with TBI because of their special significance to diagnosing TBI:

- Eye opening is a basic indicator of the level of consciousness.

- Orientation is another indicator of the level of consciousness.

- Attention suggests an improved level of consciousness.

- Agitation may be associated with disorientation and confusion.

- Confusion is typically an acute stage assessment target.

- Motor responses to verbal and nonverbal stimuli suggest the level of consciousness.

- Memory impairments may be assessed kinds.

- Thinking, abstract reasoning, and planning skills may be assessed somewhat later than the other skills.

- Verbal behavior is a good indicator of a variety of other impairments.

- Dysarthria may be assessed more or less intensively.

- Dysphagia may be assessed as the need arises.

The *Glasgow Coma Scale* (GCS; Teasdale & Jennett, 1976) is a commonly used assessment scale to evaluate the patient's condition at this time. It is a subjective rating scale whose results should be interpreted with caution and supplemented with systematic behavioral observations. This scale evaluates three categories of behavior: eye opening, motor responses, and verbal responses. Under each category, a higher score means better response (less severe damage).

- **Eye opening.** The scale evaluates the following: (a) spontaneous eye opening (maximum score of 4); (b) eye opening when verbally commanded (score of 3); (c) eye opening only in response to pain (score of 2); and (d) no response (score of 1).

- **Motor responses.** The scale evaluates the following responses with the specified scores: (a) obeying verbal commands (score of 6); (b) attempting to pull examiner's hand away from painful stimulation (score of 5); (c) pulls the body part in response to pain (score of 4); (d) flexes body part in response to pain (score of 3); (e) extends limbs or increases rigidity in response to pain (score of 2); (f) does not respond (score of 1).

- **Verbal responses.** The scale evaluates the following responses with specified scores: (a) conversing with good orientation (score of 5); (b) conversing though disoriented (4); (c) using intelligible words without engaging in conversation score of (score of 3); (d) producing unintelligible words (score of 2); giving no response (score of l).

The total score on the *GCS* can range from 3 to 15. Based on the scores, brain injury is classified as:

Coma: A score of 8 or less

Severe head injury: 3 to 8

Moderate head injury: 9 to 12

Mild head injury: 13 to 15

The different levels of scores obtained on the *GCS*, administered 6 hours postaccident, may help predict the outcome or extent of recovery. However, the test is relatively insensitive because it does not allow scoring of untestable behaviors. For instance, a patient may be unable to open his or her eyes because of a bandage onthem or unable to move a limb because of injury. Another patient may be unable to respond verbally because of intubation. Therefore, the test may overestimate the severity of injury.

The **Glasgow Outcome Scale** (GOS; Jennett & Teasdale, 1981) is useful in evaluating outcome for, or course of recovery from, TBI. The scale describes five potential outcomes for patients with TBI.

1. *Death.*

2. *Vegetative state.* As noted previously, patients in vegetative state give no meaningful responses although they may open their eyes, track moving stimulus visually, and have sleep/wake cycles.

3. *Severe disability.* With this outcome, patients are conscious, but are dependent on caregiver assistance for all daily activities. Cognitive and physical functions may be relatively preserved.

4. *Moderate disability.* With this outcome, although they have persistent disabilities, the patients are relatively independent. Patients may continue to work; the level of responsibility they assume may be somewhat lower than those of the premorbid period, however.

5. *Good recovery.* With this outcome, patients return to their premorbid functional levels without significant limitations. Mild and persistent neurobehavioral deficits do not affect their work and living activities.

The **Rancho Los Amigos Scale of Cognitive Levels** (RLAS; Hagen, 2000) is a widely used assessment procedure to evaluate the cognitive and behavioral levels of patients with TBI. The revised scale (Hagen, 2000) helps rate behaviors at 10 levels.

1. *No response, total assistance.* The patient does not respond to auditory, visual, kinesthetic, pain and other stimuli; needs total assistance.

2. *Generalized response, total assistance.* The patient gives nonspecific and aimless response to stimuli; gives delayed response to pain stimuli; needs total assistance.

3. *Localized response, total assistance.* The patient blinks, turns toward or away from sound, tracks a visual stimulus that is within the visual field, gives a specific response to sensory stimulation, and may respond to family members, but not to others.

4. *Confused-agitated, maximal assistance.* The patient is highly distractible, but pays attention to environmental stimuli; alert and responds to simple commands; easily agitated; exhibits inappropriate or incoherent verbal responses; may be uncooperative of treatment efforts.

5. *Confused-inappropriate-nonagitated, maximal assistance.* The patient is alert, relatively calm, though may be agitated when stimulated; confused and still disoriented to time, place, and persons; shows improved attention; has severely impaired recent memory; tries to use everyday objects inappropriately.

6. *Confused-appropriate, moderate assistance.* The patient is inconsistently oriented to place and persons; vaguely recognizes staff; consistently follows simple directions; has impaired recent memory; exhibits some self-care behaviors with assistance and supervision.

7. *Automatic-appropriate, minimal assistance.* The patient is consistently oriented to place and person although may not be to time; attends to familiar tasks for about 30 minutes; performs daily routines with minimal assistance; lacks insight into one's condition, overestimates personal abilities, fails to plan for the future; may be oppositional and uncooperative.

8. *Purposeful-appropriate with standby assistance.* The patient is oriented to person, place, and time; exhibits generally appropriate and normal behavior; may exhibit low stress threshold and difficulty with abstract reasoning skills; attends to a familiar task for about an hour; can recall past and recent events; can learn new information and generalize it; aware of one's impairments; may be depressed, irritable, easily frustrated.

9. *Purposeful and appropriate, standby assistance on request.* The patient can work for two hours at a stretch; capable of shifting back and forth between tasks; completes most familiar tasks but may request help with unfamiliar tasks; aware of impairments; low frustration tolerance, irritability, and depression may still be evident.

10. *Purposeful and appropriate, modified independent.* The patient can handle most tasks with periodic breaks; can initiate and carry out most daily activities, although may need some extra time. Because the patient knows and anticipates problems, he or she can plan and use compensatory strategies. The patient's social and emotional behaviors are consistently appropriate.

The *RLAS* scores cannot precisely predict prognosis for patient recovery. Generally, the longer the patient stays in the earlier levels, the poorer the prognosis for recovery.

The **_Galveston Orientation and Amnesia Test_** (GOAT; Levin, O'Donnell, & Grossman, 1979) is used to evaluate patients who are coming out of coma. It consists of ten questions designed to assess the patient's orientation to time, place, and persons (including self) and memory for events preceding and succeeding the injury. Sample questions include:

Biographic information. Questions asked of the patient include "What is your name?" "When were you born?" "Where do you live?" and "How did you get here?"

Orientation. Questions include "Where are you now?" "What time is it now?" "What is the month?" and "What is the year?"

Memory. Questions include "What is the first event you can remember *after* the injury?" "Can you describe in detail (e.g., time, date, companions) the first event you can recall *after* injury?" "Can you describe the last event you recall *before* the accident?" and "Can you describe in detail (e.g., date, time and companions) the first event you recall before the injury?"

The patient is awarded 100 points at the beginning of the test administration and points are deducted for incorrect responses. The scores are interpreted as follows:

- *Average:* 80 to 100
- *Borderline cases:* 66 to 79
- *Impaired:* 0 to 65

Several other tests are available to assess consciousness, cognition, and memory skills. These include the Disability Rating Scale (DAS; Rappoport & Associates, 1982) and the Comprehensive Level of Consciousness Scale (CLOCS; Stanczak & Associates, 1984). The DAS is more comprehensive and more sensitive to change than the Glasgow Outcome Scale. The DAS rates eye opening, communication ability, motor responses, feeding, toileting, grooming, level of functioning (dependency), and employability. The CLOCS is more comprehensive than the Glasgow Coma Scale and helps assess behaviors in eight categories: posture, resting eye position, spontaneous eye opening, other ocular movements, pupillary reflexes, motor activities, responsiveness, and communicative effort.

Assessment of Memory and Reasoning Skills

In patients with TBI, nonverbal skills (e.g., memory, aspects of perception, drawing, construction, reasoning) tend to be impaired more than verbal skills (e.g., naming, repetition). Some of the communication deficits of patients with TBI may be due to attention, perceptual, and memory deficits. Therefore, it is essential to understand these impairments to plan for effective rehabilitation programs.

- **Assessment of memory impairments.** Memory skills have been categorized and broken down into smaller components in numerous ways. The following kinds of memory may be impaired to varying extents in patients with TBI:
  - *Amnesia* is a term typically used in medical settings, suggests a failure to remember. Generally, classic amnesic syndromes are associated with damage to medial temporal lobes and hippocampus and involve profound memory

loss with relatively intact cognitive functions. Such damage may be uncommon in patients with TBI. Therefore, the term *amnesia* is not frequently used to describe the memory impairments of people with TBI.

○ *Retrospective memory* is memory for past events. This memory component may be subdivided into *declarative memory* and *procedural memory*. Declarative memory is remembering what has been learned in the past about things, places, and events in general. The clinician can assess declarative memory by asking questions that test general knowledge. For instance, the clinician may ask a series of questions to test the patient's knowledge of historic, geographic, political, academic, and social events. *Procedural memory* is remembering how to perform actions, including driving, shaving, cooking, and so forth. The clinician may assess procedural memory by asking the patient to describe how he or she would mail a letter, cook a meal, fix a leaking faucet, prepare a lecture outline, send e-mail messages, plant flowers in the garden, and so forth.

○ *Prospective memory* is remembering to do certain things at particular times. Keeping appointments and checking the mail at a certain time of the day are examples of prospective memory. The clinician can assess this skill by asking questions about such upcoming events as dinner time, doctor's appointment or bedside visits, medication times, scheduled rehabilitation activities, and so forth.

○ *Posttraumatic memory loss* (anterograde amnesia) is difficulty remembering events following the TBI. The clinician can assess this skill by asking client-specific questions about known events that took place after the injury. For instance, the clinician can ask about who brought the patient to the hospital, what was done to him or her soon after arrival in the hospital, activities that followed admission, events of the day, and so forth. Interview of family members or police and rescue staff who brought the patient to the hospital will help corroborate the patient's descriptions.

○ *Pretraumatic memory loss* (also known as *retrograde amnesia*) is difficulty remembering events that preceded the trauma. The clinician can assess this skill by asking questions about known events that preceded the injury. For instance, the patient may be asked where he or she was or what he or she was doing before the injury. Once again, interviews of individuals associated with the patient (e.g., family members) and those associated with the events surrounding the trauma (e.g., other passengers in a car involved in the accident and police or rescue staff who arrived on the accident scene) may provide corroborative evidence.

○ *Impaired visual memory* is difficulty in recalling what is seen for a brief duration. To assess this, clinicians show various geometric forms for a brief duration (e.g., a triangle or a circle drawn on a card) and then ask the patient to draw it from memory.

• **Assessment of thinking, reasoning, and planning skills.** Impaired thinking, reasoning, and planning skills may be assessed informally as well as with standardized instruments. For example:

- ○ The clinician may assess *verbal abstract reasoning skills* by asking the patient to state the meaning of such proverbs as *a stitch in time saves nine*. The clinician also may ask the patient to state the differences and similarities between objects or words (e.g., "How are *pencils* and *pens* similar?" "How are they different?" "What is the difference and similarity between a *cabbage* and a *cucumber*?"). Several standardized tests or subtests of other tests also may be used to assess verbal reasoning skills. For instance, some tests of intelligence contain items to assess reasoning skills, ability to detect verbal absurdities, and so forth. These items may be administered to the patient. Tests that ask the patient to arrange pictures to tell a story are also useful.

- ○ The clinician may assess *nonverbal abstract reasoning skills* by administering several available tests. A commonly administered test is the Standard Progressive Matrices (Raven, 1960). This test consists of black and white incomplete geometric designs and several choices to complete the pattern; the patient selects a pattern that completes the pattern. A colored version of the test is also available. Another test that may be administered is the Wisconsin Card Sorting Test (Berg, 1948) in which the patient is asked to sort cards on which one or all four symbols (a triangle, a cross, a star, and a circle) are printed. The patient is told "right" or "wrong" at each attempt.

The extent to which reasoning and thinking skills are assessed will depend on the needs of the patient. Extensive assessments of cognitive functions with such standardized instruments as tests of intelligence are performed by a psychologist. Several test batteries, more or less comprehensive in their coverage, are available to assess cognitive and reasoning skills patients with TBI. These include the Brief Test of Head Injury (BTHI; Helm-Estabrooks & Hotz, 1991), the Ross Information Processing Assessment—Second Edition (Ross, 1996), the Scale of Cognitive Ability for Traumatic Brain Injury (Adamovich & Henderson, 1992), and the Woodcock-Johnson Psychoeducational Battery III (Woodcock, McGrew, & Mather, 2001). These and other tests help evaluate memory skills, orientation, reasoning and thinking, and so forth.

Assessment of Communicative Deficits Associated with TBI

Patients with severe brain injury experience lasting communication deficits, which include word retrieval problems that result in paraphasic and circulocutionary speech. These deficits, however, may not be apparent on simple language measures. While phonologically and syntactically correct, language productions of those who have sustained significant brain injury in the past may have subtle problems that are difficult to detect or problems that the traditional tests of speech and language fail to sample (Murdoch & Theodoros, 2000). Timed tests are sometimes useful as the patient tends to do worse under time pressure. Discourse analysis may reveal some of these problems more efficiently than standardized tests.

In assessing communicative deficits of patients with TBI, tests of aphasia have not proven especially useful. However, some clinicians may use certain subtests of aphasia test batteries (e.g., a confrontation naming test, a word fluency test, measures of reading and reading comprehension, and language comprehension test) to sample responses of interest. Most of the communicative deficits found in patients with TBI require samples of social communication to make a discourse analysis to assess pragmatic communicative deficits that predominate in these patients. Repeated samples of conversational exchanges will be more useful than standardized tests of language skills in assessing the pragmatic deficits as well as deficits in comprehending abstract or complex information and difficulties in understanding humor, proverbs, and implied meanings of statements. A patient's conversation with people other than the clinician is likely to provide more valid information than structured test items (Gillis, 1996).

Assessment of Dysarthria Associated with TBI

Initially, most clinicians may administer a bedside screening test to evaluate speech intelligibility and note the types and frequency of speech production errors. If dysarthria is extensive and persistent after the initial acute stage, clinicians make a detailed assessment. In evaluating dysarthria, clinicians may use both specialized dysarthria test batteries and traditional tests of articulation. Speech samples will be useful as well. Two commonly used tests are:

- *The Frenchay Dysarthria Assessment* (Enderby, 1983). This test helps evaluate respiration, articulation, resonance, phonation, and reflexive aspects of the motor speech mechanism. Altogether, the test evaluates 28 aspects of the motor speech system including the functioning of the lips, jaw, palate, and the larynx. The sampled skills and the neuromuscular system are rated on a 9-point rating scale, with 9 being normal and 1 being severe dysfunction.

- *Assessment of Intelligibility of Dysarthric Speech* (Yorkston & Beukelman, 1981). This test helps evaluate articulation skills and the resulting speech intelligibility, assessed through recorded productions of selected single words and sentences. The recordings are submitted to independent judges who help evaluate speech intelligibility, rate of speech, intelligible and unintelligible words produced per minute, and a communication efficiency ratio calculated by dividing the intelligible words per minute by 190 (which is the normal speech rate).

Articulation skills of patients with TBI also may be assessed with the traditional tests of articulation that typically sample single word productions and limited sentences. The traditional tests, however, may not accurately reflect the articulatory skills of patients with TBI, as the tests tend not to give credit for distorted sounds that are still intelligible. Moreover, judges who know the test words may overestimate the patient's articulatory proficiency (Yorkston, Beukelman, & Traynor, 1988).

A thorough analysis of dysarthria involves a more detailed assessment of the motor speech system than many standardized tests allow for. In addition to evaluating articulation and speech intelligibility, the clinician should make a detailed assessment of:

- *The respiratory system.* The clinician should assess the respiratory support for speech, the smoothness of the inhalation-exhalation cycles, the degree of forced exhalations, respiratory pressure and flow, and so forth.

- *The phonatory system.* The clinician should assess the laryngeal muscle function and phonation. Laryngeal muscle weakness may be evident when the patient is asked to cough or produce glottal stops. Such voice quality problems as hoarseness, harshness, and strained and strangled voice should be noted.

- *Resonatory system.* This involves an assessment of the adequacy of the velopharyngeal structures and the resonance aspects of speech production. Hypernasality, hyponasality, and nasal escape of air during speech production should be noted.

A detailed description of the motor speech evaluation is beyond the scope of this chapter. Therefore, the clinicians should consult one of several sources available on diagnosis and evaluation of dysarthria (Duffy, 2005; Freed, 2000; Murdoch & Theodoros, 2001; Yorkston, Beukelman, Strand, & Hakel, 2010.

Assessment of Language Skills

As summarized in Chapter 12, various neurobehavioral effects of TBI complicate language deficits. Inattention, confusion, perceptual problems, impulsiveness, emotionality, lack of judgment, reasoning problems, and difficulty with abstract concepts affect their communication skills. Also, as noted, many standardized tests of language skills, especially those used to assess patients with aphasia, do not capture the unique pragmatic communication deficits of patients with TBI. Because of the changing nature of the patient's physical and behavioral condition, assessment should be continuous and adaptive.

Assessment should include systematic and continuous analysis of the patient's physical and behavioral condition, communication and cognitive functions, and general improvement or lack of it. Initial language assessment will be brief and informal, and subsequent assessment will be in-depth and both informal and formal.

- *Systematic and continuous analysis.* The initial condition of the patient may be coma, confusion, or various levels of consciousness. Systematic and continuous analysis of the patient's actions will help document the changing condition of the patient's general behavior, attention and alertness, and communicative attempts. Depending on the results of observation, various aspects of language assessment may be implemented.

- *Analysis of language and communication in the initial stages.* In the initial stages, and especially when the patient recovers from coma or altered levels of consciousness, the patient may be mute or may exhibit confused language. However, as the patient's physical condition improves, the mute patient may begin to talk and confused language may get cleared up. Frequent observation; attempts at simple conversation; and questions about orientation to time, place, and persons will help document the initial communicative status of the patient and subsequent changes.

- *Assessment of language comprehension (receptive language).* During the acute stage of injury when the patient may be confused, simple conversational exchanges may give an idea of the patient's comprehension of spoken language. As the patient's confusion subsides and alertness improves, formal assessment of language comprehension will be productive. The clinician may administer the Peabody Picture Vocabulary Test-Third Edition (Dunn & Dunn, 1997) to assess comprehension of single words. Conversational exchanges may be continuously used to assess improvement in language comprehension. The original Token Test (DeRenzi & Vignolo, 1962) and the Revised Token Test (McNeil & Prescott, 1978) may be used to assess language comprehension. Token tests give a series of commands to assess language comprehension. Although not standardized on adults, the Test for Auditory Comprehension of Language, Third Edition (Carrow-Woolfolk, 1999) may be useful in assessing significant impairments in language comprehension. A reading test, passages from newspapers or magazines, or printed stories—all specifically selected for the given patient—may be used to assess comprehension of silently or orally read material.

- *Assessment of verbal expression.* Various aspects of verbal expression, including naming, word fluency, picture description, and story narration may be assessed either with client-specific procedures or standardized tests. (See Chapter 8 on assessment of aphasia for some of the tests.) Conversational speech samples may be recorded to make an analysis of such pragmatic skills as turn taking, topic initiation, appropriate topic selection, topic maintenance, conversational repair, social appropriateness of speech, rambling, logical sequencing of events, appropriate use of gestures, and so forth. A writing sample will help analyze difficulties in letter formation and word and sentence writing.

Assessment of Dysphagia

Although assessment of dysphagia in patients with TBI is a primary responsibility of speech-language pathologists, space here will not permit a detailed description of the procedures; the reader should consult other sources (Murdoch & Theodoros, 2001). It may be noted that the assessment may require both a clinical bedside evaluation of swallowing and radiological procedures. An initial bedside evaluation will take note of any problem the patient has in swallowing by conducting a few feeding trials and observing the patient during typical feeding times.

Among several formal procedures, the **videofluoroscopy (videofluoroscopic swallowing study)**—a radiological method for examining the physiological processes involved in swallowing—is the most useful and commonly used procedure. In this procedure, the patient is asked to drink or swallow various boluses of foods impregnated with barium (to enhance contrast on X-ray pictures). The swallowing movements and any problems (especially aspiration) are noted and the reasons for the problems are analyzed (Logemann, 1998; Murdoch & Theodoros, 2001).

Ethnocultural Considerations in Assessment

There is little or no research on ethnocultural issues in the assessment of patients with TBI. However, the issues are not likely to be different from those raised in the assessment of aphasia or any other disorder of communication. General guidelines available in the literature on the assessment of clients with varied ethnocultural background apply (Battle, 2002; Screen & Anderson, 1994).

Suggestions offered in the assessment of aphasia in ethnoculturally diverse clients are applicable for patients with TBI. A client-specific approach; minimal dependence on standardized tests that may not be relevant to the patient's ethnocultural background; detailed information on the family's ethnic, cultural, and linguistic background; an understanding of the patient and the family's view of the disability; expectations of the patient and the family regarding rehabilitation will help make an appropriate assessment of an ethnoculturally diverse patient with TBI. See Chapter 8 for details.

Postassessment Counseling

At the end of the assessment session, discuss the results of your assessment with the client and the family members. Most adult clients and their family members want to know your tentative diagnosis, treatment recommendations, and prognosis. They may have additional questions about such topics as the duration of treatment and the availability of TBI support groups.

Describe Your Findings

Begin your counseling by summarizing the results of everything you have learned about the client. Your impressions probably will be based on information from the medical chart, conversations with other medical professionals, formal or informal assessment tools, and your own clinical observations:

- Describe the type of head injury experienced by the client and the areas of the brain affected by the injury, including whether the damage was focal or diffuse.

- Provide an estimate of severity—mild, moderate, or severe.

- Describe the types of assessments you conducted and summarize the results in clear, nontechnical language.

- Describe in general terms the cognitive and behavioral consequences of this type of brain injury—stressing, if appropriate, that you cannot predict whether these cognitive and behavioral issues will appear in this client.

- Describe in general terms the stages of progression for clients with head injury— again stressing that you cannot make a firm prediction of how this client's rehabilitation will proceed. The Rancho Scale may be a good guide for indicating the typical progression of some clients with head injuries.

- Explain your recommendations for treatment, including which cognitive, language, speech, and behavioral deficits may be the primary targets of intervention. Explain the rationales for these treatment targets if there are questions about why they were chosen.

- Provide information on the rehabilitation facility that will be providing the services and describe the other medical professionals that may be involved in the rehabilitation process. It may be useful to include specific information on what each member of the rehabilitation team will be doing with the client on a daily basis.

- Give the client and family plenty of time to ask questions about your findings.

Make Recommendations

Recommending treatment for a head injury is usually appropriate in most cases. Even if the client's head injury is a mild concussion that seems to be resolving spontaneously, a single session that provides reassurance and education about the condition is fully justified. The recommendation for treatment in cases of moderate and severe head injuries should be made promptly after the assessment is complete.

Suggest Prognosis

It is difficult to make a prognosis in cases of TBI, especially in the early stages of rehabilitation. It usually is impossible to predict the outcome of rehabilitation with any degree of certainty. This is because each head injury is a unique and complex disorder, varying in severity, type of injury, and extent of damage. Medical doctors typically use severity and length of coma, in conjunction with size and location of lesions, to make a general prognosis for recovery. Overall, the shorter the severity and length of the coma, the better the client's chances for significant progress in rehabilitation. An explanation of the relationship between coma and rehabilitation may be beneficial to the family as they seek information on the outcome of the recovery process.

Answer Frequently Asked Questions

Mostly because of the many Web sites that offer information on head injury, clients and their families may be fairly knowledgeable about the basics of the disorder. They may ask specific questions about complications, type of head injury, extent of the brain damage, and treatment. The answers clinicians give to the clients' questions should be direct and scientifically based.

The clinician should answer all questions the clients and their caregivers ask. While it is not possible to list all kinds of questions clients may ask, a few commonly encountered questions and potential answers follow. You may need to modify the terms you use to suit the education, prior knowledge, and the judged sophistication of clients and families in formulating your answers.

What types of behaviors might we see when he is home? It is impossible to accurately predict how a client will adjust to the home environment after he or she is discharged from a hospital. This is because there are so many factors that influence a TBI patient's actions, including the severity of the injury, the area of the brain damaged, the personality of the client before the injury, and the dynamics of the family relationships. Nevertheless, the typical behaviors that might occur can be summarized according to severity:

- Mild head injury—fatigue, memory impairment, irritability, headaches, dizziness, and problems with concentration
- Moderate and severe head injury—depression, apathy, childlike egocentricity, anxiety, a quickness for frustration and anger, significant memory deficits, changes in personality, impulsiveness, suspiciousness, dependency, poor judgment, lack of insight, decreased speed of thinking, attention problems, sleeping disturbances, difficulty learning new materials, and fatigue

What are some of the treatment options? The type and intensity of treatment varies with the severity of the injury. In cases of a concussion, the recommended treatment just may be reassurance and education. (For example, clients and families will be reassured to learn that full recovery is possible following a concussion. They also will need to know that the short-term consequences of a concussion include headaches, distractibility, modest memory deficits, fatigue, and irritability, all of which are likely to diminish over time in most cases. They also need to understand the importance of preventing the reoccurrence of another concussion and how the effects of repeated concussions are cumulative.)

Treatment for moderate and severe TBI is much more involved and usually requires the participation of numerous medical professionals. In general, TBI treatment addresses the client's cognitive, language, speech, and behavioral deficits either by enhancing residual skills or by teaching strategies that can compensate for the deficits. The ultimate goal of treatment is assist the client to be as successful as possible in daily activities—at home, school, or work.

How long will treatment take? It depends on several factors. In many cases of concussion, full recovery can occur in hours or days, so treatment beyond reassurance and education usually is not needed. For individuals with moderate and severe head injuries, treatment starts in the acute stages of hospitalization and continues during inpatient and outpatient rehabilitation. In moderate and severe TBI cases, treatment usually takes months (and sometimes years). Family involvement in the rehabilitation process can facilitate rehabilitation by helping to ensure that treatment gains in the treatment sessions are carried over to the home environment. For the most severely injured individuals, long-term in-home care or at a residential facility likely will be needed.

What types of support groups are available in our area? The clinician should be ready to provide the family with a list of supportive organizations or activities that specialize in clients with TBI, including those that offer support for caregivers. Many families may not be interested in such opportunities during the acute and inpatient rehabilitation stages of treatment because of the overwhelming challenges they face during those times. However, once the client is discharged and is living at home, these types of resources and opportunities can be quite helpful in assisting the family with the daily process of caring for a brain-injured loved one.

References

Adamovich, B., & Henderson, J. (1992). *Scales of Cognitive Ability for Traumatic Brain Injury (SCATBI)*. Chicago, IL: Riverside.

Andrews, B. T. (2000). Prognosis in severe head injury. In P. R. Cooper & J. G. Golfinos (Eds.), *Head injury* (4th ed., pp. 555–565). New York, NY: McGraw-Hill.

Battle, D. (2002). Communication disorders in multicultural society. In D. Battle (Ed.), *Communication disorders in multicultural populations* (3rd ed., pp. 3–31). Boston, MA: Butterworth.

Berg, E. A. (1948). A simple objective technique for measuring flexibility in thinking. *Journal of General Psychology, 39*, 15–22.

Beukelman, D., Burke, R., & Yorkston, K. (2002). Dysarthria and traumatic brain injury. In K. Hux (Ed.), *Assisting survivors of traumatic brain injury* (pp. 135–168). Austin, TX: Pro-Ed.

Bigler, E. D. (Ed.). (1990). *Traumatic brain injury.* Austin, TX: Pro-Ed.

Carrow-Woolfolk, E. (1999). *Test for Auditory Comprehension of Language* (3rd ed.). Austin, TX: Pro-Ed.

DeRenzi, E., & Vignolo, L. A. (1962). The Token Test: A sensitive test to detect receptive disturbances in aphasics. *Brain, 85,* 665–678.

Duffy, J. R. (2005). *Motor speech disorders: Substrates, differential diagnosis, and management* (2nd ed.). St. Louis, MO: Elsevier Mosby.

Dunn, L. M., & Dunn, L. M. (1997). *Peabody Picture Vocabulary Test–Third Edition.* Circle Pines, MN: American Guidance Service.

Enderby, P. (1983). Frenchay dysarthria assessment. San Diego, CA: College-Hill Press.

Folstein, M. F., Folstein, S. E., & McHugh, P. R. (1975). "Mini-Mental-State." A practical method for grading the cognitive state of patients for the clinician. *Journal of Psychiatric Research, 12,* 189–198.

Freed, D. (2000). *Motor speech disorders: Diagnosis and treatment.* Clifton Park, NY: Cengage Delmar.

Gillis, R. J. (1996). *Traumatic brain injury: Rehabilitation for speech-language pathologists.* Boston, MA: Butterworth-Heinemann.

Graham, D. I., & Gennarelli, T. A. (2000). Pathology of brain damage after head injury. In P. R. Cooper & J. G. Golfinos (Eds.), *Head injury* (4th ed., pp.133–153). New York, NY: McGraw-Hill.

Hagen, C. (2000). *Rancho Levels of Cognitive Functioning–Revised.* Presentation at TBI rehabilitation in a managed care environment: An interdisciplinary approach to rehabilitation, Continuing Education Programs of America, San Antonio, TX.

Harrington, T., & Apostolides P. (2000). Penetrating brain injury. In P. R. Cooper & J. G. Golfinos (Eds), *Head injury* (4th ed., pp. 349–360). New York, NY: McGraw-Hill.

Helm-Estabrooks, N., & Hotz, G. (1991). *Brief Test of Head Injury* (BTHI). Odessa, FL: Psychological Assessment Resources.

Jennett, B., & Teasdale, G. (1981). *Management of head injuries.* Philadelphia, PA: F. A. Davis.

Jeremitsky, E., Omert, L., Dunham. C. M., Protetch, J., & Rodriguez, A. (2003). Harbingers of poor outcome the day after severe brain injury: Hypothermia, hypoxia, and hypoperfusion. *Journal of Trauma, 55*(2), 388–389.

King, W. J., MacKay. M., Sirnick, A., & The Canadian Shaken Baby Study Group. (2003). Shaken baby syndrome in Canada: Clinical characteristics and outcomes of hospital cases. *Canadian Medical Association Journal, 168*(2), 155–159.

Kraus, J. F., & McArthur, D. L. (2000) Epidemiology of brain injury. In P. R. Cooper & J. G. Golfinos (Eds.), *Head injury* (4th ed., pp. 1–26). New York, NY: McGraw-Hill.

Levin, H. S., O'Donnell, V. M., & Grossman, R. (1979). The Galveston Orientation and Amnesia Test. *The Journal of Nervous and Mental Disease, 167*(11), 675–684.

Logemann, J. A. (1998). *Evaluation and treatment of swallowing disorders* (2nd ed.). Austin, TX: Pro-Ed.

McNeil, M. R., & Prescott, T. E. (1978). *Revised Token Test.* Austin, TX: Pro-Ed.

Murdoch, B. E., & Theodoros, D. G. (2001). *Traumatic brain injury: Associated speech, language, and swallowing disorders.* Albany, NY: Singular Thomson Learning.

Rappaport, M., Hall, K., Hopkins, K. Belleza, T., & Cope, D. (1982). Disability rating scale for severe head trauma patients: Coma to community. *Archives of Physical Medicine and Rehabilitation, 63,* 118–123.

Raven, J. C. (1960). *Guide to the standard progressive matrices sets A, B, C, D, and E.* London, UK: H. K. Lewis.

Ross-Swain, D. (1996). *Ross Information Processing Assessment–Second Edition* (RIPA–2e). San Antonio, TX: Pearson.

Screen, R. M., & Anderson, N. B. (1994). *Multicultural perspectives in communication disorders.* San Diego, CA: Singular.

Stanczak, D. E., White III, J. G., Gouvier, W. D., Moehle, K.A., Daniel, M., Novack, T., & Long, C. J. (1984). Assessment of level of consciousness following severe neurological insult: A comparison of the psychometric qualities of the Glasgow Coma Scale and the Comprehensive Level of Consciousness Scale. *Journal of Neurosurgery, 60,* 955–960.

Teasdale, G., & B. Jennett. (1976). Assessment and prognosis of coma after head injury. *Acta Neurochir (Wien), 34*(1–4), 45–55.

Tien, R., & Chesnut, R. M. (2000). Medical management of the traumatic brain-injured patient. In P. R. Cooper & J. G. Golfinos (Eds.),

Head injury (4th ed., pp. 457–482). New York, NY: McGraw-Hill.

Woodcock, R. W., McGrew, K., & Mather, N. (2001). *Woodcock-Johnson Tests of Cognitive Abilities and Tests of Achievement* (3rd ed.). Rolling Meadows, IL: Riverside.

Yorkston, K. M., & Beukelman, D. R. (1981). *Assessment of intelligibility of dysarthric speech.* Austin, TX: Pro-Ed.

Yorkston, K. M., Beukelman, D. R., Strand, E. A., & Hakel, M. (2010). *Management of motor speech disorders in children and adults.* Austin, TX: Pro-Ed.

Yorkston, K., Beukelman, D., & Traynor, C. (1988). Articulatory adequacy in dysarthric speakers: A comparison of judging formats. *Journal of Communication Disorders, 21,* 351–361.

CHAPTER 14

Assessment of Traumatic Brain Injury (TBI): Protocols

- Overview of TBI Protocols
- Assessment of TBI: Interview Protocol
- TBI Assessment Protocol 1: Orientation and Memory
- TBI Assessment Protocol 2: Perception and Reasoning Skills
- TBI Assessment Protocol 3: Communication Skills

Overview of TBI Protocols

Assessment protocols provided in this chapter help assess TBI disorders in adults in an efficient manner. The protocols offer ready-made formats that clinicians can use in structuring their client and family interviews and assessing various parameters of TBI and its disorders.

The protocols offered in this chapter also are available on the accompanying CD. The clinician may print the needed protocols in evaluating his or her clients. The clinician may combine these protocols in suitable ways to facilitate the evaluation of an adult's TBI.

In assessing adults with multiple disorders, the clinician may combine these protocols with protocols from other chapters. For example, the clinician may combine the TBI assessment protocols with dysarthria assessment protocols (Chapter 6) or aphasia assessment protocols (Chapter 8).

The protocols given in this chapter are specific to TBI disorders in adults. To complete the assessment on a given client, the clinician should combine these disorder-specific protocols with the common assessment protocols given in Chapter 2:

- The Adult Case History
- Orofacial Examination and Hearing Screening Protocol
- Diadochokinetic Assessment Protocol for Adults
- Adult Assessment Report Outline

Assessment of TBI: Interview Protocol

Name _____ DOB _____ Date _____ Clinician _____

Individualize this protocol on the CD and print it for your use. 💿

Preparation

- Review the guidelines given under *The Initial Clinical Interview* in Chapter 1.
- Arrange for comfortable seating and lighting.
- Record the interview on audio or video.
- Initially interview the client alone and then have the accompanying person join the interview.
- Review the case history ahead of time and take note of areas you want to explore during the interview.

Introduction

☐ Introduce yourself. Describe the assessment plan and tell the client the time it will take.

Example: "Hello Mr./Mrs. [*client's name*]. My name is [*your name*] I am the speech-language pathologist who will be assessing you today. I would like to start by reviewing the case history and asking you a few questions. After we finish talking, I will work with you. Today's assessment should take about [*estimate the amount of time you plan to spend*]."

Interview Questions

The questions are generally directed toward the adult client. When interviewing the client and the accompanying person together, it is essential to pose the same, but reworded, question to the accompanying person. A few examples are shown within the brackets; the clinician may use this strategy whenever necessary.

- What is your main concern following your head injury? [What do you think is his (her) main problem?]
- How would you describe this (speech, language, memory, attention) problem? [How would you describe her (his) problem?]
- When did you first notice that your (speech, language, memory, attention) was different? [When did you notice that his (her) abilities were different?]
- [Have you noticed any changes in behavior or personality since the injury?]
- Has your (speech, language, memory, attention) changed over time? If so, how?

(continues)

Assessment of TBI: Interview Protocol (continued)

- What does your family doctor say about your (speech, language, memory, attention) problem?

- Did your family doctor refer you to other specialists?

- What did the doctor(s) tell you?

- Have you seen a speech-language pathologist before? What was the advice?

- Did you follow the advice? Have you received speech therapy before?

- Besides a (speech, language, memory, attention) problem, are you concerned with any other aspects of your speech, memory, or attention abilities?

- How would you describe these other problems? [How would you describe his (her) overall speech?]

- Are there times when your (speech, language, memory, attention) is better or worse? For example, is it better in the morning than in the evening? [Do you also think her (his) (speech, language, memory, attention) varies throughout the day?]

- Do you believe that your (speech, language, memory, attention) problem is affecting your social interactions? Would you describe how?

- Do you think that your (speech, language, memory, attention) problem is affecting your job performance? How is it affected?

- Do you have any other chronic health conditions or concerns?

- Are you currently on any medications?

- Is there anything you would like to add about your problem?

- It looks like I have most of the information I wanted from you. Do you have any questions for me at this point?

- Thank you for your information. It will be helpful in my assessment. I will now work with you to better understand your problem. When we are done, we will discuss our findings.

Review the case history again and ask additional questions if needed.

TBI Assessment Protocol 1: Orientation and Memory

Name _____ DOB _____ Date _____ Clinician _____

Individualize this protocol on the CD and print it for your use. 💿

Ask the client each of the following questions. Score the responses as:

$$0 = \textit{Incorrect} \qquad 1 = \textit{Partially Correct} \qquad 2 = \textit{Correct}$$

Discontinue the questioning in any section if the client appears to be anxious or frustrated with his or her performance. Describe the discontinuation in the "Clinician's summative statement" section at the end of protocol. Before scoring the recent and remote memory subtest, talk to a family member, friend, or caregiver for correct answers if that information is not in the client's medical chart.

Orientation	Scoring
How old are you?	0 1 2
What year is this?	0 1 2
What month is this?	0 1 2
What day of the month is this?	0 1 2
What day of the week is this?	0 1 2
What is your birthday?	0 1 2
What city are we in right now?	0 1 2
What building are we in right now?	0 1 2
What time of day is it right now?	0 1 2
Short-Term Memory	
Repeat these numbers back to me: 7-2-9	0 1 2
Repeat these numbers back to me: 5-1-8-6	0 1 2
Repeat these numbers back to me: 4-9-2-6-8-3	0 1 2
Recent Memory	
What is my name?	0 1 2
What did you have for breakfast this morning?	0 1 2
Who is the president of the United States?	0 1 2
Who is the governor of this state?	0 1 2
What kind of shirt (blouse) did you wear yesterday?	0 1 2

(continues)

TBI Assessment Protocol 1: Orientation and Memory (continued)

Remote Memory	Scoring
Where did you go to high school?	0 1 2
What was the name of your high school?	0 1 2
Do you have brothers or sisters? What are their names?	0 1 2
What was the first car you owned? (Or where was the first house you owned?)	0 1 2
How did you meet your wife (husband)?	0 1 2
Judgment	
What would you do if you found a lady's purse on the sidewalk?	0 1 2
What would you do if you had a flat tire while driving on a freeway?	0 1 2
What would you do if a fire alarm went off in your house late at night?	0 1 2
What would you do if a Girl Scout asked you to buy some cookies?	0 1 2
Attention	
I'm going to say a list of words. I want you to tap your hand on the table each time you hear the word "green."	
Water, sleep, many, green, look, raise	0 1 2
Open, market, baseball, face, candy, green	0 1 2
Fall, story, blue, point, green, snow	0 1 2
Rug, grass, record, purple, green, paper	0 1 2
Clinician's summative statement:	

TBI Assessment Protocol 2: Perception and Reasoning Skills

Name _____ DOB _____ Date _____ Clinician _____

Individualize this protocol on the CD and print it for your use. ⊙

Perception of Colors and Visual Searching

Instructions: Ask the client to point to objects in the room that have distinctive colors. The objects might include a white lab coat, a brown-colored wall, a green rug, and so forth. The verbal instructions are, "Show me something in the room that is white." If there is no response, give a verbal and gestural cue

	Score 0 = Incorrect 1 = Correct with cue 2 = Correct w/o cue
1. Color: _____	0 1 2
2. Color: _____	0 1 2
3. Color: _____	0 1 2
4. Color: _____	0 1 2
5. Color: _____	0 1 2
6. Color: _____	0 1 2
7. Color: _____	0 1 2
8. Color: _____	0 1 2
Clinician's summative statement:	

(continues)

TBI Assessment Protocol 2: Perception and Reasoning Skills (continued)

Perception (Matching Letters)

Instructions: Copy the letters on the following table onto separate pieces of paper. Show the letters one at a time, and ask the client to find its match in the set of 10 letters on the next page. If the client is unable to match a letter, provide a verbal and gestural cue that indicates which horizontal row the item is in (e.g., "It is in this row.").

	Score 0 = Incorrect 1 = Correct with cue 2 = Correct w/o cue
1. U	0 1 2
2. R	0 1 2
3. M	0 1 2
4. O	0 1 2
5. E	0 1 2
6. B	0 1 2
7. H	0 1 2
8. P	0 1 2
9. A	0 1 2
10. F	0 1 2
Clinician's summative statement:	

URMOE

BHPAF

(continues)

TBI Assessment Protocol 2: Perception and Reasoning Skills (continued)

Perception (Recognizing Shapes)

Instructions: Show the diagram with the geomeiric shapes (on the following page), and ask the client to point to the items using the phrase, "Show me the _____." If the client is unable to identify a shape, provide a verbal and gestural cue that indicates which horizontal row the item is in (e.g., "It is in this row.").

	Score 0 = Incorrect 1 = Correct with cue 2 = Correct w/o cue
1. Circle	0 1 2
2. Square	0 1 2
3. Triangle	0 1 2
4. Rectangle	0 1 2
5. Oval	0 1 2
6. Cylinder	0 1 2
7. Arrow	0 1 2
8. Cross	0 1 2
Clinician's summative statement:	

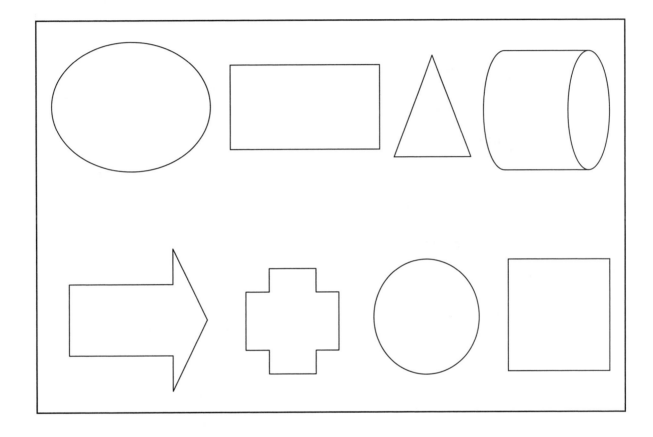

(continues)

TBI Assessment Protocol 2: Perception and Reasoning Skills (continued)

Reasoning (Semantic Categories)

Instructions: "I am going to say a list of words. All of the words are related to each other, except for one. I want you to tell me which word does not belong with the other ones."

	Score 0 = Incorrect 1 = Correct
1. Magazine, sky, newspaper, book	0 1
2. Waterfall, engine, truck, gasoline	0 1
3. Clock, time, hour, minute, hose	0 1
4. Music, knife, spatula, spoon, fork	0 1
5. Sofa, chair, ottoman, rug, table	0 1
6. Sock, glasses, shirt, pants, shoes	0 1
7. Daisy, rose, cactus, tulip, iris	0 1
8. Frog, deer, raccoon, bear, chipmunk	0 1
Clinician's summative statement:	

Reasoning (Inductive)

Instructions: *"I am going to say a word, and I want you to say a word that means the opposite. For example, if I say 'hot,' you would say, 'cold.'"*

	Score 0 = Incorrect 1 = Correct
1. Fast (slow)	0 1
2. Soft (hard)	0 1
3. Poor (rich)	0 1
4. Subtract (add)	0 1
5. Break (fix or repair)	0 1
6. Interesting (boring)	0 1
7. Anonymous (famous)	0 1
8. Graceful (clumsy)	0 1
Clinician's summative statement: 	

(continues)

TBI Assessment Protocol 2: Perception and Reasoning Skills (continued)

Reasoning (Deductive)

Instructions: "I am going to describe something, and I want you to tell me what it is."

	Score 0 = Incorrect 1 = Correct
1. It is round. It is often made of rubber. It will bounce. Children play with it. (ball)	0 1
2. It is far away. It is in the sky. You can see it at night. It sometimes is full. (moon)	0 1
3. It is flat. It is made from wood. It often is white. People write on it. (paper)	0 1
4. You hold it in your hand. It uses electricity. It will ring. People talk on it. (phone)	0 1
5. It is food. It is made of wheat. It usually is sliced. (bread)	0 1
6. It is sharp. It usually is made of metal. You hold it. It is often used in the kitchen. (knife)	0 1
7. People wear them. They have a frame. They sit on your nose. They have lenses. (glasses)	0 1
8. It grows in the ground. It has a trunk. It usually is tall. It can provide shade. (tree)	0 1
Clinician's summative statement:	

Reasoning (Divergent Thinking)

Instructions: "I am going to tell you a word that can have more than one meaning. I want you tell me at least two meanings of each word. For instance, if I said, "bat," you might say, 'It's an animal that flies at night, and it's a stick used in baseball.'"

	Score 0 = Incorrect 1 = Correct
1. Carp (a fish or complain)	0 1
2. Jack (a man's name, or a tool to raise a car)	0 1
3. Palm (a type of tree [plant], or the center of your hand)	0 1
4. Kid (a child, or to tease or joke with someone)	0 1
5. Firm (something that is hard [solid], or a business, such as a law firm)	0 1
6. Bank (the side of a river, or a place to store money)	0 1
7. Fast (something that is quick, or to go without food)	0 1
8. File (a place to store papers, or a tool to shape metal)	0 1
Clinician's summative statement:	

(continues)

TBI Assessment Protocol 2: Perception and Reasoning Skills (continued)

Reasoning (Figurative Language)

Instructions: "I am going to tell you a saying that means more than what it says. For example, "Save it for a rainy day" really means that people should save money for hard times. I want you to tell me the deeper or real meaning of these sayings. Note: These are American idioms and should only be used with native English speakers."

	Score 0 = Incorrect 1 = Correct
1. A Piece of Cake (something that is easy)	0 1
2. To Bend Over Backwards (very willing to help or satisfy)	0 1
3. Can't Cut the Mustard (someone who is not good enough to do something)	0 1
4. To Drive Someone Up the Wall (something that is very annoying or aggravating)	0 1
5. Go Out on a Limb (to take a risky chance to help someone or do something)	0 1
6. Haste Makes Waste (doing something too quickly will result in a poor result)	0 1
7. Know the Ropes (to understand all the details of something)	0 1
8. Pulling Your Leg (someone is joking)	0 1
Clinician's summative statement:	

TBI Assessment Protocol 3: Communication Skills

Name _____ DOB _____ Date _____ Clinician _____

Individualize this protocol on the CD and print it for your use. 💿

Assess Confrontation Naming

Ask questions after presenting a picture. Write down the incorrect responses; take note of the missing article. Score the self-corrections as:

No = *No attempt*   S = *Successful*   UnS = *Unsuccessful*

Clinician's Questions	Correct Response	Incorrect Response	Self-Corrections
What is this?			No S UnS
What is this?			No S UnS
What is this?			No S UnS
What is this?			No S UnS
What is this?			No S UnS
What is this?			No S UnS
What is this?			No S UnS

Assess Responsive Naming

Ask questions with no physical stimulus presentation. Write down the incorrect responses.

Clinician's Questions	Correct Response	Incorrect Response
What do people wear to see better?	"Glasses"	
What is that you are sitting on?	"Chair"	
What do you use to unlock a door?	"Key"	
What do you use to cut vegetables?	"Knife"	
What do you do when you are sleepy?	"Sleep"	
What do you use to write?	"Pen"	
What do you want when you are thirsty?	"Water"	
What do you want when you are hungry?	"Food"	

(continues)

TBI Assessment Protocol 3: Communication Skills (continued)

Assess Categorical Naming (Word Fluency Test)

Give 1 minute for each category. Write down the responses or the number of responses given. Normative studies have shown that non-brain-damaged individuals generate an average of 17 animals in 1 minute. For words beginning with F, A, and S, they average approximately 37 total items (FAS scores combined) (Tombaugh, Kozak, & Rees, 1999).

Clinician's Questions	Client's Responses
"Tell me the names of all the animals you can think of."	
"I will say a letter of the alphabet. I want you to tell me all the words you can think of that start with that letter. Ready? Let's start with the letter 'F.'"	
"Now the letter 'A.'"	
"The last one is letter 'S.'"	

Defining Words

Ask the client to define or describe the following words. Correct responses must contain complete sentences and include the underlined word or words in the correct response column. If a response is incorrect, write it in the Incorrect Response column.

Clinician's Questions	Correct Response	Incorrect Response
What is a pencil?	"It's something to <u>write</u> with."	
What is a telephone?	"You <u>talk</u> to people on it."	
What is a key?	"It's used to <u>open</u> (or <u>unlock</u>) a door."	
What is a camera?	"You use it to <u>take pictures</u>."	
What is a cello?	"It's used to make <u>music</u>" or "It's a musical <u>instrument</u>."	
What is a sailboat?	"It's a boat the uses the <u>wind</u> to go."	
What is an umbrella?	"It's something to keep <u>rain</u> (or <u>water</u>) off of you."	
What is a triangle?	"It's a shape with <u>three sides</u> (or <u>three lines</u>)."	

(continues)

TBI Assessment Protocol 3: Communication Skills (continued)

Reading for Comprehension (Single Sentences)

The clinician shows the client a sentence with the final word omitted; the client reads the sentence and chooses the correct final word in a field of three.

Sentences	A	B	C
Put the key in the _____.	cover	candy	door
I enjoyed reading the _____.	book	shoes	cotton
He plays music on his _____.	tooth	guitar	lamp
While sleeping, he often will _____.	run	snore	flower
The boy missed school because he was _____.	cable	picture	sick
The old movie was in black and _____.	purple	red	white
My doctor is a general _____.	practitioner	contractor	military
Why save money for a rainy _____?	morning	night	day
It is hard to learn a new _____.	language	day	friend
When I was gone, she cleaned the _____.	bathroom	event	better

Reading for Comprehension (Paragraph)

The client reads the following paragraph and then answers multiple choice questions about it. The client can respond either by verbally producing the answer or by pointing to it. Do not let the client see the paragraph while answering the questions.

A fox was taking her babies out for a walk one beautiful morning. As she came to a stream, the fox encountered a lioness with her cub. "Why such airs over one solitary cub?" sneered the fox, "Look at my healthy and numerous litter of five, and imagine, if you are able, how a proud mother should feel." The lioness gave her a squelching look, and lifting up her nose, walked away, saying calmly, "Yes, just look at that wonderful collection. What are they? Foxes! I've only one, but remember that one is a lion." Quality is better than quantity.

Clinician's questions	Choice A	Choice B	Choice C
What time of day were they out walking?	morning	afternoon	evening
Which animal had only one baby?	fox	lion	rabbit
The fox had how many babies?	three	four	five
What was the weather like in the story?	hot	cold	nice
Where did the fox encounter the lion?	on the grass	near the hill	at the stream

Writing the Names of Pictured Items

The clinician presents pictures of single objects or actions and asks the client to write the name of the pictured item. Use color photographs of common objects or activities as the stimuli.

Pictured Items	Correct	Incorrect
Item _____		
Item _____		
Item _____		
Item _____		
Item _____		
Item _____		
Item _____		
Item _____		
Item _____		
Item _____		

Writing Sentences

The clinician asks the client to watch carefully as he or she performs an action. The client is asked to write a complete sentence that describes the action. A correct response contains correct spelling for all words and is a complete sentence (e.g., You snapped your fingers.).

Clinician's actions	Correct	Incorrect
Snap your fingers.		
Rub your chin.		
Knock once on the table.		
Clear your throat.		
Rub your hands together as if you were cold.		
Stretch your arms and yawn.		
Write something on a piece of paper.		
Stand up and sit down.		

Reference

Tombaugh, T. N., Kozak, J., & Rees, L. (1999). Normative data stratified by age and education for two measures of verbal fluency: FAS and animal naming. *Archives of Clinical Neuropsychology, 14,* 167–177.

PART VII

Assessment of Fluency Disorders

CHAPTER 15

Assessment of Fluency Disorders: Resources

- An Overview of Fluency and its Disorders in Adults
- Epidemiology of Stuttering in Adults
- Definition and Measurement of Stuttering
- Additional Features of Stuttering
- Diagnostic Criteria for Stuttering
- Assessment of Stuttering
- Neurogenic Stuttering
- Cluttering
- Assessment of Quality of Life and Functional Communication
- Postassessment Counseling

An Overview of Fluency and its Disorders in Adults

A group of speech disorders is characterized mainly by impaired fluency. A basic feature of fluency disorders is an increased rate of dysfluencies that disrupts the relatively easy, smooth, flowing, and rhythmic nature of speech. Each fluency disorder has several additional features that help distinguish one from the other. In subsequent sections, we will take a look at both the common and unique aspects of each of the fluency disorders.

Specific fluency disorders include stuttering, neurogenic stuttering, and cluttering. Fluency also may be impaired in certain neurological conditions, especially in nonfluent aphasias, but it is not diagnosed as stuttering of any kind. Of these varieties of fluency disorders, stuttering has received the most research and clinical attention because it is the fluency disorder clinicians typically assess and treat in both children and adults.

Assessment of Fluency Disorders in Adults May be Complicated

Assessment and diagnosis of fluency disorders in adults may be more challenging than they are in children. Impaired fluency in adults may have more causal variables than it typically does in children. In children, clinicians frequently diagnose stuttering of early onset as the dominant form of fluency disorders. To a lesser extent, clinicians may diagnose cluttering. In adults, however, a fluency disorder may be diagnosed as stuttering or cluttering as in the case of children, but also as neurogenic stuttering.

To complicate the diagnostic efforts even more, fluency is impaired in many other clients who have sustained neurological damage (e.g., strokes resulting in nonfluent aphasia) or have a neurodegenerative disease (e.g., dementias). Such fluency impairments are not necessarily diagnosed as stuttering or neurogenic stuttering, though they pose differential diagnostic challenges. Therefore, a clinician assessing adults for a potential fluency disorder needs to make a differential diagnosis among several possibilities. The clinician should be fully knowledgeable about the varieties of fluency disorders, their associated clinician conditions, and potential etiological factors.

Epidemiology of Stuttering in Adults

In this book, the term *stuttering* implies that the disorder began during the childhood years, often during the preschool years. Therefore, adults who seek clinical services for their stuttering will have had the disorder for many years, even decades. Their stuttering may have changed over the years. Stuttering severity may have increased over the years. And with that increase, the clients may have developed many additional features, including anxiety and other negative emotional reactions associated with speech, speaking situations, and certain conversational partners. In some individuals, stuttering may have decreased in severity, but is still a communication problem. In others, the problem may have remained relatively stable for decades.

Many adults who seek services will have had therapy for varying durations. Therefore, most adults who seek help are doing so because of either poor outcomes of past therapies or poor maintenance of initially satisfactory outcomes. In either case, the clinician works with many adults who are "experienced" clients. They will have experienced different assessment and treatment approaches.

Epidemiological studies document the distribution of a disease or disorder (incidence and prevalence) in various populations within and across national boundaries. A good knowledge of epidemiological facts about stuttering is essential to assess and counsel the clients, their family members, or both. Generally replicated research has established several observations about the prevalence and incidence of stuttering in general and specific populations (Bloodstein & Ratner, 2008; Culatta & Goldberg, 1995; Guitar, 2006; Yairi & Ambrose, 2005; Van Riper, 1982). The basic concepts, research methods used in studies, and the results obtained, include the following:

- **Incidence and prevalence are two related but different epidemiological concepts.** *Incidence* refers to the appearance of new cases of a disease or disorder during the past 12 months in children or adults who have been free from it. A researcher who states that "one percent of the general population stutters" is describing an incidence. It helps predict the number of children born in a year might begin to stutter. *Prevalence*, on the other hand, is a measure of the number of individuals who currently stutter in a county, state, or region. A head-count type of statement that, "there are 200 children and adults who stutter in the Fresno school district" is a statement of prevalence. Incidence and prevalence figures may be derived from each other when one knows the total population for which an either statement is applicable.

- **The longitudinal and the cross-sectional are the two commonly used methods of research.** In the *longitudinal method*, investigators select a small number of study participants and observe them over a period of time, often for several months or years. The participants selected will be free from the disorder or disease under study. The investigators evaluate the participants on a regular basis (e.g., every two weeks or once a month) to find out how many of them ("normal" at the outset) begin to exhibit the disorder being studied; any such number specifies the incidence of the disorder studied. In the *cross-sectional method*, on the other hand, investigators sample participants from different strata of a defined population (e.g., all elementary school children in a given school district). The strata in this case are the different grades. The investigator may find, for example, that an X number of children in each grade stutter. A total number of children who stutter may be calculated for the entire school district; these numbers specify the prevalence of the disorder. A simpler and more straightforward method of establishing the prevalence of a disorder is to find out the number of children who have been diagnosed with stuttering in educational and clinical facilities in a region or state.

- **Stuttering in adults will have begun in their early childhood years.** Children in their preschool years are especially vulnerable to stuttering. Therefore, assessment of stuttering in adults needs to take into consideration a relatively long history with that disorder.

- **Onset of stuttering is rare in teenagers and adults.** There is a progressive decrease in the number of new cases from preschool years to preteen years. Onset in teenagers is rare and it is rarer still in adults. When an adult is reported to have a sudden onset of stuttering, and it is verified that there was no prior stuttering, the clinician should consider the possibility of neurogenic stuttering or psychiatric stuttering. A more gradual onset reported in an adult may be a relapse of early-onset stuttering that was in remission for years.

- **Stuttering is more common in males than in females.** The reported male:female ratios depend on the age at which they are observed. In the general population, it is close to 3:1 (male:female). In preschoolers, the male:female ratio is closer, perhaps 1.4 to 1. This means that stuttering is more common in preschool or early elementary grade girls than in adult females. But more girls who begin to stutter recover from it, and as a consequence, fewer adult females than males stutter.

- **Roughly 1% of the general U.S. population stutters.** This is a measure of stuttering that persists into adulthood; in a certain number of children, stuttering lasts a few months or years. Therefore, if the transitory stuttering is included in the calculation, the prevalence of stuttering must be higher than 1%, perhaps as high as 5% in the preschool and early elementary grade levels. Between 5% and 10% of the population may have stuttered at one time or another in their lifetime; this is known as the *lifetime incidence* of stuttering.

- **Slightly more than 1% of the European populations stutter.** By and large, European studies report a slightly higher incidence than their American counterparts; the reasons are not entirely clear.

- **Stuttering is found in varied cultures and societies.** Proving the negative is difficult if not impossible, and therefore, it is difficult to show that stuttering *does not* exists in a given society, because a more intensive or extensive observation may uncover the problem. Johnson's (1944) claim that Native Americans do not stutter has since been rejected because stuttering is prevalent among them (Zimmerman, Liljeblad, Frank, & Cleeland, 1983). In most societies, investigators have found people who stutter, although there may be variations in incidence rates (Van Riper, 1982).

- **Family history and gender influence the prevalence rates.** Familial incidence of stuttering is higher than the 1% found for the general population. Nearly half of all individuals who stutter may have a blood relative who also stutters or has stuttered. Females who stutter further increase the risk of stuttering among their descendents.

- **The concordance rates for identical (monozygotic) twins is higher than that for ordinary siblings.** This means that if one member of an identical twin pair stutters, the other member has an increased risk of stuttering. Fraternal twins also have a higher concordance rate than ordinary siblings; this suggests that concordance rates may partly be due to environmental factors (e.g., more similar reactions to twins than to ordinary siblings).

- **Stuttering may be slightly more prevalent in African, including the Caribbean, populations than in whites.** In some African and Caribbean countries, a prevalence rate of 2.5 or higher has been reported. Stuttering in the Hispanic and Asian populations may be roughly comparable to that found in European or American populations (Robinson & Crowe, 2002).

- **Adults who stutter may have any level of intelligence as measured through IQ tests.** An adult who stutters may have normal, below normal, or superior IQ. Stuttering has not prevented many persons from outstanding artistic, scientific, and professional achievements.

- **The prevalence of stuttering may be slightly higher in adults with diagnosed intellectual disabilities** (Bloodstein & Ratner, 2008). In people with Down syndrome, the prevalence is reported to be as high as 53%; even the lowest prevalence level reported, 15%, is much higher than that for the general population (about 1% to 1.5%).

- **Spontaneous recovery is less common in adults than in children.** From an assessment and treatment standpoint, spontaneous recovery is not a significant issue in adults who stutter, while it may be in the case of children. Adults who have been stuttering for years—typically since their early childhood days—most likely need to be assessed and treated.

Definition and Measurement of Stuttering

There is no universally agreed upon definition of stuttering. Varied definitions are a function of differing theoretical orientations. Researchers and clinicians who hold different views on the nature and causation of stuttering define the disorder differently. Nonetheless, theoretical differences have not been a serious impediment to diagnosing stuttering in adults, although a differential diagnosis among stuttering of early onset, cluttering with stuttering, and neurogenic stuttering can be problematic. Difficulties emerge when the clinician has to determine the potential etiologic factors that distinguish the different forms of stuttering (i.e., the different types of dysfluencies that constitute stuttering). Such causal factors often have to be inferred from indirect evidence. Most clinicians diagnose stuttering at a practical level: They evaluate the pattern of behaviors or symptoms and their interrelationships. It is interesting to note that in most cases—adults and children included—family members or the adult clients themselves will have made a diagnosis long before they even make their first contact with a speech-language pathologist (SLP). Clinicians typically confirm the diagnosis based on their assessment.

It is not useful to catalogue the varied definitions of stuttering. Nonetheless, it is essential for clinicians to be aware of some major types of definitions that they are likely to find in research articles, assessment procedures, and treatment manuals.

Stuttering as Avoidance Behavior

Some definitions consider dysfluencies—regardless of their type or frequency—as normal aspects of speech. Stuttering, within these definitions, refers to avoidance behaviors. Two classic definitions, both offered by Johnson, illustrate this kind of definition.

- **Stuttering is an anticipatory, apprehensive, hypertonic, avoidance reaction** (Johnson & Associates, 1959). Johnson considered stuttering to be a reaction developed to avoid the negative consequences of normal dysfluencies. Stuttering emerges as an avoidance reaction because some overly concerned parents diagnose a disorder (stuttering) based on normal nonfluencies that all children exhibit. Faced with the parental criticism of their normal nonfluencies that cannot be avoided, the child then begins to learn various responses that help avoid or mitigate the parental negative reactions. These avoidance reactions are stutterings, not the nonfluencies, or in our term, dysfluencies.

- **Stuttering is what a person does to avoid stuttering.** This alternative definition (Johnson, et al., 1967) underscores the importance of avoidance, not increased frequency or severity of dysfluencies. Therefore, under both the Johnsonian definitions, dysfluencies play a relatively minor role in the assessment and diagnosis of stuttering.

That stuttering is an avoidance behavior is based on the theory that there is no difference in the dysfluency rates of individuals who do and do not stutter. We will see in a later section that this is not the case.

Definitions in Terms of Unspecified Behaviors

Some definitions do not specify the behaviors that imply stuttering. Such definitions characterize stuttering in some molar or global terms.

- **Stuttering is a *moment* that an expert judges it as such.** With this definition, stuttering is assessed subjectively by an expert who judges that a time duration in a speaker's speech contained what he or she considers *stuttering*. Specific types of behaviors that should be considered in the assessment are not precisely described.

- **Stuttering is an *event* so recognized by an expert.** This is essentially similar to the *stuttering is a judged moment* in speech concept. Those who advocate that stuttering is a moment also advocate that it is an event so recognized by an expert. The properties or characteristics of the event are left unspecified, as in the definition of stuttering as a moment in speech.

Definitions that do not specify behaviors that constitute stuttering create problems for objectively measuring stuttering during assessment or treatment. They also pose difficulties in teaching new clinicians to measure stuttering.

Definitions Limited to Certain Dysfluency Types

Definitions that limit stuttering to specific kinds of dysfluencies make a categorical distinction between *stuttered* versus *nonstuttered* types of dysfluencies. A *categorical distinction* implies that certain kinds of dysfluencies are present in the speech of people who stutter and that they are absent in the speech of normally fluent speakers.

- **Some types of dysfluencies are abnormal, hence stuttered, whereas other types are normal.** Several definitions of stuttering are based on the concept that certain kinds of dysfluencies are normal enough to be of no clinical significance and certain other kinds are abnormal enough to be considered stuttering. Normal types of dysfluencies are found in all speakers, whereas the stuttering types are found only in those who stutter. The abnormal types may be described as *stuttering*, *stuttering-like*, or *within-word* dysfluencies. Generally considered to be abnormal are part-word repetitions and speech sound prolongations, although one could add silent prolongations and broken words to this list. All other kinds of dysfluencies (e.g., word and phrase repetitions, pauses, interjections) are considered normal.

- **Stuttering and nonstuttering types of dysfluencies distinguish people who stutter from those who do not.** The distinction is justified on the basis of the observation that stuttering (abnormal) types of dysfluencies are less common in the speech of normally fluent speakers and the nonstuttering types are more common. The distinction is also justified on the basis of some classic listener reaction studies in which lay people were more likely to label speech samples with part-word repetitions and speech sound prolongations as *stuttered* whereas those with other kinds of dysfluencies as *nonstuttered* (Sander, 1963; Williams & Kent, 1958). Unfortunately, these classic studies were biased; the speech samples presented to listeners for their judgment contained more part-word repetitions and sound prolongations than the other kinds. The studies did not show that when speech samples contained other kinds of dysfluencies (e.g., word repetitions or interjections) at certain high frequencies, would not be considered stuttered.

- **There is no complete agreement on the types of dysfluency that are stutterings.** Investigators do not uniformly classify dysfluencies into stuttered versus nonstuttered (or any other) categories (see Bloodstein & Ratner, 2008 and Yairi & Ambrose, 2005 for a discussion of research studies). Some researchers consider only part-word repetitions and speech sound prolongations as stuttering. Others might add silent prolongations. A few include what they describe as blocks—a dysfluency type difficult to define. Some consider single-syllable repetitions as stuttering, but not multisyllabic word repetitions. Still others believe that any whole word repletion, including repetitions of multisyllabic words, is stuttering (Bloodstein & Ratner, 2008; Conture, 2001; Guitar, 2006; Van Riper, 1982; Yairi & Ambrose, 2005). There is yet another distinction between within-word and between-word dysfluency; only the former is considered stuttering, but the repetition of monosyllabic words, which is neither a within-word nor a between-word dysfluency is also considered stuttering (Conture, 2001). Some may consider *tense pauses* as stuttering although others reject all kinds of pauses as clinically nonsignificant (Yairi & Ambrose, 2005). There is also a suggestion that different kinds of dysfluencies may be evaluated as "probably normal," "questionable," and "probably abnormal" (Culatta & Goldberg, 1995). It is not clear how clinicians should evaluate *questionable* dysfluencies. It is also not clear why broken words (within-word pauses) or silent prolongations (silent articulatory postures), which are probably more abnormal than part-word repetitions, should be excluded from the list of stuttered dysfluencies.

The distinction between stuttering versus nonstuttering types of dysfluencies is categorical. Categorical distinctions, however, need clarity. In practice, what appears to be categorical is not at all so because all kinds of dysfluencies may be found in all speakers to a more or less extent. Therefore, counting the presence of only certain kinds of dysfluencies to diagnose stuttering is problematic, as enumerated next.

Definition Based on Quantitative Criteria

A *quantitative criterion* of dysfluencies is based on the assumption that while all dysfluencies may be found in all speakers, the amount will differ. This criterion will also admit that some kinds of dysfluencies may be generally lower in all speakers and other kinds of dysfluencies may be generally higher in people who stutter, but the dysfluency types are not categorically (exclusively) distributed in the two groups (the normal versus the fluency-impaired).

The quantitative (frequency) criterion may help define stuttering in an empirical and practically useful manner. There is enough empirical support and even some consensus among researchers that *frequency* of dysfluencies is important in diagnosing stuttering (e.g., Culatta & Goldberg, 1995; Conture, 2001; Guitar, 2006; Yairi & Ambrose, 2005).

- **No dysfluency type is exclusive to either people who stutter or those who speak normally fluently.** Most if not all researchers agree on this (see Bloodstein & Ratner, 2008, for a review of research and perspectives). There is no dysfluency type, including those considered abnormal (e.g., part-word repetitions or speech sound prolongations) that is totally absent in normally fluent speakers (Bloodstein & Ratner, 2008). Studies have shown, and researchers agree, that most normally fluent speakers will produce, at least on certain occasions, dysfluencies that some categorize as stuttering (Bloodstein & Ratner, 2008; Boey, Wuyts, Van de Heyning, De Bodt, & Heylen, 2007; Carlo & Watson, 2002; Johnson & Associates, 1959; Natke, Sandrieser, Pietrowski, & Kalveram, 2006; Pellowski & Conture, 2002; Roberts, Meltzer, & Wilding, 2009; Silverman, 1972; Silverman, 2004; Westby, 1979). The frequency of part-word repetitions and sound prolongations may be lower in normally speaking individuals than it is in those who stutter; but all people who stutter do not necessarily have a very high frequency of just those two types of dysfluencies. If one ignores the frequency criterion and adheres to a strict categorical distinction between stuttered and nonstuttered dysfluencies, then all speakers are stutterers, at least on occasions when they produce part-word repetitions and speech sound prolongations. This unacceptable position is avoided only when we consider that it is the increased *frequency* of dysfluencies that trigger the diagnosis, not a certain baserate found in most speakers.

- **Frequency, not the presence or absence of some form of dysfluency, distinguishes the clinical and the nonclinical groups.** In people who stutter, frequency of most types of dysfluencies, not just the stuttering-type, increases. The classic study by Johnson and Associates (1959) has documented that children who stutter exhibited all types of dysfluency (except for revisions) at a higher frequency than those who did not stutter. The nonstuttering speech samples had a dysfluency rate of 7.28% whereas the stuttering samples had a rate of 17.91%. Subsequent research, as summarized in various sources has confirmed that people who stutter exhibit a higher frequency of dysfluencies compared to those who speak normally fluently (Bloodstein & Ratner, 2008; Culatta & Goldberg, 1995; Conture, 2001; Yairi & Ambrose, 2005).

- **Researchers who make categorical distinctions agree that frequency is important.** In fact, those who advocate that only certain kinds of dysfluencies are stuttered do so mainly because in the speech of people who do not stutter, their frequency is lower, but *not at zero* (see, for example, Culatta & Goldberg, 1995; Conture, 2001; Guitar, 2006; Yairi & Ambrose, 2005). Therefore, on any type of dysfluency, a categorical distinction (presence in one group of speakers and absent in another) is unsustainable. When all the research on dysfluencies in individuals who do and do not stutter is carefully evaluated, it becomes evident that frequency of dysfluencies of all kinds is the key factor in separating those who do and those who do not stutter.

- **Excessive frequency of any dysfluency may signal a fluency disorder.** Several listener evaluation studies have shown that even word repetitions or schwa interjections—traditionally considered as nonstuttering—may be judged by lay listeners as *dysfluent* or *stuttered*, and in need of therapy, when their frequency exceeds 5% of the words spoken (DeJoy & Jordan, 1988; Hegde & Hartman, 1979a, 1979b). Any kind of dysfluency, when it is excessive in frequency, may raise concerns in listeners, leading to a request or recommendation for intervention.

- **Increased frequency of dysfluencies creates a fluency disorder.** We do not necessarily need a categorical distinction among dysfluencies to justify that stuttering is indeed a disorder. This needs to be stated because some who make a categorical distinction between stuttering and normal types of dysfluency do so to underscore the importance of diagnosing stuttering as a disorder (e.g., see Yairi & Ambrose, 2005). Presumably, a categorical distinction helps reject the invalid Johnsonian assumption that people who stutter do not have a disorder based on dysfluencies, because they just do (more of) what nonstuttering people do. A diagnosis of stuttering based on increased frequency of dysfluencies (e.g., 5% or more of the words spoken) rejects that Johnsonian notion just as forcefully as the diagnosis based on an unsustainable categorical distinction.

- **That something in excess may be a disorder is well established.** Several behavior (psychiatric) disorders illustrate this logic. For example, to diagnose an anxiety disorder in some people, it is neither necessary nor possible to show that "normal" people do not experience anxiety at any level; an increased level of anxiety beyond a certain point is sufficient to diagnose the disorder. There is no categorical distinction between people who are clinically anxious and those who are not in the sense that anxiety is absent in one set of people and it is present in the other set—a categorical distinction. Similarly, a diagnosis of phobia in some people does not necessitate an absence of fear reactions in the nonphobic normal population. Furthermore, a categorical distinction is not the only means to show that stuttering is *qualitatively* different from normally fluent speech, with all its dysfluencies. New characteristics emerge when a behavior of low (and thus normal) frequency turns into a behavior of high (and abnormal) frequency. Once anxiety, phobia, or dysfluencies increase beyond a certain normal limit, the clinical picture becomes more complex.

- **An increased frequency of all or any type of dysfluency adds additional features.** Increased frequency of dysfluencies does not occur in isolation; it brings about additional changes, which may seem like qualitative changes. All qualitative changes are indeed quantitative changes, some of them more easily measured than others. As described in subsequent sections, increased frequency of dysfluencies—all types combined—is associated with increased muscle tension; more rapid and forceful rate of repetitions; increased number of iterations per repetitions; increased duration of dysfluencies, especially prolongations; negative emotional reactions; avoidance behaviors; negative self-evaluations; unfavorable social, educational, and occupational consequences; feelings of lack of control over dysfluencies; and other effects. Increased frequency of dysfluencies along with all such changes, taken together, may be seen as a qualitative distinction between people who stutter and those who do not. Each changed aspect (e.g., muscle tensions or emotional reactions associated with speech and speaking situations) has its normal level from which it increases to an abnormal level. The manner in which increased frequency of dysfluencies creates additional problems and sets the person apart from normally fluent speakers in specific ways is similar to how an increase in normally felt anxiety to clinically significant levels sets someone apart from people not diagnosed with clinical anxiety.

- **Listeners may judge some dysfluency types as abnormal at lower frequency than other types.** Although all types of dysfluency, when emitted at high frequency, may alert the listeners to a fluency disorder (DeJoy & Jordan, 1988; Hegde & Hartman, 1979a, 1979b), the classical view that part-word repetitions and speech-sound prolongations have something special about them, may be valid. What is special about them is not their ability to categorically distinguish persons who stutter from those who do not, however. Their special feature is that they may alert listeners to a fluency disorder at a *lower frequency* than all other types found in a speaker's speech. Possibly such other dysfluency types as broken words (tensed pauses within words) and silent prolongations (prolonged articulatory postures in the absence of voicing) also might alert listeners to a fluency problem at low frequencies. Two listener evaluation studies showed that part-word repetitions, speech-sound prolongations, and broken words (Hegde & Dansby, 1988; Hegde & Stone, 1991) evoke judgment of *stuttered* speech at 3% of the words produced, whereas other types of dysfluencies (e.g., word repetitions and schwa interjections) need to be at 5% or more to be so judged. These results suggest that listeners have a lower level of tolerance for the dysfluency types that are traditionally considered stuttering, and a higher level of tolerance for other types. This differential listener tolerance threshold may be at the heart of the traditional distinction between stuttered or nonstuttered types of dysfluency (DeJoy & Jordan, 1988; Hegde & Hartman, 1979a, 1979b; Hegde & Dansby, 1988; Hegde & Stone, 1991). It may be noted, however, that the differential listener tolerance thresholds for different dysfluency types do not support a categorical distinction between them; they support a distinction based only on frequency, because all dysfluencies cross the threshold of tolerance beyond a certain frequency.

- **Dysfluency durational criterion may be valid in some cases.** As noted, to diagnose stuttering, a criterion of 3% of words stuttered may be acceptable when counting only part-word repetitions, speech sound prolongations, broken words, and silent prolongations. A 5% criterion, however, may be used when all kinds of dysfluencies are counted (including those held at 3%). Nonetheless, what does a clinician do when the dysfluency rates are below even 3%, but there is enough concern about the fluency of a speaker? Such a concern may emanate from dysfluencies that are of low frequency, but more abnormally long in duration than the duration found even in most people who stutter. For instance, most people who stutter because of a high frequency of their dysfluencies may prolong their sounds for about 1 second. What if a person prolongs a sound for 5 seconds but does so only on 2% of the words spoken? There may be justification to diagnose this person as a stutterer. In the first author's clinical and clinical supervisory experience with several hundred children and adults who stutter, this has not occurred, however. A person who exhibits duration of dysfluencies that are longer than what is found in most people who stutter also exhibits a high frequency of dysfluencies. Frequency and duration are possibly correlated; just a high duration but low frequency is unusual at best. Nonetheless, it is practical and prudent to keep the criterion of abnormally long duration as one means of diagnosing stuttering. It should be noted that this criterion of abnormal dysfluency durations references others who stutter, not normally fluent speakers.

- **The number of repetition iterations affects judgments of severity, not the diagnosis of stuttering.** The higher the number of iterations (e.g., t-t-time versus t-t-t-t-t-time), the greater the severity of stuttering. Most clinicians, however, do not precisely measure the number of units of repetition to diagnose stuttering; they depend on the frequency. It is not evident in the literature that a speaker will repeat parts of a word many times, while the frequency of such repetitions remains very low. It is likely that multiple units of repetitions occur in the context of an abnormally high frequency of those dysfluencies. Thus, the frequency criterion might capture the dysfluency durations as well.

As described in the next section, there are other features of stuttering that are important in its diagnosis. Most are not as well quantified as the frequency of dysfluencies. Some of the features may be assessed through standardized tools, while others are clinically observed and described.

Additional Features of Stuttering

While a quantitative criterion specifies the essential conditions for a diagnosis of stuttering, it is important to understand the additional features, that when present, further justify a diagnosis of stuttering. These additional features create significant individual differences in the clinical picture that need to be assessed. The features also have treatment implications. Among the multitudes of additional features found in specific individuals, associated motor behaviors, negative emotional reactions, and mismanagement of airflow are significant.

Associated Motor Behaviors

Stuttered speech may often be associated with a variety of nonspeech motor behaviors. Increased *muscle tension* is an essential feature of these motor behaviors. Most adults who stutter exhibit what appears to be a *struggle* to get the sounds out, prompting Bloodstein (1995) to characterize stuttering as an *anticipatory struggle response*. Increased tension may be most obvious on the face of the person who stutters. Not only the speech muscles, but other muscles, some indirectly related and others not related, may be tensed as well. For instance, muscles of the shoulders, chest, feet, hand, and thigh may be tensed. This tension is typically associated with stuttered speech and may be absent or negligible when the person speaks fluently. Extraneous movements of such tensed muscles during stuttering is called *associated motor behaviors*. Some of the common associated motor behaviors to be noted in a diagnostic session are listed in Table 15–1.

Table 15–1. Varieties of Associated Motor Behaviors Observed in Persons who Stutter

Rapid and tense eye blink
Tensed and prolonged shutting of the eyelids
Rapid upward, downward, or lateral movement of the eyes
Knitting of the eyebrows
Nose wrinkling and flaring
Pursing or quivering of the lips
Tongue clicking
Teeth clenching, grinding, and clicking
Tension in facial muscles
Wrinkling of the forehead
Clenched jaw, or jerky or slow or tensed movement of the jaw
Jaw opening or closing unrelated to target speech production
Tension in chest, shoulder, and neck muscles; including twitching and extraneous movements
Head movements including turns, shakes, jerks, and lateral, upward, and downward movements
Tensed and jerky hand movements including fist clenching and hand wringing
Tensed and jerky arm movements including tapping on the thighs or pressing against the sides of the abdomen
Tensed and jerky leg movements including kicking motions
Tensed and jerky feet movements including grinding, pressing, rubbing, or circular movements on the floor
Generally tense body postures

Assessment of Associated Motor Behaviors

Although muscular tension and associated motor behaviors have been measured in research studies, most clinicians do not routinely measure them. Instead, the clinicians take note of them and describe them in their diagnostic reports. Chapter 16 and the accompanying CD offer a protocol to assess *Motor Behaviors Associated with Stuttering*. The protocol lists the typically observed associated motor behaviors; before printing the protocol, the clinician may add to the list or delete what is not observed in the assessed client. The clinician may rate the frequency of associated motor behaviors on a 3-point scale (1 = Not observed; 2 = Infrequent; 3 = Frequent).

Negative Emotional Reactions

It is well documented that people who stutter experience a variety of unpleasant emotions because of their speech difficulty. Soon after the onset, children begin to experience negative emotions, but their emotional reactions may get stronger and varied as they continue to stutter and grow older. More severe stuttering that persists longer and results in more unfavorable social and personal consequences to the speaker will produce the most profound negative emotional reactions.

The term *negative attitudes* is often used to describe the negative emotional reactions and the associated behavioral tendencies. Negative attitudes are inferred from verbal descriptions of negative feelings and measurable avoidance reactions. For example, a man who stutters might say that he "finds ordering in restaurants very unpleasant" and that he "would rather have someone else order" for him. Such statements may be ascertained during the clinical interview or with the help of a questionnaire. From such statements, the clinician also might infer that the man has a negative attitude toward ordering in restaurants. Therefore, the standard method of indirectly measuring attitudes is to assess negative emotions and avoidance reactions. Some clinicians may consider it sufficient to measure emotional and avoidance reactions and refrain from *inferring* attitudes from what is measured.

Intensity and frequency of negative emotional reactions differ across individuals, but generally they include:

- **Fear, anxiety, or apprehension is a common emotional reaction.** At the least, most adults who stutter tend to be apprehensive of their speech; most are anxious when they expect to speak, and some dread it altogether.

- **The clients feel frustrated at self-expression.** Most will report that they feel frustrated in not being able to speak fluently. Adults who stutter may express their exasperation verbally or nonverbally.

- **The clients make negative statements about themselves.** Often described as "negative self-image," self-reported negative statements about themselves, especially related to themselves as competent speakers, are quite common in people who stutter.

- **Lacking in self-confidence is a common experience.** Most adults who stutter will report a lack of self-confidence in speaking situations. They also may claim that their stuttering is due to their lack of self-confidence in their ability to speak.

The real causality may be reversed: They lack self-confidence in speaking situations because in the past, they have stuttered while speaking in those situations.

- **The clients report unpleasant feelings about speech in general.** That speech is a pleasant experience for most speakers may not hold good for many who stutter. Because of their stuttering, many may find their speaking experience strongly unpleasant.

- **The clients may believe that listeners negatively react to their stuttering.** Some persons who stutter believe that their listeners are impatient, critical, or unsympathetic. Although most people are generally patient, uncritical, and sympathetic, persons who stutter may experience unfavorable reactions from a few individuals who do respond negatively. Some listeners may not be sure of how to react to a person who stutters. Such experiences of people who stutter may be generalized to most listeners.

- **The clients feel embarrassed in social situations.** Most adults who stutter will describe their embarrassment, even feelings of humiliation, when they stutter.

- **The clients feel they lack control over their stuttering.** Some adults who stutter may express the belief that their stuttering may be due to some external, uncontrollable, and inexplicable force. They feel and express a sense of helplessness when they are stuck with stuttering and are thus unable to move forward with fluent expressions. Some experts also believe that stuttering is an involuntary (uncontrollable) response.

Avoidance Behaviors

Persons who stutter tend to avoid specific words, particular speaking situations, and certain conversational partners. This well-established feature of stuttering may be more numerous and pronounced in adults than in children who stutter, although even pre-schoolers who stutter may have significant avoidance behaviors (Hegde & Pomaville, 2008). Each adult who stutters will have a pattern of avoidance reactions that may be unique to that person. Typically observed avoidance reactions in persons who stutter include:

- **The clients may avoid saying specific words.** It may indeed be an effort to avoid stuttering on certain *sounds* at the beginning of words because stuttering is highly correlated with the first sounds on certain words (Bloodstein & Ratner, 2008). Persons who stutter substitute synonyms to avoid stuttering on words that begin with specific sounds. Adults who stutter often can make a list of words or sounds they try to avoid saying.

- **Avoidance of various speaking situations is a common occurrence.** Typically avoided because of their prior history of increased stuttering in them include talking over the phone, ordering in restaurants, speaking in front of formal audiences, introducing self, asking for directions when lost, buying something at a counter, and so forth.

- **Certain conversational partners may be typically avoided.** Although there are individual differences that depend on their past history with stuttering, conversational partners typically avoided may generally include one or both the parents, strangers, authority figures, supervisors or bosses, and persons of the opposite sex.

- **Verbal interactions may be generally minimized.** Minimizing conversation in general, especially initiating conversation, is an often observed avoidance. Persons who stutter may say less or be unusually brief. Some of them may be especially reluctant to talk about their speech problem.

- **During stuttering, the client may avoid eye contact.** Adults who stutter may look away from the listener's face, especially when they stutter.

Avoidance behaviors are conditioned responses. They are reinforced because they reduce such negative emotions as anxiety associated with stuttering. For example, the instant a person who stutters avoids the production of a dreaded word, his or her anxiety is likely to subside; the avoidance in this case is negatively reinforced (becomes stronger). The next time, when the same dreaded word is expected to be produced, he or she will substitute it with another, fluently produced, word. In this manner, avoidance of specific words and speaking situations is perpetuated. During treatment, it is essential to monitor the avoidance reactions of people who stutter. Increased fluency due to treatment should be associated with decreased avoidance. If specific avoidance reactions persist in certain speaking situations, treatment should be extended to those situations.

Mismanagement of Airflow

Stuttered speech in adults may be associated with mismanaged airflow. This problem has been studied in the past as potential respiratory abnormalities, although the conclusions from those studies are that people who stutter do not have inherent respiratory problems (Bloodstein & Ratner, 2008). Airflow mismanagement may be evident during stuttered speech production, but absent during fluent speech. In some individuals, such mismanagement may be a dominant part of the stuttering symptom complex, requiring special attention during treatment. Specific ways in which persons who stutter mismanage their airflow during stuttering include the following:

- **Persons who stutter may try to speak with an insufficient air supply.** They may attempt to speak on limited or shallow inhalation. Consequently, they tend to run out of air at the end of phrases and sentences. Sometimes, the speaker appears to be squeezing the last bit of air from his or her lungs to continue speech production.

- **The clients may attempt speech during exhalation.** Unlike people who speak normally fluently, persons who stutter may speak while they exhale air; the speech thus produced is often stuttered.

- **Impounding inhaled air in the lungs may be an additional problem.** The person who stutters may hold the inhaled air by suddenly closing the glottis. The person may appear to make an attempt to speak while the air is impounded.

- **The airflow may suddenly stop during speech production.** The person may suddenly stop the airflow in the middle of speech production, causing silent prolongations or "blocks."

- **Respiration may be dysrhythmic.** Inhalations and exhalations may disrupt each other.

- **The airflow may be noisy.** Audible inhalation, exhalation, or both may be evident in some individuals.

- **The airflow may be uneven.** Persons who stutter may have difficulty maintaining an even airflow throughout an utterance.

Diagnostic Significance of Additional Features

Individuals widely differ in the number and severity of additional features. These features are more likely the result, not causes, of stuttering. For instance, a person who avoids speaking on the telephone does so because of his or her past history of stuttering on the telephone. Fear may be a part or cause of this avoidance, but neither the fear of, nor the avoidance of speaking on the telephone preceded stuttering when it began in early childhood. To claim causality, it is essential to demonstrate such precedence in preschoolers in whom stuttering typically begins. Similarly, it is only because of the past stuttering that a person feels anxious in certain speaking situations.

Although it is important to assess the additional features, a diagnosis of stuttering does not depend on them. The burden of diagnosis falls on the core behaviors of stuttering: increased frequency of dysfluencies that then caused the additional features. In the absence of speech disruptions, none of the described additional features would lead to a diagnosis of stuttering (Yairi & Ambrose, 2005). For example, a nose wrinkle, fear of speaking situations, avoidance of talking on the phone, in the absence of increased speech dysfluencies, would not be a basis to diagnose stuttering. Such reactions may be associated with (or caused by) other clinical conditions as well. Some people, for example, may avoid speaking situations because of their audience phobia, not stuttering. Others may wrinkle their noses when they fluently express disapproval or disgust. A person may be reluctant to talk on the telephone because of his or her severe apraxia, spasmodic dysphonia, global aphasia, or severe dementia.

Diagnostic Criteria for Stuttering

Even though a total consensus is difficult to achieve, there are trends in data and threads in the thinking of most experts that frequency of dysfluencies with a differential consideration of types as well as the duration of dysfluencies, will give a reasonable basis to diagnose stuttering in adults and children. Therefore, we define stuttering as **a fluency disorder characterized by excessive frequency or duration of dysfluencies, with consequent and variable additional features.** Accordingly, stuttering may be diagnosed when:

- dysfluencies of all types exceed 5% of the words spoken

- part-word repetitions, speech-sound prolongations, and broken words exceed 3% of the words spoken

- measured duration of any dysfluencies are clinically judged to be abnormal, regardless of the frequency of dysfluencies

In most adults who stutter, additional features, summarized in the previous section, may support the diagnosis of stuttering. In the presence of an increased dysfluency rate, mismanaged airflow, associated motor behaviors, anxiety about speech and speaking situations, and avoidance of speech and speaking situations will help confirm the diagnosis and suggest treatment targets. The described diagnostic criteria may be adhered to, even when the additional features are minimal. Table 15–2 describes the dysfluencies that are measured in the assessment of stuttering in adults.

Table 15–2. Types and Examples of Dysfluencies Measured in Assessing Stuttering in Adults

Dysfluency types	Examples

Repetitions
    Part-word repetitions
    Whole-word repetitions
    Phrase repetitions
	"What t-t-t-time is it?"
	"What-what-what are you doing?"
	"I want to-I want to-I want to do it"

Prolongations
    Sound/syllable prolongations
    Silent prolongations
	"Lllllet me do it"
	A struggling attempt to say a word when there is no sound.

Interjections
    Sound/syllable interjections
    Whole-word interjections
    Phrase interjections
	"um . . . um I had a problem this morning."
	"I had a well problem this morning."
	"I had a you know problem this morning."

Silent Pauses A silent duration between words and sentences considered too long	"I was going to the (pause) store."
Broken Words A silent pause within words (intralexical pause)	"It was won (pause) derful."
Incomplete Phrases A production that includes an incomplete phrase	"He wanted to—I think I will not say any more."
Revisions A production that involves word changes	"I will take a taxi, . . . a cab."

Assessment of Stuttering

Assessment of stuttering in adults is a multifaceted activity. The clinician needs to assess the dysfluency rates in conversational speech. To establish a reliable percentage of dysfluencies, the clinician needs an extended speech sample; in most cases, more than one sample may be needed. To calculate the percent dysfluency rate, the clinician should count the number of words or syllables, as preferred. It is recommended that the percent dysfluency rates be established based on the number of words spoken, because the calculation based on syllables produced inflates fluency. The clinician also needs to assess associated motor behaviors, emotional reactions, and avoidance behaviors. A thorough case history and interview with the client and his or family members will help assess the onset and development of stuttering along with its effects on the client's life and work. All clinicians will also include such standard assessment procedures as a hearing screening and orofacial examination. Table 15–3 gives an overview of assessment of stuttering in adults.

Common assessment protocols, including an *Adult Case History* and *Orofacial Examination and Hearing Screening*, are provided in Chapter 2. Therefore, in this section, we will consider the assessment of the core behaviors that constitute stuttering: dysfluencies and their clinical measurement for diagnosing stuttering.

Assessment of Dysfluency Rates

It was suggested earlier that whether only certain kinds of dysfluencies are considered to be stutterings or whether all kinds may be so considered, the frequency of dysfluencies has to be measured to diagnose stuttering. Once the frequency of all kinds of dysfluencies is measured, clinicians are free to diagnose stuttering on the basis of some or all types.

Table 15–3. An Overview of Stuttering Assessment

1. History of the client, family, and stuttering
2. Interview of the client and his or her family members
3. Orofacial examination
4. Hearing screening
5. Speech and language sampling
6. Assessment of stuttering: Measuring dysfluency rates in conversational speech and oral reading
7. Assessment of associated motor behaviors
8. Assessment of avoidance and emotional reactions
9. Measurement of speech rate, word output, and the percentage of dysfluency in conversational speech and reading
10. Recommendations and report writing

Clinicians should strive for both *intraobserver* and *interobserver* reliability. By repeatedly measuring dysfluencies in the same sample of the same client and achieving consistency of scores, the clinician can establish intraobserver reliability. By having another clinician measure dysfluencies in the same speech sample and comparing the measure with one's own, the clinician can establish interobserver reliability. Both are essential to make valid judgments about the presence of stuttering, the extent of its severity, and its improvement under treatment.

Stuttering (dysfluency rates) in adults may vary across days. Therefore, it is essential to get repeated speech samples. To achieve an adequate speech sample and to reliably measure dysfluencies, the clinician may take the steps that follow.

- **Audio- or videorecord one or more conversational speech samples.** With adult clients, the clinician can use various conversational topics of interest to audio- or videorecord naturalistic conversations. The initial clinical interview affords an excellent opportunity to record naturalistic conversational speech samples. During this interview, the clinician has an opportunity to raise varied topics that help sample dysfluency rates as the clients talk about their stuttering problem, how it started and developed, and what effects it had on their life and work. The clinician also can record another sample of conversation with a family member, friend, or other informant.

- **Audio- or videorecord an oral reading sample.** An oral reading sample may reveal a certain pattern of dysfluencies that may not be easily detected in conversational speech. A dysfluency rate that is higher in oral reading than in conversational speech may suggest that the client tends to stutter on specific sounds and words that cannot be avoided in oral reading, but can be in conversation by word substitutions and circumlocution.

- **Tape-record a monologue.** Ask the client to speak on a topic of interest for a few minutes. Keep your interruption to a minimum. Dysfluency rates may be lower in monologues than in conversation.

- **Obtain taped speech samples from home.** Adult clients may be asked to bring a taped speech sample for the assessment session or they may bring one for the next appointment. Ask the client to audio- or videotape two or three samples with different conversational partners, recorded on different days.

- **Listen to the samples once without counting dysfluencies.** This action helps you get familiarized with the client's speech, the types and patterns of dysfluencies, speech and language skills, and any idiosyncratic expressions. This step may be skipped if the clinician is experienced or is familiar with the client. Familiarity with speech helps measure dysfluencies efficiently and reliably.

- **Count and record all types of dysfluencies.** This is done either on the first or second listening. Repeat the measurement within a week if unsure of your count or any two of your measures differ widely. At the least, two of the three measures should be close to each other. Use the guidelines given in Table 15–4 to measure dysfluencies. *Use the Dysfluency Measurement Protocol* given in Chapter 16 (also on the CD) to record the frequency of dysfluencies.

Table 15–4. Guidelines on Measuring Dysfluencies

Dysfluency	Counting
Sound repetitions	Count them as one instance, regardless of the number of units of repetitions in an instance (e.g., *t-time* or *t-t-t-t-time* are both counted as one instance of part-word repetition). Consider the number of units if judging severity of stuttering.
Syllable repetitions	Count them as either word repetitions or part-word repetitions (e.g., *I-I-I* contains a word repetition whereas *t-t-t-time* contains a part-word or sound repetition).
Sound prolongations	Count as one instance, regardless of their length. If judging the severity of stuttering, take note of the durations. A prolongation of 1 second is clinically significant, but even that of 500 ms may be so.
The same type of dysfluency that is separated by another dysfluency or a period of fluency	Count the same type twice (e.g., *um . . . wha, wha . . . um what time is it?* has two interjections separated by a part-word repetition)
Silent pauses	Judge the appropriateness of pauses at their junctures.
Silent prolongations (articulatory postures with no voicing)	Count them as separate from sound prolongations.
A chain of mixed dysfluencies in which one form of dysfluency is followed by another with no fluent productions in between	Count the different types of dysfluencies in the chain separately (e.g., *I-I-I um IIIIlike to-to-to um d-d-do this this this mmmethod*).

- **Count and record the number of dysfluencies in oral reading.** Use the same guidelines given in Table 15–4. You may use the *Dysfluency Measurement Protocol* given in Chapter 16 (and on the CD) to record the dysfluencies. Alternatively, use a double-spaced printed copy of the passage the client reads orally and make notations of dysfluencies on it. Write abbreviations for different forms of dysfluencies on top of the word (e.g., *pwr* for part-word repetitions, *pro* for sound prolongations) or write abbreviations in between words (e.g., *si* for sound interjection, *pi* for phrase interjections).

Analysis of the Speech Sample

To diagnose stuttering based on a quantitative criterion, it is essential to calculate the percent dysfluency rate for different kinds of speech tasks (conversational speech, monologue, oral reading, and home speech sample). The rate should be calculated separately for each of the speech tasks. The *Dysfluency Measurement Protocol* given in Chapter 16 (and on the CD) facilitates this task. To accomplish this, the clinicians should do the following.

- **Calculate the total number of dysfluencies.** Use the *Dysfluency Measurement Protocol* to record the total number of dysfluencies for the different kinds of speech and reading samples. Next, derive the grand total of dysfluencies observed in the various samples collected.

- **Count the number of words spoken or read in a sample.** Use the following guidelines:
  - Exclude all interjected sounds, syllables, words, and phrases—they are counted as dysfluencies (e.g., do not add *ums* and *you know* to the word count; they are added to the dysfluency count).
  - Count the single-syllable words as one word (e.g., the pronoun *I* is counted as a single word).
  - Count the whole word as one word, disregarding the part that is repeated (e.g., t-t-t-time is counted as one word).
  - Determine the total number of words for each speech sample and oral reading sample separately.

- **Calculate the percent dysfluency rate.** Use the following formula to calculate the percentage separately for each speech and oral reading sample:

$$\frac{\text{The total number of dysfluencies in the sample}}{\text{The total number of words in the sample}} \times 100 = \% \text{ dysfluency rate}$$

- **If necessary, obtain additional samples.** As noted earlier, additional samples and measurement of dysfluencies in them may be necessary if any two samples show widely discrepant dysfluency rates.

- **Diagnose stuttering and write a report.** Summarize and integrate all data, diagnose stuttering if data support it, and write a clinical report. Use the *Assessment Report Outline* given in Chapter 2 and on the CD.

Assessment of Stuttering Variability

It is important to assess how stuttering varies across speaking situations. Typically, clients may stutter more or less in certain speaking situations. Situational variability in stuttering has treatment implications. If a client's stuttering is more frequent and more severe in certain situations, treatment effects may not readily generalize to those situations. The clinician or a trained caregiver may have to give informal therapy in those difficult situations associated with higher rates of stuttering.

A behavioral questionnaire is the most efficient method of assessing variability in stuttering across speaking situations or speech tasks. The clinician may use the *Stuttering Variability Assessment Protocol* in Chapter 16 and on the CD to complete this assessment task.

Assessment of Negative Emotional Reactions

To what extent and how formally clinicians assess negative emotional reactions depend on whether they take one or the other of the two perspectives that exist on the role the negative emotions play in the origin and treatment of stuttering. One perspective holds that negative emotions are *causes* of stuttering; the other perspective holds that negative emotions are the *results* of stuttering. Obviously, these two perspectives have different consequences for assessment and treatment of stuttering.

Clinicians who believe that negative emotions are causally related to stuttering assess emotional reactions in greater detail and depth than those who consider them as consequences of stuttering. They may use standardized instruments that help assess negative emotional reactions. Negative emotions (e.g., anxiety about stuttering on a word, in a situation, or in front of a certain person) are conditioned reactions that lead to avoidance behaviors (see the next section for details). Therefore, most assessment instruments evaluate both negative emotions and avoidance behaviors. Generally, the method is that of rating scales that contain questions about speech and speaking situations. Persons who stutter rate each item that describes a speech situation, emotional reactions, or avoidance behaviors (from which negative emotions may be inferred).

There are several rating scales to measure negative emotions or attitudes. For instance, the S-Scale (Erickson, 1969), designed to measure speech-related attitudes with 39 items, consists of such statements as *"I dislike introducing one person to another,"* to which the person who stutters responds *True* or *False*. A shorter and more reliable version of the S-Scale with only 24 items was developed by Andrews and Cutler (1974).

Brutten and Vanryckeghem (2003) have published a *Behavior Assessment Battery* (BAB) that is both comprehensive and well researched for reliability and validity. The test battery includes the following 3 subtests:

- *BigCAT: A Communication Attitude Test for Adults.* This subtest consists of 35 items that include such statements as: "There is something wrong with the way I speak" and "Some people make fun of the way I talk." Most of the statements are about how a person who stutters thinks about his or her speech.

- *Speech Situation Checklist.* This subtest describes 51 speaking situations. Examples include *talking on the phone* or *selling a product*. It has two sections on which the items are repeated. One section, called the *Emotional Reaction (SSC-ER)*, helps assess such negative emotions as anxiety, concern, tension, and worry experiences in speaking situations. The persons who stutter rate their negative emotions on a 5-point scale (*none* to *very much*) experienced in the described speaking situations. The other section, *Speech Disruption (SSC-SD)*, helps assess the degree of speech disruption experienced in the same 51 speaking situations with a 5-point scale (*not at all* to *very much*).

- *Behavior Checklist (BCL).* This subtest is a checklist of behaviors that persons who stutter exhibit in an effort to terminate or avoid their stuttering; the authors consider them *coping strategies*. Most of the listed behaviors are associated motor behaviors (e.g., "wrinkle your forehead" or "move your arm"). Other behaviors listed are verbal (e.g., "hum before speaking" or "add a sound to a word"). Some are avoidance reactions (e.g., "omit a particular word or words" or "substitute one word for another.")

The *Overall Assessment of the Speaker's Experience of Stuttering* (Yaruss & Quesal, 2006) is another instrument that helps assess emotional and cognitive aspects of stuttering. It uses a 5-point rating scale and consists of four sections:

- *Section I. General Information.* It helps assess the extent of knowledge the person who stutters has about stuttering (e.g., "stuttering in general" or "factors that affect stuttering") and feelings about ability to communicate stuttering treatment (e.g., "your speaking ability" or "techniques for speaking fluently").

- *Section II. Your Response to Stuttering.* This section helps assess feelings (e.g., "helpless," "angry"); tension, associated motor behaviors, and avoidance; and the views persons who stutter hold about their speech and stuttering (e.g., "I do not want people to know that I stutter" or "I cannot accept the fact that I stutter").

- *Section III. Communication in Daily Situations.* This section helps assess the degree of difficulty in various speaking situations (e.g., "talking while under pressure," or "using the telephone at work").

- *Section IV. Quality of life.* This sections helps assess the degree to which stuttering affects a person's life and work in general (e.g., "relationship with family," or "sense of self-worth or self-esteem").

Several other rating scales are available and clinicians who wish to use them may consider other sources (e.g., Bloodstein & Ratner, 2008). Before using any of the available tests, clinicians should examine the reliability and validity data the authors present for their assessment tools.

Assessment of Avoidance Behaviors

The clinical interview is an excellent vehicle to assess avoidance behaviors of clients who stutter. During the interview, clinicians may ask questions about avoidance behaviors a client might exhibit. In addition, the clinician may take note of word substitutions and circumlocutions that suggest potential avoidance of certain words. An efficient method of assessing avoidance behaviors is to use a behavioral questionnaire that lists most commonly observed avoidance reactions. In the form of such a questionnaire, Chapter 16 and the accompanying CD offer a protocol to assess *Avoidance Behaviors Associated with Stuttering.*

Some standardized assessment batteries include subtests or specific items that help assess avoidance. For instance, the *Behavior Checklist* subtest of the *Behavior Assessment Battery for Adults* (Brutten & Vanryckeghem, 2003) contains several items related to avoidance. When the entire battery is administered, the clinicians will have assessed various aspects related to the experience of people who stutter, including avoidance reactions.

Assessment of Airflow Mismanagement

Most clinicians assess mismanagement of airflow informally and symptomatically. Throughout the assessment session, the clinician may take note of whether the client attempts speech while the airflow is being exhausted, while inhaling air, or whether the flow of air abruptly stops during speech production.

When a person who stutters exhibits multiple and serious airflow problems during stuttered speech, it may be necessary to address them in treatment. An airflow management program may then be a part of the treatment plan for such an individual (Hegde, 2007).

Neurogenic Stuttering

Neurogenic stuttering or *acquired stuttering* is associated with neurological disorders. The term *acquired stuttering* may not necessarily help distinguish neurogenic stuttering from stuttering of early childhood onset because the latter is also acquired (neither strictly inherited in all cases nor congenital). Unlike the more typical stuttering of early onset, neurogenic stuttering has its onset in adulthood (Duffy, 2005; Hegde, 2008a, 2008b; Helm-Estabrooks, 1999).

Neurogenic stuttering is often associated with several neurological disorders, including (Duffy, 2005; Hegde, 2008a, 2008b; Helm-Estabrooks, 1999):

- strokes with or without aphasia

- apraxia of speech with its underlying neuropathology

- extrapyramidal diseases (especially Parkinson's disease)

- brain tumor

- encephalitis

- dementia associated with Alzheimer's disease and dialysis dementia (in patients who receive dialysis over 3 to 4 years for their renal failure)

- anorexia nervosa

- drug toxicity (especially those prescribed for asthma, depression, and convulsion disorders)

- bilateral brain damage and multiple lesions of a single hemisphere (causing persistent stuttering)

- unilateral brain lesions (typically causing transient neurogenic stuttering)

Neurogenic stuttering may be characterized by all forms of dysfluency. There are some diagnostic features that may help distinguish neurogenic stuttering from stuttering of early childhood onset. The features that help distinguish the two forms of stuttering are presented in Table 15–5.

Assessment of neurogenic stuttering will be based on the differential symptoms listed in Table 15–5 as well as the results of neurodiagnostic techniques. A documented neuropathologic condition is essential for the diagnosis. A *Neurogenic Stuttering Assessment Protocol* is presented in Chapter 16 (and on the CD) for clinical use.

Cluttering

Another disorder of fluency, cluttering is characterized by rapid and irregular speech rate, indistinct articulation, and possibly some language and thought disorders. It is also known as *tachyphemia*. Cluttering gives the impression of hurried speech even under normal or relaxed conditions. Cluttering is associated with stuttering. This means that people who clutter tend to stutter as well, although those who stutter do not have a higher-than-normal chance of cluttering.

Table 15–5. The Features that Help Distinguish Neurogenic Stuttering from Stuttering of Early Onset

Neurogenic Stuttering of Adult Onset	Stuttering of Early Childhood Onset
Presence of neurological symptoms	Absence of neurological symptoms
Late onset, often in older people	Early onset, especially in preschool and early grade-school years
Repetitions of medial and final syllables in words	Absent or uncommon
Dysfluent production of function words	May be present in children who stutter, but uncommon in adults who have been stuttering from their childhood years
Dysfluencies even in imitated speech	Less likely
Dysfluencies during whispered speech	Whispered speech is typically fluent
Rapid speech rate or unpredictable rate	Both uncommon
The adaptation effect, minimal or negligible	Significant adaptation effect
Lack of muscular effort associated with stuttering	Presence of muscular effort, associated with stuttering
Few or infrequently observed associated motor behaviors although facial grimacing and foot tapping may be observed	Several and frequently observed associated motor behaviors
Less evident tension and anxiety associated with stuttering	More evident tension and anxiety associated with stuttering
Lack of improvement in stuttering under shadowing, unison speaking, delayed auditory feedback, and masking	Improvement in stuttering under shadowing, unison speaking, delayed auditory feedback, and masking
Problems in copying and drawing, block designs, sequential hand positions, and tapping out rhythms (all nonverbal symptoms of brain injury)	No clinically significant problems in copying and drawing, block designs, sequential hand positions, and tapping out rhythms
Presence of such other problems as dysphagia, seizures, paresis, or paralysis	Absence of such other problems
Other behavioral symptoms that are typically associated with brain injury (e.g., attention deficit, impulsive behavior)	Such symptoms are typically absent or nonsignificant

Much of the early information on cluttering was published in German. Probably underdiagnosed in the United States, the prevalence rate of cluttering in the United States is not well established. Publications in English on cluttering have been on the increase (see review of literature by Daly, 1986; Daly & Burnett, 1999; Myers & St. Louis, 1992).

The causes of cluttering are not well understood. No particular gene or genes have been identified. Nonetheless, the importance of genetic variables is underscored by the observed familial tendency to clutter (Myers & St. Louis, 1992). In about 50% of people who clutter, studies have documented deviant electroencephalographic (EEG) findings.

The distinguishing features of cluttering include the following (Daly, 1986; Daly & Burnett, 1999; Myers & St. Louis, 1992):

- **Rapid speech rate is a basic characteristic.** An abnormally fast rate that may progressively accelerate (*festinating* rate of speech). Increased rate may be evident even within multisyllabic words. Periodically, the speech may be highly rushed, compressed, and telescoped. The rapid rate, especially its compressed nature, leads to articulatory breakdowns. It is the rapid and indistinct speech that distinguishes cluttering, because some speakers are capable of speaking rapidly, yet clearly.

- **Articulatory breakdowns are related to the rapid speech rate.** Although a person who clutters may have an independent articulation disorder, articulatory breakdowns evident in most who clutter are due to their hurried speech. In their urgency to move fast with their speech production, people who clutter omit sounds, syllables, and even words. They may reduce consonant clusters to singletons, transpose sounds within words, and invert the order of sounds. The result is greatly reduced speech intelligibility.

- **Increased frequency of dysfluencies is common.** People who clutter repeat longer words and phrases, frequently revise their sentences, and interject with extraneous words and phrases. While pausing at inappropriate junctures, they may fail to pause at appropriate junctures (e.g., between sentences).

- **Features that characterize stuttering may be somewhat diminished.** Struggle during dysfluent speech productions, associated motor behaviors, word substitutions and circumlocutions, or anxiety about speech and speaking situations that typically accompany stuttering of early onset may be diminished or absent in people who clutter. People who clutter as well as stutter may have these features as prominently as their cluttering features.

- **Fluency may improve under demanding conditions.** Unlike people who stutter, those who clutter may be more fluent under stressful or demanding conditions. Drawing attention to dysfluencies might decrease them. People who clutter may be more fluent while giving short answers, talking in a foreign language, and speaking after interruption.

- **Language difficulties are possible.** Variable across individuals who clutter, language problems may be significant in some. Disorganized syntactic structures, run-on sentences, and incorrect use of prepositions and pronouns have been noted in some individuals. In addition, poor narrative skills (improper sequencing of ideas or events), inappropriate interjections of topics, and poor topic maintenance; word-finding problems; generally inadequate language formulation; poor listening skills and short attention span; a general verbosity; tangential expressions; and poor eye contact also have been noted.

- **Prosodic problems may be evident.** Possibly due to their festinating speech rate, people who clutter have impaired rhythm of speech.

- **Some may have voice problems.** Loud to begin with, the voice may fade toward the end of sentences. The voice may be monotonous as well.

- **Thinking may be disorganized.** These difficulties are inferred from language impairments and include short attention spans, lack of self-monitoring, and an inability to take into account the perspective of the listener, and a lack of appreciation of the listener's difficulty in understanding one's own speech.

- **Motor incoordination may be an additional feature.** People who clutter may be hasty, clumsy, and uncoordinated in their movements. Their sequencing of complex actions may be impaired and they may have difficulty imitating simple rhythmic patterns. Their poor motor control may affect their handwriting.

- **Some may have reading difficulty.** What starts out as normal oral reading may soon deteriorate. There may be numerous mistakes in oral reading.

- **Some may have writing problems.** People who stutter may write in a disintegrated fashion, characterized by poor spelling, sentence fragments, run-on sentences, omission and transposition of letters; and omission of words.

- **People who clutter may be unconcerned about their speech problem and its effects.** Unlike those who stutter, people who clutter seem to be unaware of, less aware of, or unconcerned about, their speech problem and its effects on listeners. Believing that somehow their listeners have some kind of difficulty understanding them, people who clutter are less willing to seek treatment than those who stutter.

- **Some may be accomplished in mathematics or science.** Some who clutter may excel in specific areas in spite of their communication problems. Exceptional mathematical and scientific accomplishments have been noted in some clients.

Clinicians may use the *Cluttering Assessment Protocol* presented in Chapter 16. They may individualize the same protocol given on the accompanying CD for their clinical use.

A valid diagnosis of cluttering requires that the clinician distinguish it from independent disorders of stuttering, articulation, or language. If there is evidence of an independent disorder of articulation, the clinician may analyze the speech sample to describe them. It is essential, though, that the person who clutters should be asked to say individual words at a slow rate to detect an independent disorder of articulation. Articulatory breakdowns in rapid connected speech are not evidence of an independent disorder of articulation, as that feature is indeed diagnostic of cluttering. Syntactic and morphologic disorders, however, may be assessed through language and writing samples. A coexisting stuttering may be assessed with all the stuttering assessment protocols given in Chapter 16 and on the CD.

Assessment of Quality of Life and Functional Communication

Quality of life and functional communication skills are two other concerns in assessing fluency disorders. Although all fluency disorders may negatively affect the quality of life, functional communication may be differentially affected by the different fluency disorders.

Compared to those with severe forms of aphasia, apraxia of speech, or dementia, functional (basic) communication may be less problematic for most adults with stuttering or cluttering. Unless there is a coexisting language problem or an intellectual disability, people who stutter or clutter tend to have normal or even superior language skills, though their fluency disorder may impede communication in specific situations (e.g., ordering in restaurants or buying a ticket at a counter). Generally, a measure of functional communication is obtained when clinicians assess variability of stuttering and avoidance of speech, speaking situations, and specific communication partners. Still, clinicians who wish to make an independently assessment of functional communication may use the general *Functional Communication Assessment Protocol* provided in Chapter 2 and on the accompanying CD.

Functional communication may be problematic for individuals with neurogenic stuttering. Because of their associated neurological disorder, their communication skills may have deteriorated; consequently, their basic communication may have been affected. If this is the case, the clinician may administer the general *Functional Communication Assessment Protocol* (Chapter 2 and the CD).

The quality of life assessment, on the other hand, may be relevant for all clients with fluency disorders. Every form of fluency disorder may negatively affect the quality of life. Stuttering, cluttering, or neurogenic stuttering may restrict social participation, limit occupational choices, affect personal communication, force social isolation, and make it difficult to hold a job. Unfortunately, quality of life assessment studies on people who clutter or have neurogenic stuttering is limited; there is some research on quality of life in people who stutter (Yaruss & Quesal, 2006). Section IV of the *Overall Assessment of the Speaker's Experience of Stuttering* (Yaruss & Quesal, 2006), described in a previous section, has several questions that help assess the quality of life of individuals who stutter. Clinicians may administer this instrument to assess not only the quality of life, but also feelings, reactions, and daily communication of people who stutter.

In Chapter 16, we provide a simplified *Fluency Quality of Life Assessment Protocol*. Clinicians may individualize this on the CD and print it to administer. From this protocol, clinicians may find the general areas of life that have been negatively affected by the fluency disorder. Aspects of communication that the client rates as *Somewhat Dissatisfied* or *Dissatisfied* would suggest negative quality of life.

Postassessment Counseling

At the end of the assessment session, discuss the results of your assessment with the client and the family members. Most adult clients and their family members would want to know your tentative diagnosis, treatment recommendations, and prognosis. Most have additional questions about the causes of the disorder, treatment options, cost and duration of treatment, and so forth.

Make a Tentative Diagnosis

Begin your counseling by summarizing your observations. Describe your main impressions that are based on your observations. At this point, even if you have not had a chance to analyze the speech samples, you will be in a position to say whether the client stutters, clutters, or has neurogenic stuttering. Justify your diagnosis by pointing out the main characteristics of the disorder you have observed.

If your diagnosis is cluttering, differentiate it from stuttering to help the client and the family understand the difference. If the diagnosis is neurogenic stuttering, help the client and the family understand the differences between the two forms of stuttering. Point out the unique features of each.

Make Recommendations

You may almost always recommend treatment for adults whose stuttering began in their childhood. Obviously, there has been no spontaneous recovery, and therefore, treatment is essential. The adult clients probably have had prior treatment that has failed. Therefore, you may have to justify the kind of treatment you offer and explain why the outcome may be better than those of prior treatments the client will have received.

If the diagnosis is neurogenic stuttering, you may recommend treatment in the context of the overall health as well as the additional communication disorder the client exhibits. Whether the neurogenic stuttering in the client is transitory or relatively permanent might also need to be considered. You may suggest that all communication treatment be delayed until the client's physical status is stabilized. Treatment priority in some cases may be on the other communication disorder the client has—aphasia or apraxia, for example. Because of limited treatment research on neurogenic stuttering, your recommendations may be more tentative than those offered to adults with early-onset stuttering.

You may recommend treatment for those who clutter, though you may have to discuss the difficult issue of the client's motivation for treatment and improved speech. Complicating issues are whether the client believes he or she has a disorder that needs treatment and whether the person is committed to receiving sustained treatment. You may offer treatment that is similar to that offered for stuttering. A self-monitored slower speech rate may help improve the client's speech intelligibility—the main target of treatment.

Suggest Prognosis

Prognosis for improved fluency is good for most, if not all individuals, with stuttering of early onset. Maintenance of fluency in adults, however, may require frequent follow-ups and possible booster therapy over a period of several years. Some forms of treatment, especially fluency shaping (airflow management and slow speech) require constant self-monitoring of speech—something you need to discuss with the client in the context of long-term maintenance of fluency.

You may point out that poor prognosis is often a result of several factors, including ineffective, inefficient, or improperly administered treatment; a lack of follow-up and booster treatment; or failure to complete an effective treatment program. You may emphasize that to realize a favorable prognosis, the client and the family should complete the recommended treatment program, implement the maintenance program at home, keep in touch with you to schedule follow-ups, and receive booster treatment when stuttering tends to increase. You may reassure the client that a family history of stuttering or a severe stuttering does not necessarily mean poor prognosis for improvement.

Predicting prognosis for neurogenic stuttering is more difficult than it is for stuttering of early onset. We lack sufficient data on treatment and its outcome with a significant number of individuals. Therefore, your recommendation may be to offer a period of trial therapy, evaluate the outcome, and make decisions on continued treatment in light of observed progress.

You may take a similarly cautious approach in predicting prognosis for adults who clutter. A large experimental treatment database on adults who clutter is not available. As suggested earlier, prognosis may depend greatly on the client's self-evaluation of the disorder and the motivation for treatment. You may need to discuss these issues in offering a cautious prognosis, provided the client receives regular and sustained treatment and agrees to take necessary steps to maintain fluency.

Answer Frequently Asked Questions

Mostly because of many Web sites that offer various kinds of information on stuttering, adult clients and their families are now more knowledgeable about fluency disorders than ever. They also ask specific questions about the causes and cures for stuttering. The answers clinicians give to the clients' questions should be direct and scientifically based.

The clinician should answer all questions the clients and their caregivers ask. While it is not possible to list all kinds of questions clients may ask, a few commonly encountered questions and potential answers follow. You may need to modify the terms you use to suit the education, prior knowledge, and the judged sophistication of clients and families in formulating your answers.

> ***What causes stuttering or cluttering?*** Research suggests several potential
> causes, though it is not possible to point out a cause for stuttering in a given
> individual. Scientific knowledge about the potential causes applies to groups,
> not individuals. For instance, we know that in the families of 45% to 50% of
> people who stutter or clutter, there may be other blood relatives with a similar
> disorder. This suggests the influence of genetic factors, although environmental
> influence cannot be totally ruled out. Attempts at finding a gene that causes
> stuttering of early onset and cluttering continue, though no specific gene has
> been identified to date. Even in those cases where a family history is positive,
> environmental factors may be important as well. Negative reaction to stressful
> speaking situations, a tendency to experience anxiety associated with speech,
> traumatic emotional experiences, and reactions to negative criticism may all
> play a role, although research is not definitive about such environmental
> factors.
>
> We know more about how stuttering gets exacerbated than we do about its
> origin. For example, stuttering typically increases while talking to strangers,
> speaking under stressful situations, talking to authority figures, talking in a
> hurry, ordering in restaurants, talking over telephones, and so forth. Stuttering
> typically decreases when talking to close friends or family members, especially to
> infants and small children. Singing and talking while assuming the role of
> someone else may also increase fluency. Fortunately, most fluency problems can
> be effectively treated regardless of their original causes.
>
> When there is no history of stuttering, but it appears after a stroke or brain
> tumor, most researchers assume that the stuttering is caused by the neurologic
> problem. Various kinds of brain trauma or disease can cause stuttering in adults.

How long does it take to treat stuttering effectively? It depends on several factors. Generally, it takes less time to treat a young child than it does to treat an adult who has been stuttering for many years. Progress will be faster if family members follow up on suggestions to hold informal treatment sessions at home, support and help sustain fluency, and informally monitor fluency and stuttering in naturalistic speaking situations. Generally, about 6 to 12 months of treatment, offered twice a week, may be needed to experience substantial improvement in most cases.

How effective are some of the gadgets promoted on the Internet? Some of the gadgets, especially those that delay auditory feedback of speech, feed mechanical noise to the ears, or provide rhythmic metronome-like auditory stimuli tend to decrease stuttering. There also are many variations of these devices, but some of them are not experimentally tested. We should avoid devices whose effects have not been established through scientific research. Good news is that stuttering can be effectively treated without mechanical devices. Therefore, investment in costly instruments is often unnecessary. Unfortunately, many kinds of devices in the past have not succeeded in the market place. Because of bankruptcy of manufacturers, expensive instruments, once bought, may be unserviceable; if they run on a computer, it may be impossible to upgrade the hardware or the software, rendering the unit useless.

What about maintenance of fluency following treatment? This too, depends on the individual. Generally, young children who receive effective treatment maintain fluency better than adults who do. Some evidence suggests that certain treatment procedures may promote better maintenance than other treatments, although we need much research data to be certain. Adults who are treated with a slow and prolonged speech method tend to experience a relapse of stuttering sooner or later, although the same treatment, offered as the need arises over a period of time, will help stabilize fluency. It is generally a good strategy to seek treatment if stuttering returns; such a return is not an indication of failed treatment. A schedule of regular follow-up and prompt treatment when stuttering increases will eventually help wean a person away from treatment. To get booster treatment that will help maintain fluency, it is important for you to contact me or another clinician when there is an increase in stuttering. Booster treatment can be just a few sessions. In some cases, an extended telephone conversation may be all that is needed. A treated person who continues to monitor his or her fluency is more likely to maintain fluency than the one who does not self-monitor.

What are some of the treatment options? There are various well-researched treatment options for adults who stutter. Slow speech almost always induces more fluent speech, although it may not sound very natural; it may also be difficult for most people to maintain a consistently slow speech. Many electronic instruments marketed for people who stutter induce slower speech. We can teach someone to speak slowly and thus reduce stuttering without any gadgets. We can then gradually shape a faster rate and more natural sounding speech while still keeping stuttering under check.

In recent years, there have been alternatives to slower speech that have proven effective. These alternatives avoid the undesirable effects of slow speech —mostly the unnatural sounding speech. In one effective procedure, we simply ask the persons to stop talking when a stuttering is imminent, in progress, or just occurred. The person pauses for a brief duration and then continues to talk. We usually select a technique that is best for the individual.

When do we start treatment? As soon as you are ready. It is better to start treatment sooner rather than later. We can set up a date now or you can call me or the clinic office later to begin treatment. [*Depending on the service setting, the clinician offers additional information on when and how to begin a treatment program for the client.*]

References

Andrews, G., & Cutler, J. (1974). Stuttering therapy: The relation between changes in symptoms level and attitude. *Journal of Speech Hearing Disorders, 39,* 312–319.

Bloodstein, O. (1995). *A handbook on stuttering* (5th ed.). Clifton Park, NY: Thomson-Delmar.

Bloodstein, O., & Ratner, N. B. (2008). *A handbook on stuttering* (6th ed.). Clifton Park, NY: Cengage Delmar.

Boey, A. R., Wuyts, F. L., Van de Heyning, P. H., De Bodt, M. S., & Heylen, L. (2007). Characteristics of stuttering-like disfluencies in Dutch-speaking children. *Journal of Fluency Disorders, 32,* 310–329.

Brutten, G. J., & Vanryckeghem, M. (2003). *Behavior Assessment Battery: A multidimensional and evidence-based approach to diagnostic and therapeutic decision making for adults who stutter.* Destelbergen, Belgium: Organization for the Integration of Handicapped People.

Carlo, E. J., & Watson, J. B. (2002). Disfluencies of 3- and 5-year old Spanish-speaking children. *Journal of Fluency Disorders, 28,* 37–53.

Conture, E. G. (2001). *Stuttering: Its nature, diagnosis, and treatment* (2nd ed.). Boston, MA: Allyn & Bacon.

Culatta, R., & Goldberg, S. A. (1995). *Stuttering therapy: An integrated approach to theory and practice.* Needham Heights, MA: Allyn and Bacon.

Daly, D. A. (1986). The clutterer. In K. O. St. Louis (Ed.), *The atypical stutterer: Principles and practices of rehabilitation.* Orlando, FL: Academic Press.

Daly, D. A., & Burnett, M. L. (1999). Cluttering: Traditional views and new perspectives In R. F. Curlee (Ed.), *Stuttering and related disorders of fluency* (2nd ed., pp. 222–254). New York, NY: Thieme.

DeJoy, D. A., & Jordan, W. J. (1988). Listener reactions to interjections in oral reading versus spontaneous speech. *Journal of Fluency Disorders, 13,* 11–25.

Duffy, J. R. (2005). *Motor speech disorders* (2nd ed.). St. Louis, MO: Mosby.

Erickson, R. L. (1969). Assessing communication attitudes among stutterers. *Journal of Speech and Hearing Research, 12,* 711–724.

Guitar, B. (2006). *Stuttering: An integrated approach to its nature and treatment* (3rd ed.). Baltimore, MD: Lippincott Williams & Wilkins.

Hegde, M. N. (2007). *Treatment protocols for stuttering.* San Diego, CA: Plural.

Hegde, M. N. (2008a). *Hegde's pocketguide to communication disorders.* Clifton Park, NY: Cengage Delmar.

Hegde, M. N. (2008b). *Hegde's pocketguide to assessment in speech-language pathology* (2nd ed.). Clifton Park, NY: Cengage Delmar.

Hegde, M. N., & Dansby, E. (1988). Differential listener threshold of tolerance for different forms of dysfluencies [abstract] *Asha, 30*(10), 141.

Hegde, M. N., & Hartman, D. E. (1979a). Factors affecting judgments of fluency: I. Interjections. *Journal of Fluency Disorders, 4,* 1–11.

Hegde, M. N., & Hartman, D. E. (1979b). Factors affecting judgments of fluency: I. Word repetitions. *Journal of Fluency Disorders, 4,* 13–22.

Hegde, M. N., & Pomaville, F. (2008). *Assessment of communication disorders in children: Resources and protocols.* San Diego, CA: Plural.

Hegde, M. N., & Stone, D. M. (1991). Listener tolerance thresholds for phrase repetitions and part-word repetitions [abstract]. *Asha, 33*(10), 118.

Helm-Estabrooks, N. (1999). Stuttering associated with acquired neurological disorders. In R. F. Curlee (Ed.), *Stuttering and related disorders of fluency* (2nd ed., pp. 255–268). New York, NY: Thieme.

Johnson, W., Brown, S. F., Curtis, J. F., Edney, C. W., & Keaster, J. (1967). Speech handicapped school children. New York: Harper & Row.

Johnson, W. (1944). The Indians have no word for it. I. Stuttering in children. *Quarterly Journal of Speech, 30,* 330–337.

Johnson, W., & Associates (1959). *The onset of stuttering.* Minneapolis, MN: University of Minnesota Press.

Myers, F. L., & St. Louis, K. O. (1992). *Cluttering: A clinical perspective.* Kibworth, England: Far Communications.

Natke, U., Sandrieser, P., Pietrowski, R., & Kalveram, K. T. (2006). Disfluency data of German preschool children who stutter and comparison children. *Journal of Fluency Disorders, 31,* 165–176.

Pellowski, M. W., & Conture, E. G. (2002). Characteristics of speech disfluency and stuttering behaviors in 3- and 4-year-old children. *Journal of Speech, Language, and Hearing Research, 45,* 20–35.

Roberts, P. M., Meltzer, A., & Wilding, J. (2009). Disfluencies in nonstuttering adults across sample lengths and topics. *Journal of Communication Disorders, 42,* 414–427.

Robinson, T. L. & Crowe, T. A. (2002). Fluency disorders. In D. E. Battle (Ed.), *Communication disorders in multicultural populations* (pp. 267–297). Boston, MA: Butterworth-Heinemann.

Sander, E. K. (1963). Frequency of syllable repetition and "stutterer" judgments. *Journal of Speech and Hearing Disorders, 28,* 19–30.

Silverman, E. M. (1972). Generality of disfluency data collected from preschoolers. *Journal of Speech and Hearing Research, 5,* 84–92.

Silverman, F. H. (2004). *Stuttering and other fluency disorders* (3rd ed.). Long Grove, IL: Waveland Press.

Van Riper, C. (1982). *The nature of stuttering.* Englewood Cliffs, NJ: Prentice-Hall.

Westby, C. E. (1979). Language performance of stuttering and nonstuttering children. *Journal of Communication Disorders, 12,* 133–145.

Williams, D. E., & Kent, L. R. (1958). Listener evaluations of speech interruptions. *Journal of Speech and Hearing Research, 1,* 124–131.

Yairi, E., & Ambrose, N. G. (2005). *Early childhood stuttering.* Austin, TX: Pro-Ed.

Yaruss, J. S., & Quesal, R. W. (2006). Overall assessment of the speaker's experience of stuttering (OASES): Documenting multiple outcomes in stuttering treatment. *Journal of Fluency Disorders, 31,* 90–115.

Zimmerman, G. N., Liljeblad, S., Frank, A., & Cleeland, C. (1983). The Indians have many terms for it: Stuttering among the Bannock-Shoshoni. *Journal of Speech and Hearing Research, 26,* 315–318.

CHAPTER 16

Assessment of Fluency Disorders: Protocols

- Overview of Fluency Assessment Protocols
- Interview Protocol
- Dysfluency Measurement Protocol
- Stuttering Variability Assessment Protocol
- Associated Motor Behaviors Assessment Protocol
- Avoidance Behaviors Assessment Protocol
- Neurogenic Stuttering Assessment Protocol
- Cluttering Assessment Protocol
- Fluency Quality of Life Assessment Protocol

Overview of Fluency Assessment Protocols

Assessment protocols provided in this chapter help assess fluency disorders in adults in an efficient manner. The protocols offer ready-made formats that clinicians can use in structuring their client and family interviews, measuring dysfluencies, recording associated motor behaviors, noting avoidance behaviors, assessing neurogenic stuttering, and evaluating cluttering.

The protocols given in this chapter also are available on the accompanying CD. The clinician may print the needed protocols in evaluating their clients. The clinician may combine these protocols in suitable ways to facilitate the evaluation of an adult's fluency problems.

In assessing adults with multiple disorders of communication, the clinician may combine these protocols with protocols from other chapters. For example, the clinician may combine these fluency assessment protocols with voice assessment protocols (Chapter 18).

The protocols given in this chapter are specific to stuttering, neurogenic stuttering, and cluttering. To complete the assessment on a given client, the clinician should combine these disorder-specific protocols with the **common assessment protocols** given in Chapter 2:

- The Adult Case History
- Orofacial Examination and Hearing Screening Protocol
- Diadochokinetic Assessment Protocol for Adults
- Adult Assessment Report Outline

Interview Protocol

Name _____ DOB _____ Date _____ Clinician _____

Have the client complete the *Adult Case History Form* given in Chapter 2. Let the client's case history guide your interview.

Note that your interview of the client, family members, or both is mainly concerned with getting additional information that supplements and clarifies what is given on the case history form. Details about associated clinical conditions or communication disorders, occupational difficulties, and personal and social consequences of stuttering also may be explored during the interview.

End the assessment with the postassessment counseling outlined in Chapter 15.

Individualize this protocol on the CD and print it for your use. 💿

Preparation

- [ ] Review the guidelines given in the Initial Clinical Interview described in Chapter 1.
- [ ] Make sure the setting is comfortable with adequate seating and lighting.
- [ ] Record the interview with the client; this will serve as an extended speech sample for analyzing the dysfluency rates.
- [ ] Find out the client's preferences about how to be interviewed. If the client prefers to be interviewed alone, do so first; then conduct a separate interview of the family member. Finally, conduct a joint interview with both the client and the family member.
- [ ] Review the case history ahead of time, noting areas you want to review or obtain more information about.

Introduction

- [ ] Introduce yourself. Briefly review your assessment plan for the day and give an estimate of the duration of assessment.

    Example: "Hello Mr./Mrs. [*client's name*]. My name is [*your name*]. I am the speech-language pathologist who will be assessing you today. I would like to start by reviewing the case history and asking you a few questions. After we finish talking, we will complete a few procedures to assess your speech problem. Today's assessment should take about [*estimate the amount of time you plan to spend*]."

(continues)

Interview Protocol (continued)

Interview Questions

Ask the following kinds of questions to get clarifications or additional information. Skip or rephrase questions as found appropriate. Some clients or their family members need to be questioned in greater detail about the kinds of dysfluencies the client exhibits because they only describe the problem in general terms; others give more specific descriptions. Note that many answers the clients or family members give to the initial question may require additional follow-up questions not specified in the outline. Although the outline shows the questions that need to be asked and answered, avoid relentless questioning. Frequently, paraphrase what the clients and informants say by way of answers to your questions. Ask about the views, thoughts, or feelings of the client as well as the informants. If appropriate, express approval of what they say. Note that it is not just the clinician who asks questions; clients and their informants also will have questions that the clinician needs to answer. If they have questions about the typical features of stuttering, causes of the problem, treatment options, and so forth, answer briefly and promise more detailed information later. Note that the questions are addressed to the adult client, but rephrase them if you are addressing an informant. Depending on the answer you get for a question, modify the following question or skip it if it is unnecessary.

- ☐ What is your primary concern regarding your speech?
- ☐ Can you describe the problem?
- ☐ So you think you stutter. What exactly do you do when you stutter?
- ☐ Do you repeat sounds, like *t-t-time*? What sounds do you repeat often?
- ☐ Do you repeat the first syllable in words? Do you remember some of the syllables you typically repeat?
- ☐ Do you prolong the sounds of speech? Any examples from your own speech?
- ☐ Do you repeat words and phrases? Can you give examples of words you typically repeat?
- ☐ Do you start a sentence and not finish it? Can you give some examples?
- ☐ Do you revise something you begin to say? For example, do you sometime say things like "I want juice, water"? We all revise, but do you do it very frequently?
- ☐ What about such interjections as "um" and "you know" and "OK" and "I mean?" Once again, all speakers say them, but do you interject them too frequently?
- ☐ Do you sometime pause too much when others perhaps don't expect you to pause? For example when a stranger asks "What's your name?" Do you take a bit too much time to say your name?
- ☐ Do you sometimes pause in between words?
- ☐ I think what you have described is typical of most people who stutter. They repeat sounds and words, prolong sounds, interject extraneous materials, say incomplete sentences, and drop an idea and revise repeatedly. Is there any other behavior that concerns you? For instance, do you show any facial expressions that draw attention to your speech difficulty? Can you describe some of them?

☐ Do you make any hand or feet movement when you stutter?

☐ What other kinds of extraneous movements do you make when you stutter?

☐ Let us now talk a little bit about how it all started. You may have heard your parents say something about how you started to stutter. When do you think your problem was first noticed? Do you know who noticed it?

☐ Do you know why someone thought you stuttered?

☐ Did your patents or someone mention something unusual or some special event that they thought was associated with the beginning of your stuttering?

☐ Do you remember your reaction when someone told you that you stutter? What is the earliest recollection of your stuttering, how you felt about it, and how people reacted to it?

☐ Did anyone during your early days of stuttering suggest that you do something to avoid stuttering? What kind of suggestions? For example, did anyone suggest that you speak slowly or think before you talk?

☐ Any other suggestions that you remember?

☐ Do you remember how you reacted to those suggestions? Did you follow them? Did they help? Which ones helped you speak more fluently?

[*Ask follow-up questions about the strategies suggested and employed, their effects, the client's reaction, and the additional steps the family members took to help the client speak more fluently.*]

☐ How did your stuttering change over the course of time? Did it get worse, improve, or stabilize?

☐ Does your stuttering vary over time and situations? How does it vary?

☐ Under what conditions are you more fluent than usual?

☐ When or under what conditions do you stutter more than usual?

☐ Has your stuttering become stable across situations and time? When did your stuttering become more stable?

☐ Once again, what you have told me is typical of most people who stutter. Stuttering tends to vary across time and situations. Now I want to discuss some associated problems that may be a reaction to stuttering. For instance, do you have difficulty saying certain words? Can you think of some examples?

☐ What do you do when you don't want to say certain words because you stutter on them? Do you use similar words, use vague words, or describe instead of naming something?

☐ Do you avoid speaking to certain individuals? Can you think of some specific individuals you would rather not speak to because of stuttering?

☐ Do you freely speak to some individuals? In other words, whom do you not avoid speaking to because you are typically more fluent while talking to them?

☐ Do you appear frustrated when you can't get the words out?

(continues)

Interview Protocol (continued)

☐ How do you express your frustration?

☐ What is your earliest recollection of how your parents, other children, or teachers reacted to your stuttering? What kind of reactions were they?

[Ask follow-up questions about the client's emotional reactions and feelings associated with stuttering and other avoidance reactions.]

☐ Do you feel that your stuttering has affected your social interactions? Can you describe how?

☐ Do you feel that your stuttering has affected your interaction with your family members? Can you describe how?

[Ask follow-up questions about spousal relationship, spousal reactions, support, or lack thereof if the client is married.]

☐ Do you feel that your stuttering is affecting [has affected] your education through the years? Can you describe how?

☐ Do you think your stuttering affected [will affect] your occupational choice?

[Ask follow-up questions on occupational choice the client has made or is expected to make and how stuttering is a factor in his or her choice.]

☐ Do you feel that your stuttering is affecting [will affect] your job performance? Can you describe how?

☐ What do you think of your colleagues' or supervisors' reactions to stuttering? Do you think they are supportive of you or critical?

☐ Do you think your stuttering has affected your reading and writing skills? Would you describe how?

☐ Compared to your typical conversational speech, do you stutter more while reading aloud? Do you know why?

☐ What kind of concerns have you heard from your teachers, colleagues, or supervisors?

[Ask follow-up questions about the effects stuttering had on the client's social, academic, and personal life.]

☐ Do you have any language problems that you are concerned with?

☐ Did you have any problems producing the speech sounds correctly? Are there any English speech sounds you think you don't produce too well?

☐ What do you think of your voice? Do you have any concerns about your voice?

[Ask follow-up questions about other communication disorders the client may have.]

☐ What is your first language?

☐ What other language or languages do you speak? What is the language routinely spoken at home? [Skip the next three questions if the client is monolingual.]

☐ Do you speak the two languages equally well? If not, which language is stronger?

☐ If you speak two languages, do you know in what language you began to stutter?

☐ If you speak two languages, do you feel you stutter to the same extent in both the languages? If not, in what language do you stutter less?

☐ Did you have any brothers or sisters who stutter or have ever stuttered? If they ever did, do they still stutter? Was treatment ever received?

☐ Do you know of any other member of your family—on both your mother's and father's sides—who ever stuttered?

[*Ask follow-up questions about the family history of stuttering, treatment received by other members of the family, and the current status of their stuttering.*]

☐ Would you tell me some of your ideas as to why you stutter? What do you know about the causes of stuttering in general?

☐ Do you know of any treatments for stuttering? How did you learn about them?

[*Discuss the client's beliefs about stuttering, its causes, and its treatment; answer any questions the client or the family members may have about the causes and remedies for stuttering, and tell them that you will offer more information later.*]

☐ Do you have hearing problems?

☐ Have you ever had a hearing test? If so, when and where? What were the results?

☐ Has you seen any other specialists for your stuttering? If so, who and when? What were their recommendations? How have you followed up on this?

☐ In the past, have you received therapy for your stuttering? When and where?

☐ What kind of therapy did you receive? Can you describe the types of activities that you and your clinician did during your therapy sessions?

☐ How did you respond to your initial therapy? Do you feel the therapy was helpful? Why or why not?

☐ If the therapy was helpful, how long did you maintain fluency? When did stuttering return?

☐ Would you please describe any repeated therapies you may have had? What were the outcomes?

☐ Did you receive any other kind of speech therapy?

[*Ask follow-up questions about previous treatment for stuttering or any other communication disorder and the nature and effects of such treatment.*]

☐ Why are you seeking therapy now? What is your goal in seeking therapy?

☐ What do you want to get out of therapy now?

☐ Do you believe you have the time and commitment to continue therapy on a regular basis?

☐ Do you think you will be able to complete the tasks that we may assign you? For example, we may want you to self-monitor your speech most of the time or conduct home therapy sessions with one of your family members.

☐ Are there any other kinds of concerns you have about your speech that you wish to let me know?

(continues)

Interview Protocol (continued)

> [*Ask follow-up questions about any other problem the client or the informant may mention; may include behavior problems, interpersonal or marital difficulties, intellectual disabilities, neuromotor limitations, academic difficulties, occupational problems, and so forth.*]

Before concluding the interview, review the case history and follow up with any additional questions you need to ask. Fill in any "blanks" in the medical, social, educational, and occupational histories.

Close the Interview

Before you close the initial interview, summarize the major points you have learned from the interview, allowing the client and the informant an opportunity to add or correct information. Close the interview with the following:

☐ You have given me sufficient information to begin my assessment. I know that you repeat sound, syllables, and words; prolong sounds; interject syllables and words; and do other things as you have described to me. Now, do you have any questions for me at this point?

☐ Thank you very much for you input. The information has been very helpful.

☐ Now, I will work with you to complete the assessment. When we are finished, we will discuss the findings. I will also answer your questions about stuttering and its treatment.

Dysfluency Measurement Protocol

Name _____ DOB _____ Date _____ Clinician _____

Individualize this protocol on the CD and print it for your use. ⬯

Dysfluency Types	Frequency			
	Speech	Monologue	Oral reading	Home speech

Repetitions
  Part-word
  Whole-word
  Phrase				

Prolongations
  Sound/syllable
  Silent				

Interjections
  Sound/syllable
  Whole-word
  Phrase				

Silent Pauses				
Broken Words (intralexical pauses)				
Incomplete Phrases				
Revisions				
Total of dysfluencies/ Number of words				
Percent dysfluency rate				

Comments: _____

_____

_____

Stuttering Variability Assessment Protocol

Name _____ DOB _____ Date _____ Clinician _____

Place a check mark in the boxes to let us know if you **typically stutter,** **speak fluently,** *or* **experience tension and anxiety** *in the described situation or task.*

If an item is not relevant to you, please write NA next to it.

In the situation or while performing the speech task	I *typically* stutter	I *typically* speak fluently	I typically experience tension and anxiety
1. Telephone conversation	☐	☐	Yes ☐ No ☐
2. Self-introduction	☐	☐	Yes ☐ No ☐
3. Speaking to my boss or supervisors	☐	☐	Yes ☐ No ☐
4. Conversation with friends	☐	☐	Yes ☐ No ☐
5. Having a heated discussion on a controversial topic	☐	☐	Yes ☐ No ☐
6. Talking to infants and babies	☐	☐	Yes ☐ No ☐
7. Justifying my actions to someone	☐	☐	Yes ☐ No ☐
8. Narrating a personal experience	☐	☐	Yes ☐ No ☐
9. Giving directions	☐	☐	Yes ☐ No ☐
10. Asking for directions	☐	☐	Yes ☐ No ☐
11. Saying something in a hurry	☐	☐	Yes ☐ No ☐
12. Clarifying something I said	☐	☐	Yes ☐ No ☐
13. Ordering in a restaurant	☐	☐	Yes ☐ No ☐
14. Giving a quick answer to a question	☐	☐	Yes ☐ No ☐
15. Singing a song	☐	☐	Yes ☐ No ☐
16. Buying a ticket at a counter	☐	☐	Yes ☐ No ☐
17. Talking to pet animals	☐	☐	Yes ☐ No ☐
18. Raising a question in a group discussion	☐	☐	Yes ☐ No ☐

In the situation or while performing the speech task	I *typically* stutter	I *typically* speak fluently	I typically experience tension and anxiety	
19. Answering questions in a job interview	☐	☐	Yes ☐	No ☐
20. Asking for a specific product at a store	☐	☐	Yes ☐	No ☐
21. Talking with my spouse	☐	☐	Yes ☐	No ☐
22. Giving a formal lecture to a group	☐	☐	Yes ☐	No ☐
23. Quickly interjecting my comment in a group discussion/conversation	☐	☐	Yes ☐	No ☐
24. Returning my phone calls	☐	☐	Yes ☐	No ☐
25. Talking with my children	☐	☐	Yes ☐	No ☐
26. Conversation with a member of the opposite sex	☐	☐	Yes ☐	No ☐
27. Asking for a pay raise	☐	☐	Yes ☐	No ☐
28. Reading aloud in front of a group	☐	☐	Yes ☐	No ☐

Please also complete the following lists:

List 1. I typically stutter while saying the following words:

List 2. I typically stutter on the following speech sounds:

Associated Motor Behaviors Assessment Protocol

Name _____ DOB _____ Date _____ Clinician _____

Individualize this protocol on the CD and print it for your use. ◌

Rate each behavior: 0 = Not observed   1 = Infrequent   2 = Frequent

Associated Motor Behaviors Checklist	Rating *(0, 1, or 2)*
Rapid and tense eye blink	
Tensed and prolonged shutting of the eyelids	
Rapid upward, downward, or lateral movement of the eyes	
Knitting of the eyebrows	
Nose wrinkling and flaring	
Pursing or quivering of the lips	
Tongue clicking	
Teeth clenching, grinding, and clicking	
Tension in facial muscles	
Wrinkling of the forehead	
Clenched jaw, or jerky or slow or tensed movement of the jaws	
Jaw opening or closing unrelated to target speech production	
Tension in chest, shoulder, and neck muscles (e.g., twitching and extraneous movements)	
Head movements (e.g., turns, shakes, jerks, and lateral, upward, and downward movements)	
Tensed and jerky hand movements (e.g., fist clenching and hand wringing)	
Tensed and jerky arm movements (e.g., tapping on the thighs or pressing against the sides of the abdomen)	
Tensed and jerky leg movements (e.g., kicking motions)	
Tensed and jerky feet movements (e.g., grinding, pressing, rubbing, or circular movements on the floor)	
Generally tense body postures	
Other behaviors observed or reported:	

Comments: _____

_____

_____

Avoidance Behaviors Assessment Protocol

Name _____ DOB _____ Date _____ Clinician _____

Individualize this protocol on the CD and print it for your use. 💿

Have the adult client respond to each item. Ask the client to select one of three options for each behavior by circling it:

0 = Not avoided   1 = Infrequently avoided   2 = Frequently avoided

Avoidance of Speaking Situations	Scoring
Saying one's own name	0 1 2
Responding to roll calls	0 1 2
Speaking situations (moves away from the speaking situation)	0 1 2
Ordering in restaurants	0 1 2
Speaking on the telephone	0 1 2
Introducing self	0 1 2
Giving personal phone numbers or addresses	0 1 2
Speaking in front of the class or a social group	0 1 2
Reading aloud in front of a class	0 1 2
Answering questions in the classroom	0 1 2
Saying the names of family members [specify]:	0 1 2
Asking for directions when lost	0 1 2
Other speaking situations you avoid:	
Strategies used to Avoid Stuttering	
Depending on others for communication needs	0 1 2
Gesturing instead of speaking	0 1 2
Having a family member ask for something in a store	0 1 2
Pretending not to hear a question	0 1 2
Pretending to be thinking when questions are asked	0 1 2
Pretending not to know an answer	0 1 2
Pretending ignorance of a word on which stuttering is likely	0 1 2

(continues)

Avoidance Behaviors Assessment Protocol (continued)

Strategies used to Avoid Stuttering	Scoring
Letting others finish a word or complete a sentence	0 1 2
Coughing or throat clearing before saying a difficult word	0 1 2
Whispering	0 1 2
Talking in a soft voice (sudden reduction in loudness on certain words)	0 1 2
Talking in a loud voice (sudden increase in loudness on certain words)	0 1 2
Talking in an impersonated tone (e.g., a character in a play)	0 1 2
Talking with an unusual physical posture	0 1 2
Talking with an exaggerated articulation	0 1 2
Other strategies you use to avoid stuttering:	
Avoidance of Conversational Partners	
Strangers	0 1 2
Family members [specify]:	0 1 2
Bosses and other authority figures	0 1 2
Persons of the opposite sex	0 1 2
Colleagues	0 1 2
Friends	0 1 2
Neighbors	0 1 2
Other conversational partners you avoid [specify]	
Avoidance of Certain Words	
Substitution of one word for another	0 1 2
"Beating around the bush" instead of saying something directly	0 1 2
Pretending not to know a word	0 1 2
Refusing to say a particular word	0 1 2
Saying *this thing* and *that thing* frequently	0 1 2
Other strategies you use to avoid specific words [list them]:	

Avoidance of Talking About Stuttering	Scoring
Switching topic when stuttering is mentioned	0 1 2
Leaving the room when conversation is initiated on stuttering	0 1 2
Getting upset when asked about stuttering	0 1 2
Refusing to talk about other people's reactions to stuttering	0 1 2
Refusing tot talk about colleagues' or bosses' reaction to stuttering	0 1 2
Unwilling to talk about stuttering and associated emotional experiences	0 1 2
Other strategies you use to avoid talking about stuttering [list them]:	
Avoidance of Talking in General	
Keeping quiet when a question is asked	0 1 2
Avoiding discussion on controversial issues	0 1 2
Not taking part in social conversations	0 1 2
Avoiding eye contact during conversation	0 1 2
Reducing the amount of talking in general	0 1 2
Other strategies you use to avoid talking in general [list them]:	

Comments: _____

_____

_____

Neurogenic Stuttering Assessment Protocol

Name _____ DOB _____ Date _____ Clinician _____

Individualize this protocol on the CD and print it for your use. 💿

Place a check mark to indicate the presence or absence of the feature.

Neurogenic Stuttering	Present	Absent
Significant and well-documented evidence of neuropathology: strokes, tumors, head trauma (bilateral brain damage), and multiple lesions in a single hemisphere		
Repetition of medial and final syllables (other dysfluencies similar to those found in early-onset stuttering)		
Dysfluent production of function words (more like children with early onset, and unlike adults with early onset)		
Dysfluent while whispering		
Lack of the adaptation effect		
Lack of muscular effort associated with dysfluencies		
Associated motor behaviors, less common		
Minimal or no tension and anxiety associated with dysfluencies		
No significant improvement in fluency under delayed auditory feedback, shadowing another person's speech or oral reading, unison reading, and masking noise		
Significant problems in copying and drawing, copying block designs, making sequential hand positions, tapping out rhythm, and so forth that suggest brain injury		

Comments: _____

_____

_____

Cluttering Assessment Protocol

Name _____ DOB _____ Date _____ Clinician _____

Individualize this protocol on the CD and print it for your use. 💿

Observed positive and negative signs are checked and examples are given.

Positive Signs	Negative Signs
☐ Speech rate abnormalities:	☐ Difficulty controlling the rate, even with contingent feedback
☐ Errors of articulation:	☐ Can produce the sounds under slower speech rate
☐ Dysfluencies:	☐ Repetition of sounds and sound prolongations ☐ Few or no associated motor behaviors, word substitutions and circumlocutions, minimal or no struggle during dysfluent speech
☐ Worsening of dysfluencies when relaxed and while reading familiar texts ☐ Improved fluency under stressful or demanding conditions, while giving short answers, talking in foreign language, and speaking after interruption	☐ Absence of anxiety about speech and speaking situations ☐ Unconcerned about the speech problem and its effects on listeners ☐ Unwilling to seek or continue treatment
☐ Language difficulties:	
☐ Prosodic problems:	
☐ Voice problems:	
☐ Disorganized thought processes:	
☐ Motor incoordination:	
☐ Reading difficulty:	

(continues)

Cluttering Assessment Protocol (continued)

Positive Signs	Negative Signs
☐ Writing problems:	
☐ Academic problems:	

Comments: _____

_____

_____

Fluency Quality of Life Assessment Protocol

Name _____ DOB _____ Date _____ Clinician _____

Individualize this protocol on the CD and print it for your use. 💿

Administer this to the client. Give an example of how the client should read and respond.

"I would like to know how your fluency problem has affected your life. I would like you to read the item in this manner: *With my ability to talk with my family, I am . . . Satisfied, Somewhat Satisfied, Somewhat Dissatisfied, or Dissatisfied,* and then place a check mark in the column for your answer."

With my ability to talk with:	I am				
	Satisfied	Somewhat satisfied	Somewhat dissatisfied	Dissatisfied	N/A
my family					
my friends					
my colleagues					
strangers					
my supervisors					
members of the opposite sex					
authority figures					
my neighbors					

With my ability to:	I am				
	Satisfied	Somewhat satisfied	Somewhat dissatisfied	Dissatisfied	N/A
order in restaurants					
talk over the phone					
ask for directions					
introduce myself					
give my name and telephone numbers to others					

(continues)

Fluency Quality of Life Assessment Protocol (continued)

With my ability to:	Satisfied	Somewhat satisfied	Somewhat dissatisfied	Dissatisfied	N/A
			I am		
discuss controversial social or political issues					
give a talk in front of a group					
quickly ask a question					
quickly respond to a question					
use the right words					
express my feelings and opinions					
interject my comments in a group discussion					
talk to sales persons in stores					

With my ability to:	Satisfied	Somewhat satisfied	Somewhat dissatisfied	Dissatisfied	N/A
			I am		
enjoy social relationships					
enjoy personal relationships					
achieve my educational goals					
perform my job					
achieve promotions in my job					
generally achieve my life goals					

With my:	Satisfied	Somewhat satisfied	Somewhat dissatisfied	Dissatisfied	N/A
			I am		
feelings and thoughts about myself					
level of self-confidence					
general quality of life					

PART VIII

Assessment of Voice

CHAPTER 17

Assessment of Voice: Resources

- Epidemiology and Ethnocultural Variables
- Voice Disorders in Adults
- Mutism
- Aphonias
- Dysphonias
- Spasmodic Dysphonia
- Causes of Voice Disorders
- Overview of the Assessment Process
- Clinical Assessment of Voice
- Instrumental Assessment of Voice
- Quality of Life Assessment
- Assessment of Voice in Ethnoculturally Diverse Adults
- Postassessment Counseling

Assessment and treatment of voice disorders was primarily the responsibility of medical professionals until the 1930s. It is only in subsequent decades that speech-language pathologists progressively became more involved in serving people with voice disorders (Stemple, Glaze, & Klaben, 2010). Currently, speech-language pathologists are the recognized specialists in assessing and treating voice disorders in children and adults.

Voice is *disordered* when its loudness, pitch, quality, and resonance are judged to be abnormal, inappropriate, or socially nonfunctional. Voice in a person may be judged inappropriate or abnormal because it deviates from the typically accepted (reinforced) patterns of vocal productions found in persons of comparable age and gender within the cultural community. A person with a voice disorder may fail to meet the social and occupational demands of communication. Certain kinds of voice disorders or disorders of sufficient severity may lead to social or occupational handicap. Serious and persistent voice disorders, therefore, affect the quality of life of individuals who have them.

Epidemiology and Ethnocultural Variables

Epidemiologic studies of voice disorders, especially in the adult population, are limited. Because of the varied diseases that can affect voice, it has not been difficult to determine the incidence or prevalence of voice problems in persons with several common, as well as many rare, medical conditions. While voice disorders may exist without central nervous system pathology or other disorders of communication, they also are a part of many neurological disorders and resulting communication problems (e.g., dysarthria). Voice disorders are relatively common in certain occupational groups who are described as heavy voice users (Roy, Merrill, Gray, & Smith, 2005; Roy, Merrill, Thibeault, Parsa, Gray, & Smith, 2004; Verdolini & Ramig, 2001). There has been no comprehensive study of voice disorders in all these and many other subgroups.

According to the National Institute of Deafness and Communicative Disorders, voice disorders are found in 7.5 million people in the United States. In a telephone survey of 1326 adults in the age range of 21 to 66 years living in the states of Utah and Iowa, about 30% had a voice disorder in their lifetime and 7% currently had a problem (Roy et al., 2005). In another survey with a smaller sample of 117 individuals in the age range of 65 to 94, 47% reported a voice disorder in their lifetime and 29% currently had it (Roy, Stemple, Merrill, & Thomas, 2007). It is possible that voice disorders may be more prevalent in the older population than in the younger.

It is estimated that 5% to 10% of the working people use their voice heavily in their work settings and are more prone to voice disorders (Roy, Weinrich, Gray, Tanner, & Stemple, 2003). A study by Roy et al. (2004) reported that 11% of teachers, compared with 6.2% of nonteachers, may have a voice disorder. During their lifetimes, 57% of teachers, compared with 28.8% of nonteachers may have a voice disorder. Female teachers are generally more prone to voice disorders than their male counterparts. Roy et al. (2004) concluded that "being a teacher, being a woman between 40 and 59 years of age, having 16 or more years of education, and having a family history of voice disorders were each positively associated with having experienced a voice disorder in the past" (p. 281). Among those seeking treatment in voice clinics, teachers outnumber other professionals (Titze, Lemke, & Montequin, 1997). It is estimated that people who hold such "talking professions" as acting, singing, telemarketing, selling in stores, announcing on the radio, preaching, athletic coaching, auctioning, cheerleading, and so forth may have a higher prevalence of voice disorders than the general population. Mothers who may yell at young children and loudly cheer their children's sporting accomplishments also may be at a high risk for voice disorders. Similarly, factory workers who need to speak above the ambient mechanical noise also are at high risk for voice disorders (Aronson & Bless, 2009).

Different types of voice disorders are differentially distributed in the general population. Aphonia (no voice) with no organic pathology, often described as "psychogenic," may be more prevalent in women, especially homemakers, than in men (Aronson & Bless, 2009). Spasmodic dysphonia (a strained-strangled voice quality) also may be more common in women than in men. Voice disorders due to vocal nodules may be more common than voice disorder of any other etiology; they occurred in 21.6% of patients. Vocal nodules are most common in males under 14 years of age and females in the age range of 25 to 45 years. Voice disorders occur in decreasing frequency due to edema (14.1%), polyps (11.4%), cancer (9%), vocal fold paralysis (8.1%), and with no laryngeal pathology (7.9%). Voice disorders due to laryngeal pathologies are more common in people 45 years or older, and those associated with carcinoma and vocal fold paralysis are most common in the elderly (Herrington-Hall, Lee, Stemple, Niemi, & McHome, 1988). In addition, people with a family history of voice disorders and those who are prone to frequent episodes of allergies, asthma, colds, sinus infection, and postnasal drip have a high risk for voice disorders.

Differential prevalence of voice disorders in different **ethnocultural groups** has not been researched adequately. It is known, however, that many diseases that affect voice are differentially distributed across different ethnic groups. It is expected that such differences in the prevalence of relevant diseases cause differential prevalence of voice disorders (see Holland & DeJarnette, 2002, for review of studies); some examples include the following:

- **Prevalence of laryngeal cancer is the highest among African Americans.** Progressively lower prevalence is found among Hawaiians, Hispanics, Japanese, Chinese, Filipinos, and Native Americans, in whom it is the lowest

- **Prevalence of oral cancer alone is the highest in African Americans.** In this case, there is no laryngeal or pharyngeal involvement. Prevalence of oral cancer is progressively lower in Native Americans in Alaska, Chinese, Hawaiians, Filipinos, and Mexicans. The lowest prevalence is found in Japanese Americans and American Indians.

- **Prevalence of oral and pharyngeal cancer is the highest in African American males.** White males and the Chinese have progressively lower prevalence. Nasopharyngeal cancer is especially prevalent in the Chinese.

- **Prevalence of esophageal cancer is the highest in African Americans.** Progressively lower prevalence is found in Hawaiians, Filipinos, Chinese, Japanese, and American Indians. The last two groups have roughly the same prevalence rate, whereas the Hispanics have the lowest prevalence.

- **Thyroid deficiencies are more common in whites than in African Americans.** These deficiencies can cause voice disorders.

- **Vocal nodules are more prevalent in white males than in white females.** Prevalence of nodules is more common in African American females than in African American males.

Voice Disorders in Adults

There is no agreement on how to classify voice disorders. Various classifications are both confusing and questionable. There are three main problems with the classifications of voice disorders. First, there is a confusion between etiology and symptomatology. Historically, some professionals, especially the medical, have tended to identify a voice disorder by the medical disease that caused it (Boone, McFarlane, Von Berg, & Zraick, 2010). For instance, instead of describing voice disorders, many sources describe nodules, polyps, cancer, vocal abuse, and neuropathology, as either functional, organic, or psychogenic voice disorders. Medical pathologies are causes of, not disorders of, voice.

Second, the categories of *organic* versus *functional* voice disorders muddies the definition of functional disorders. Technically, a *functional disorder* has no identifiable organic cause. That is why it is distinguished from an organic disorder that has an organic cause. Unfortunately, in voice literature, a functional disorder may be associated with an organic abnormality or a well-defined structural change in the larynx. For instance, voice disorders due to vocal fold nodules, polyps, traumatic laryngitis, Reinke's edema, diplophonia due to mass lesions—all evidencing organic changes—may still be described as functional voice disorders (Boone et al., 2010). The justification typically offered for this redefinition of *functional* voice disorders is that the observed organic pathology is due to a pattern of behavior. Nonetheless, the voice problem is still due to the laryngeal or neural organic change, and hence it is organic. Correctly defined, there only are a few functional (nonorganic) voice disorders. These include certain forms of aphonia, certain pitch disorders (as in falsetto), some loudness disorders (as in inappropriate use of breath supply for phonation), tensed voice production—all without organic pathology. Most other voice disorders traditionally considered functional (such as those caused by vocal nodules and polyps) are indeed due to tissue changes in the vocal folds, and hence, organic.

Third, the diagnostic category of *psychogenic voice disorders* lacks scientific validity. Psychogenic voice disorders also are sometimes described as *conversion reactions* or *somatization* (Aronson & Bless, 2009), although in the judgment of some clinicians, not all psychogenic voice disorders are conversion reactions (Boone et al., 2010). Once again, psychogenic disorders are *functional* in the sense that they are not associated with laryngeal organic or neural pathology. When a functional disorder is further characterized or reclassified as *psychogenic, conversion reaction*, or *somatization*, additional assumptions are made about their causation. That a voice or any other behavior disorder has its origin in the mind of a person—psychogenic—is rarely justified on evidential grounds. A conversion reaction is a Freudian term with extensive and questionable assumptions about a behavior disorder. A socially unacceptable, unresolved, and unconscious psychological conflict is supposed to have been *converted* into a disorder that is socially more acceptable than the underlying conflict. *Somatization* also implies that a nonphysical (psychological) problem has been unconsciously converted into a physical problem. Typically, however, examples of psychogenic, conversion, or somatization voice disorders cited in the literature do not demonstrate the psychodynamics of unconscious conflicts. Instead, the examples show various stressful or conflicting life situations in which a voice disorder may provide some escape from a difficult situation or an advantage to the speaker. Furthermore, Boone, at al. (2010) claim that in their extensive clinical practice, treatment of most patients with psychogenic aphonia is successful with behavioral (symptomatic) voice therapy, and that too, in a single session. Psychotherapy, presumably needed to resolve unconscious psychological conflicts, seems to be unnecessary. This treatment outcome does not support a psychodynamic (conversion) causation of functional aphonia. Furthermore, there is no efficacy data that support psychological therapy to treat voice disorders (Stemple et al., 2010).

Voice disorders presumed to have unconscious psychodynamic mechanisms may be parsimoniously described as those that are either negatively reinforced (providing certain desirable escapes) or positively reinforced (providing benefits or advantages). The hypothesis that functional (psychogenic) aphonia is a behavior disorder is consistent with how it is successfully treated with behavior therapy.

In this chapter, we call a voice disorder functional only when there is no tissue damage or neurological impairment *coexisting with the disorder*. We also prefer the term *behavioral* to *functional* because of many questionable connotations and varied definitions of the latter term in voice literature (Aronson & Bless, 2009).

Although not entirely satisfactory, voice disorders may be classified as *mutism, aphonias,* and *dysphonias*. We use this categorization, and within each of those main categories, we suggest either an organic or a behavioral origin for specific disorders.

Mutism

Mutism is absence of vocal communication, typically discussed in the context of aphonia, although there are similarities and differences between them. The similarity between the two is that there is no voice production in both mutism and aphonia. The difference is that aphonia involves whispered (nonphonated) articulation and effective communication; both are absent in mutism. Possibly, mutism is not limited to a voice disorder and may not be a voice disorder at all; if behavioral (functional), the mute person simply refuses to speak; if neurological, the mute person cannot talk. Therefore, whether the origin is neurological or behavioral, muteness is *absence of communication*. Consequently, mutism is a communication disorder in its broadest sense, not limited impaired phonation.

- **In some cases, mutism is neurophysiological.** Patients in the acute phases of aphasia, final stages of dementia, and most people who are close to death may be mute. Severe brainstem and cerebral lesions (especially frontal lobe lesions) due to traumatic brain injury or vascular lesions can cause a type of muteness called *akinetic mutism* (Aronson & Bless, 2009). Patients with akinetic mutism are alert with open eyes, but are indifferent to social interactions. Their mutism is not complete; they speak normally when verbally stimulated. The extent and duration of mutism vary across patients. Voice clinicians, however, have paid much attention to behavioral (functional) mutism.

- **Behavioral mutism is zero or near zero probability of speaking in certain social situations.** There usually is no vocal or neural pathology that prevents phonation or speech production. The term *selective mutism* is sometimes used to describe the same condition, although the evidence is often lacking to show that the individual *selects* to be mute. In any case, behavioral mutism is characterized by no voice and no silent or whispered articulation. Persons with behavioral (selective) mutism can talk, have normal voice, do talk in some situations, but do not talk in other situations. These persons, however, may communicate through gestures, facial expressions, and pulling and pushing of people around them. They may even produce limited verbalizations in a monotonous voice. Therefore, this kind of mutism is not a total loss of communication. In another kind of behavioral mutism, described as *psychogenic* or *conversion reaction* (Aronson & Bless, 2009), the person communicates with writing, has no vocal pathology, and can produce voice or vocal adduction during coughing. The client does not phonate voluntarily, but seems to be unaware of his or her own involuntary phonation.

Aphonias

Aphonia is loss of voice, an absence of phonation, though not entirely of communication. In clinical practice, individuals who are diagnosed with aphonia rarely have a total and constant loss of phonation. If they do, their diagnosis will be *mutism*, in which non-phonated articulatory movements are absent as well. Most aphonic persons produce voice during coughing, laughing, or throat clearing. Many communicate effectively with whispers, gestures, and facial expressions. Unlike persons with mutism, those who are aphonic may silently *articulate* speech sounds. Rarely avoiding communicative situations, they whisper clearly with prosodic features comparable to those of phonated speech. Some clients may speak with a faint voice with breathiness or with a weak, shrill voice.

There are several forms of aphonia. Some forms are due to neurological causes, hence considered organic. Other forms are behavioral (functional).

Neurological Aphonia

In some patients with aphonia, there is evidence of neural damage as well as other communication disorders. For instance, patients who have vocal fold paralysis also may have flaccid dysarthria. Aphonia associated with neurological involvement may be more or less intermittent. When there is no aphonia, there may be dysphonia. Two kinds of paralysis of the vocal folds often are associated with aphonia and dysphonia.

- **Periods of aphonia may be associated with unilateral vocal fold paralysis.** Caused by damage to the recurrent laryngeal nerve (a branch of the cranial nerve X, the vagus) unilateral vocal fold paralysis may be associated with dysphonia or periods of aphonia, as a part of the symptom complex of flaccid dysarthria. The left vocal fold paralysis is more common than the right-fold paralysis because of the extensive course of the left recurrent laryngeal nerve that is likely to be damaged during trauma and surgery (Boone et al., 2010).

- **Bilateral vocal fold paralysis also may result in aphonia.** In such cases, the concern is not aphonia, but the patient's survival and food intake. To produce paralysis of both the vocal folds, the lesion must occur high in the trunk of the vagus nerve. Tumors at the base of the skull, trauma, or carcinoma may cause the vagus nerve damage, leading to bilateral vocal fold paralysis (Boone et al.,

2010). The folds may be paralyzed in the abductory or adductory positions. In either case, phonation is impaired or impossible because the folds cannot move to the midline to vibrate.

Behavioral Aphonia

Behavioral (functional) aphonia exists without vocal or neural pathology. Behavioral aphonia with a sudden onset is classified as functional or psychogenic (often with a conversion connotation) if no organic causes are found for the lack of voice (Aronson & Bless, 2009; Boone et al., 2010). As noted previously, unconscious psychodynamic explanations of conversion reaction are difficult to verify, and behavioral explanations are more parsimonious and consistent with behavioral treatments that are usually successful. In assessing behavioral aphonia, the clinician may consider whether it is correlated with some stressful life situation, preceding physical disease, and such maintaining causes as positive or negative reinforcement.

- **Aphonia may be a learned reaction to stressful life situations.** About 80% of patients who exhibit this type of (conversion) aphonia are women (Aronson & Bless, 2009). In some cases *acute* or *prolonged stress* may trigger aphonia. For instance, a person may become suddenly aphonic during a courtroom testimony, offering escape from the aversive (stressful) witness stand. A behavior (in this case aphonia) that helps escape from a stressful situation (witness stand) is *negatively reinforced*—that is, it is sustained over time. Similarly, aphonia may provide escape from a dreaded public speaking assignment, promptly followed by negative reinforcement because of successful avoidance of the speaking engagement. In other cases, aphonia may be positively reinforced and maintained. For instance, a person with aphonia may be socially reinforced when communicating with whispers. As long as the communication with whispers is effective, it is inherently reinforced.

- **Aphonia may be learned reaction to physical diseases.** Some patients may become aphonic after experiencing flu, upper respiratory illness, meningitis, or other physical illnesses. If vocal rest was advised or speech was extremely limited for any reason during the illness, aphonia, even if somewhat limited, would have been present. For instance, a patient may begin to whisper when seriously ill with flu or other upper respiratory illness. The patient may then continue to whisper even after the disease condition disappears, possibly because of positive reinforcement received during the aphonic period. Another patient, who is told not to speak for a few weeks because of severe vocal nodules, may continue to be aphonic even after the nodule has disappeared. Such cases have been documented (Boone et al., 2010).

Dysphonias

Dysphonias include all disorders of voice except for aphonia. Dysphonias are deviations in vocal parameters of intensity, frequency, and quality; they are patterns of vocal behavior that are inconsistent with those found in the verbal community.

To avoid a confusion between causes and effects, voice disorders may be described exclusively in terms of voice features (e.g., loudness, pitch, and quality). Known organic or behavioral causes may then be described.

Disorders of Loudness (Intensity)

Loudness is an auditory sensation that physical sound stimulus evokes. Intensity (also called the sound pressure) is a measure of the physical properties of the sound stimulus whereas loudness is a judgment listeners make based on their auditory sensation (Raphael, Borden, & Harris, 2007). *Intensity* may be measured by a sound level meter. *Loudness*, on the other hand, is measured as responses listeners give to sound stimulus. Listeners may be asked to judge whether two sound intensities are equal in loudness, half as loud, or twice as loud, and so forth. This is a scaling procedure in which the measured unit of loudness is called a *sone*. In this measuring procedure, 1 sone equals the loudness of a 1,000 Hz tone at 40 dB (Raphael et al., 2007). Certain verbal or nonverbal responses people give to varying intensities of sound stimuli also are more common measures of loudness. These responses may be nonverbal (e.g., moving away from the source of the sound stimulus) or verbal (e.g., "That is too loud," "Please reduce the volume"). It is these kinds of responses that are implied when loudness is defined as a subjective judgment based on the intensity of the sound stimulus.

In the context of voice, loudness refers to the magnitude (amplitude) of vocal fold vibrations. The greater the amplitude of vibrations, the higher the judged loudness of the phonated sound or voice. The vibratory amplitude or the resulting vocal intensity is largely a function of the subglottic air pressure. The greater the subglottic air pressure, the higher the amplitude of vocal fold vibrations, and correspondingly louder the resulting voice (Kent, 1997).

Disorders of vocal loudness, especially the excessively soft voice may be handicapping because of its failure to meet the social and occupational needs of voice. The typical loudness of conversational speech is around 60 dB SPL at 1 meter. The softest phonated (not whispered) voice is about 40 dB, and the highest the larynx is capable of is 100 to 110 dB (Kent, 1994). Any extreme in the range of normal vocal intensity variation is a disorder of loudness and may need clinical attention. In assessing loudness deviations, the clinician generally considers the social appropriateness of vocal intensity. Socially inappropriate loudness of voice includes several varieties:

- **In some clients, the typical voice may be excessively loud.** Listeners who judge a speaker's voice to be *too loud* find the speaker more or less aversive, depending on the degree of loudness. A few factors are associated with excessive vocal loudness:
    - *Vocal hyperfunction is a factor in excessive loudness.* The term *hyperfunction* means excessive force during phonation. Excessively loud phonation may be a longstanding pattern of vocal behavior with no organic cause or tissue change.
    - *Neurological problems affect vocal loudness.* For instance, the voice of patients with dysarthria, a neurologically based speech disorder, may vary in loudness. Such variations include periodic excessive loudness, although a voice that is too weak or soft is more common.

- *Hearing loss may affect vocal loudness.* Speech that is too loud (or too soft) may be a characteristic of some people with hearing loss. Unacceptable loudness variations also may be a feature.

- **In some clients, the typical voice may be excessively soft.** A voice that is too soft is barely audible and may require additional listener effort to hear the speaker. An excessively soft voice reduces communicative effectiveness in social and occupational situations. Factors associated with this vocal problem include:

  - *Neurological diseases are a frequent cause.* Neurological diseases including amyotrophic lateral sclerosis, Parkinson's disease, and myasthenia gravis, among others, tend to negatively affect vocal loudness (Duffy, 2005; Freed, 2000). Reduced loudness and other voice problems are often a part of dysarthria, a motor speech disorder, described more fully in Chapter 5.

  - *Laryngeal pathologies may reduce vocal loudness.* Any structural abnormality of the vocal folds that reduce its capacity to adduct can negatively affect the loudness of voice. Paralysis of the folds that make it difficult to approximate may result in excessively soft voice or aphonia. In addition, such growth as vocal nodules may reduce vocal loudness because of loss of air pressure due to inadequate approximation of the folds.

  - *A softer voice may be socially conditioned in some cultures.* Though inadequately studied, a relatively softer voice may be a characteristic of some verbal communities. Some individuals speak too softly because of their family or general cultural practices. In such cultures, relatively loud speech may be thought of as impolite. Their speech then may be judged too soft in a different verbal community.

- **Monoloudness is also a disorder of loudness.** A monotonous speech, with little or no variation in loudness (as well as pitch) is a disorder of voice found in some patients, especially in patients with neurological impairments that induce dysarthria. Monoloudness may be found in patients with flaccid, spastic, and hypokinetic dysarthria as well as apraxia of speech.

- **Lack of loudness control is another loudness disorder.** This problem also is more commonly found in patients with neurological impairments. Patients with ataxic or hyperkinetic dysarthria, for instance, may show excess loudness variation in segments of speech.

Disorders of Pitch (Frequency)

The vocal pitch is related to the frequency with which the vocal folds vibrate. The frequency-pitch relationship is similar to the intensity-loudness relationship; in each case, one is the physical stimulus, the other is the individual's response. Progressively higher frequencies of vocal fold vibrations in a speaker evoke comparably higher sensations of pitch in the listener, although the relationship between frequency and pitch is not linear.

As a response to the frequency of sound vibrations, pitch is measured in terms of listener responses. People may be asked to judge whether two (tones) sounds are of the same or different pitch. The unit of pitch measurement is called a *mel*, as the unit of frequency measure per time is called the hertz (Hz). The pitch of a 1000 Hz tone is arbitrarily fixed at 1000 mels and serves as the reference pitch. If a listener judges a tone as half as high in pitch as that of this 1000 Hz tone, then the pitch of that tone is 500 mels. The pitch of a tone judged twice as high has 2000 mels (Raphael et al., 2007).

Disorders of pitch are patterns of vocal behaviors that deviate from the practices of peers in the verbal community. Age and gender typically provide reference points to consider whether the pitch of a speaker is deviant or is within normal limits. Pitch typically varies within a speaker, and lack of variation is a problem in itself, as described later. The variations, however, occur within a socially accepted range. The average frequency of vocal fold vibrations in an individual is called the *fundamental frequency* (average f_o). Among other measures, clinicians may obtain the speaking fundamental frequency (SFF) and frequency variability. The typical or *habitual pitch* of a speaker is related to the SFF, and is defined as the average pitch heard in a sample of continuous speech (Boone et al., 2010; Case, 2002). The lowest possible (basal) and the highest possible (ceiling) pitch may also be measured for a speaker. Such instruments as the Visi-Pitch help measure these aspects of vocal pitch.

Pitch disorders, evaluated against the age, gender, and cultural background of the speaker, are of several kinds. Inappropriately high pitch, pitch breaks, monopitch, and diplophonia are among the more common pitch disorders:

- **Inappropriate pitch is often too high a pitch.** Pitch may be socially and clinically judged too high for the speaker in question. It may be too high because of the age or gender of the speaker. Both males and females may be judged to have abnormally high pitch, although high pitch in the adolescent male is probably the more common high-pitched voice disorder. Known as *falsetto, mutational falsetto,* or *puberphonia,* it is characterized by unusually high vocal pitch in postpubescent males and females. Pitch is lowered in postpubertal males as well as females, although the change is greater in the males. The pitch of boys and girls is roughly the same at age 7, with an average SFF of 260 Hz, within a range of 220–310 Hz. Beginning to diverge around age 8, the pitch of 18-year-old males is 125 Hz, reduced from 400 Hz prevalent at age 1, nearly a 70% reduction. The vocal pitch of 18-year-old females, on the other hand, is 205 Hz, reduced from the same 400 Hz at age 1, only a 50% drop (Wilson, 1987). If the pitch fails to drop to its average adult levels, both boys and girls may be diagnosed with falsetto, which is considered a *functional* or *behavioral voice* disorder because of the absence of neurological or laryngeal structural abnormalities.

- **Pitch breaks may be of three varieties.** Generally, a high-pitched voice breaks lower and a low-pitched voice breaks higher. Of the three varieties of pitch breaks, the first is associated with developmental changes in the laryngeal mechanisms in adolescents. Pitch breaks, if they occur, are evident toward the end of the pubertal changes, roughly by age 16 in boys. The second variety is associated with speaking at inappropriate pitch levels, either too high or too low. An inappropriately low-pitched voice tends to break up by an octave or two. On the other hand, an unusually high-pitched voice breaks down by the same amount. The third variety of pitch breaks is associated with vocal fatigue and hyperfunction. After a prolonged period of speaking, pitch may begin to break because of vocal fatigue. Speaking with much muscular effort also may lead to pitch as well as phonation breaks (Boone et al., 2010).

- **Monopitch is lack of normal pitch variations.** Monotonous voice (lack of pitch variations) is often found in patients with dysarthria, especially those who have ataxic or hypokinetic dysarthria. Vocal fold paralysis may be associated with monopitch. Some individuals with behavioral dysphonia also may exhibit monopitch in additional to other voice problems.

- **Diplophonia is double pitch.** Diplophonia results when voice is simultaneously produced with two distinct frequencies. In some cases, the vocal folds may vibrate at different rates because the two folds vary in their mass; there may be a tissue growth on one of the folds. Other factors that might induce diplophonia include vocal fold paralysis, laryngeal web, ventricular fold vibration, inflammation of the larynx, puberphonia, muscle tension dysphonia, paradoxical vocal fold movement, and aryepiglotic vibration (Boone et al., 2010).

Disorders of Voice Quality

Vocal quality refers to the overall effect of a combination of factors on the nature of voice. Aspects of vocal quality may be measured instrumentally, as described in a later section. Often clinically judged, the quality of voice is influenced by the manner in which phonation is produced. For instance, audible air leakage during phonation affects vocal quality. Other aspects of quality refer to how listeners react to voice. Listeners may find the voice harsh, hoarse, and unpleasant. Pitch, loudness, resonance, and laryngeal tension also influence vocal quality, but quality is more than just these factors. Faulty approximation of the vocal folds may be a basic factor producing quality deviations.

- **Breathiness is air leakage during phonation.** When the vocal folds approximate inadequately, excessive air will leak through the glottis, adding noise to the phonated sound. In some cases, breathy voice may result in speech that is almost whispered. Instrumentally measured, breathiness is most highly correlated with acoustic aperiodicity and relative amplitude of the first harmonic (Case, 2002). Several organic conditions cause less than the optimum vocal fold approximation and the resulting breathiness of voice. Extraneous growth on the vocal folds, such as nodules and polyps prevent optimum approximation of the two folds. Vocal fold paralysis will have the same effect. In some individuals, a breathy voice may be behavioral; it may be learned and maintained by social or occupational reinforcement.

- **Harshness is rough voice.** Listeners tend to judge it as grating and unpleasant. The harsh voice is produced with excessive muscular tension and forceful adduction of vocal folds (hard glottal attacks). The harsh voice may also be high pitched. Harsh voice results when laryngeal vibrations are aperiodic. Neurological diseases that cause motor speech disorders (e.g., ataxic or spastic dysarthria) and laryngeal structural problems (e.g., nodules) also may be associated with vocal harshness.

- **Hoarseness is a grating and husky quality of voice.** A commonly observed dysphonia, hoarseness is a combination of breathiness and harshness. If harshness is predominant, the vocal folds are too tightly adducted. If breathiness is predominant, the folds are somewhat loosely adducted. Voice breaks, diplophonia, and low pitch complete the clinical picture of hoarseness. Spectrographic analysis may reveal an element of noise in the main formant of a vowel production, a high-frequency noise above 3000 Hz, and a loss of high-frequency harmonic component (Case, 2002). Common causes of hoarse voice include laryngitis and abusive vocal behaviors that cause nodules and polyps. Allergies and upper respiratory illnesses and neurological damage (especially lesions of the superior and recurrent branches of the Cranial nerve X) may also cause hoarseness, as well as reduced loudness and lower pitch (Duffy, 2005).

- **Tense voice involves medial compression of the folds.** In producing this kind of vocal quality, the folds are excessively adducted. Clinicians and other listeners judge the voice produced with hyperadduction as *tensed*. An organic condition, such as the cleft of the soft palate, may encourage hyperadduction as a compensatory mechanism. Tense voice also may be a vocal behavioral pattern with no organic basis.

Disorders of Resonance

Listeners do not hear the laryngeal tone as it is produced by the vocal folds because the tone is modified in various ways by the structures above the larynx. Such modifications are called *resonance*. This normal process of resonance may be impaired for various reasons, typically organic, and the result is a resonance disorder of voice. Resonance disorders are due to a lack of balance between oral resonance and nasal resonance. Oral resonance is a contribution of the oral structures when they are disconnected with the nasal structures. Normally, oral resonance predominates on oral speech sounds. Nasal resonance is a contribution of the nasal cavities, which add resonance to nasal speech sounds. There are four kinds of resonance disorders, each with a set of causative factors.

- **Hypernasality is excessive nasal resonance on oral speech sounds.** The nasal cavities add undesirable resonance on oral speech sounds because the velopharyngeal port is not fully closed when it should. Hypernasality is most evident on vowels and vocalic consonants. Difficulty in keeping the oral and nasal cavities isolated from each other during the production of oral sounds is most often due to craniofacial anomalies including the cleft of the soft palate, submucous cleft, or velopharyngeal inadequacy. A congenitally short hard palate, short velum, and deep pharynx also may create hypernasality in children or older individuals. In older adults, however, hypernasality is often due to neurological diseases that affect the cranial nerves IX, X, or XI, resulting in reduced motor control of the velopharyngeal mechanism. Hypernasality is a significant component in flaccid, spastic, hypokinetic, and hyperkinetic dysarthrias in older adults. In some cases, the velum may be paralyzed, preventing velopharyngeal closure. Adults who are deaf (as well as children) may produce hypernasal oral speech sounds.

- **Hyponasality is too little nasal resonance on nasal sounds.** In most cases, reduced nasal resonance on nasal speech sounds is due to organic causes, although it can occur in individuals who are deaf, but have normal oronasal structures. Because of lack of self-feedback, speech of people with deafness may be both hyper- and hyponasal. The organic factors most often found to be associated with hyponasality include pharyngitis and tonsillitis, diseases of the nasal cavity, allergies and upper respiratory disorders, nasal polyps and papillomas, foreign bodies in the nasal cavity, and nasal neoplasm (growth in the nasal cavity).

- **Cul-de-sac nasality is the *bottom of the sac* resonance.** Muffled or hollow-sounding oral resonance, cul-de-sac resonance gives the impression that the voice is echoing in the back of the mouth (Andrews, 2006). This type of resonance is thought to be caused by muscle hyperfunction (Deem & Miller, 2000). When the tongue is bunched up at the back of the mouth, the oral resonance is muffled. An anterior nasal obstruction with posterior opening also may cause cul-de-sac resonance. In some individuals, this type of resonance may be due to a pattern of vocal behavior, presumably learned, with no organic basis.

- **Assimilative nasality is contextual nasal resonance.** This is nasal resonance heard on oral sounds (vowels and voiced consonants) that are adjacent to the nasal sounds. A common cause is velopharyngeal deficiency. Premature opening of the velopharyngeal port while still producing the oral sounds will add nasal resonance to oral sounds that precede the nasal sounds. Failure to promptly close the velopharyngeal port soon after producing nasal sounds will add nasality to oral sounds that follow.

Spasmodic Dysphonia

A particular type of voice disorder, spasmodic dysphonia (SD) is considered a diagnostic category by itself needing separate description. It is indeed a form of dysphonia but its characteristics are a combination of many dysphonic features, as well as some unique features. Some clinicians consider its etiology mixed or varied from behavioral (psychogenic) to neurological (Aronson & Bless, 2009) while others seem to consider its origin as either unknown (idiopathic) or entirely neurological (e.g., see Boone et al., 2010; Sapienza & Ruddy, 2009; Stemple et al., 2010). Most clinicians think that SD is a type of focal dystonia, a movement disorder, in which action-induced and task-specific movement is impaired. SD forms a clinical cluster with hyperkinetic dysarthria (Boone et al., 2010), although it can occur in the absence of neural or laryngeal pathology (Aronson & Bless, 2009; Stemple et al., 2010). Even though the current opinion is that SD is a neurological disorder, no specific neuropathology has been clearly identified in all patients (Blumin & Berke, 2007). Certain neurological symptoms, such as voice tremor, deteriorating handwriting, ataxic gait, dystonia (focal or general), spasmodic torticollis (spasms of the neck muscle) may be associated with SD (Aronson & Bless, 2009).

A relatively rare disorder, SD is more common in women than in men. Onset in a majority of cases occurs between the ages of 40 and 60 years; fewer cases are reported in younger and older populations (Aronson & Bless, 2009). The disorder is associated with vocal fold spasms (hence the recently revised name from the earlier term, *spastic* dysphonia) that result in voice judged strangled and strained. The acoustic effect of voice production is thought to be due to involuntary contractions of the laryngeal muscles (spasms). These spasms are absent in nonspeech activities or during laughing, crying, or swallowing.

As detailed by Aronson and Bless (2009), SD may have the most far-reaching effects on the lives of people who have it. It may render many individuals ineffective in their jobs, forcing them to retire or apply for disability pension. The patients may begin to avoid social interactions and remain mostly silent even in their own homes. They may experience strong negative emotions, including frustration, anger, hopelessness, helplessness, and depression. Some patients may even be suicidal.

Three types of spasmodic dysphonia have been noted: adductor SD, abductor SD, and mixed.

- **Adductor spasmodic dysphonia (ADSD) is the most common type.** More than 80% of patients with SD may have this variety. The features of ADSD include:

  ○ *The voice may be most severely strained-strangled, choked, or squeezed.* These classic symptoms of SD are most prominent in the adductor type. The voice is severely hyperfunctional. Pitch breaks, voice breaks, and laryngeal spasms especially on voiced sounds may be more or less frequent. Phonation, always extremely effortful, may be almost impossible for some patients. Vowels may be initiated with hard glottal attacks. With a jerky rhythm, the speech of patients with ADSD may have a staccato and stuttering-like characteristic, although not to be diagnosed as *laryngeal stuttering*, a term used in the past. Monopitch and reduced loudness may make it nearly impossible for them to shout. These features, absent when the patient produces phonation involuntarily (as in laughing or coughing), suddenly emerge when the patient tries to talk to someone. There may be periods of normal phonation during speech, however.

  ○ *Extreme hyperadduction of vocal folds evident on endoscopic examination.* Even the false folds also may hyperadduct. The laryngeal and lower pharyngeal airway may be severely constricted. Involuntary spasms are a feature of the laryngeal adductors—thyroarytenoid and the lateral criocoarytenoid muscles.

  ○ *Laryngeal spasms may vary across speech tasks.* Speaking on the telephone may be more difficult than face-to-face conversation. Laryngeal spasms may increase while reading aloud a new passage but decrease while singing, which may even be normal.

  ○ *Patients may exhibit additional symptoms.* Many patients may report fatigue due to their constant effort to produce voice and tension in their neck, back, and shoulder muscles. Shortness of breath may be an additional symptom. Extraneous motor behaviors including head jerks, eye blinks, dysrhythmic movements of the chest and abdomen, silent lip movements when the voice is blocked, and repetitions of sounds or syllables, may remind the clinician of people who stutter.

  ○ *ADSD may be associated with an independent vocal tremor.* Consequently, the voice may sound shaky and quivering. This problem may become more evident when ADSD is reduced by treatment.

- ○ *Most patients may try to compensate for their laryngeal spasms.* Whispering, trying to speak on inhalation, avoiding speech, and trying to reduce laryngeal resistance may change the clinical picture. Individual differences in the symptom complex is an important feature.

- **Abductor spasmodic dysphonia (ABSD) is less common than ADSD.** About 15% of patients with SD may have this variety. ABSD is diagnosed when:

  - ○ *The symptoms of ABSD are opposite to those of ADSD.* Instead of involuntarily adducting, the vocal folds involuntarily and inappropriately abduct. Sudden interruption of phonation, resulting in periods of aphonia and bursts of breathiness, is the predominant feature of ABSD. The voice that gets interrupted in this manner may be normal or hoarse.

  - ○ *The abductory spasms occur mostly on unvoiced consonants.* If the patient is asked to read a passage loaded with unvoiced consonants, the spasms increase; if the passage read is loaded with voiced consonants, the spasms will decrease.

  - ○ *The posterior cricoarytenoid muscle, the laryngeal abductor, spasms in producing ABSD.* Endoscopic examination will reveal sudden and inappropriate abduction of vocal folds during speech, showing a widely open glottis that should be approximating. The air then escapes through the open glottis with no phonation being produced.

  - ○ *Emotional state may affect the frequency of spasms.* When relaxed, the patient may have fewer spasms than when tense, anxious, or angry.

- **Mixed spasmodic dysphonia (MSD) is found in some individuals.** As the name implies, the symptoms of both ADSD and ABSD may be found in these patients.

  - ○ *The vocal folds hyperadduct as well as overabduct.* The consequence is that the voice, sounding strained-strangled, will suddenly sound breathy and aphonic. Hyperadduction and overabduction may precede and be followed by each other, or may both be intermittent.

  - ○ *Some experts believe that most patients have MSD.* Most patients may have both the abductor and adductor spasms, but one may be predominant or more evident at certain times (Blumin & Berke, 2007).

Assessment and diagnosis of SD may be challenging as there are no specific instrumental tests for it. Carefully taken case history and systematic listening for the voice deviations are essential for diagnosis.

Causes of Voice Disorders

The cause of voice disorders are in many cases a chain of events, the end result being the voice disorder. A voice disorder, as noted previously, can be confused with its cause in the chain of events, as when a clinician describes vocal nodules as a *functional voice disorder*. First, the nodules are not voice problems, and second, the voice problems associated with nodules are not functional. They often are described as functional only because the immediate cause in the causal chain is skipped and a cause of the nodule—a pattern of behavior—is identified as the cause of the voice disorder. It is important to consider the entire chain of causation, but a closely preceding factor that acts as a cause should not be ignored.

The human larynx is a sensitive biological mechanism that is capable of producing a variety of sounds, but it should remain within its range of healthy vibratory patterns. Such vibratory patterns may be affected by a variety of causes. In some cases, the causes of voices disorders may remain unknown. The disorders are then described as *idiopathic*. Known causes of voice disorders may be laryngeal pathologies and trauma, neural pathologies, or unhealthy patterns of vocal behavioral.

Laryngeal Pathologies and Trauma

Benign or malignant growths, infections, and physical trauma may affect the structural integrity of the vocal folds, causing some of the common as well as rare voice disorders.

- **Laryngeal cancer is the most serious of laryngeal pathologies.** Carcinoma (cancer) may affect the vocal folds, supraglottal structures, subglottal structures, and all or a combination of these. Causes of laryngeal cancer are inferred from correlation. Factors in the history of patients that are correlated with cancer include smoking, excessive drinking, and a combination of the two that may be the most serious. A genetic predisposition is thought to play a role. Hoarseness is a predominant sign of early cancer, and may be accompanied by a lower pitch due to heavier vocal folds. Other symptoms include pain, bleeding, respiratory problems, and swallowing difficulties. When the cancer spreads, and the only treatment option is surgical removal of the vocal folds, the patient loses the typical biological source of phonation. The patient is then a candidate for alaryngeal speech assessment and rehabilitation.

- **Contact ulcers and granuloma may be benign growths.** Ulcers are often found on the medial vocal processes. Contact ulcer granulomas are protective, granulated tissue that forms over the ulcers (Boone et al., 2010). The entire approximating margins of the vocal folds may be granulated as well as inflamated. The major voice problems are vocal fatigue and hoarseness. A potential cause in many cases is laryngopharyngeal reflux. Pre- or postsurgery intubation may be another cause. Excessive slamming of the folds, excessive shouting, and talking —all vocal behavioral patterns, may cause ulcers and granuloma as well.

- **Cysts are soft lesions.** Often unilateral, sometimes bilateral or even multiple, cysts tend to occur on the superior or inferior surface of the vocal fold margins. Some may be fluid filled. They may be whitish squamous epithelial or yellowish mucous-retention type. The causes of cysts are not well understood, although poor lymphatic drainage and vocally abusive behaviors are suggested factors. Most are benign. Preferred treatment is surgical, followed by voice therapy if warranted. The voice of the patient with cysts may be low pitched, hoarse, and weak; breathiness may be evident if the cysts are large.

- **Hemangiomas are soft, blood-filled sacs.** Similar to granulomas except softer, they tend to occur on the posterior larynx. They are more common in children, but adults may also develop them. Vocal abuse, hyperacidity, and intubation-induced trauma are the most frequent causes. Hoarseness, breathiness, low pitch, or limited pitch range are the dominant vocal characteristics. The treatment is surgical, followed by voice therapy.

- **Hyperkeratosis is pinkish rough growth.** Typically leaf shaped, the keratinized (horny) cells tend to grow on the vocal folds or inner glottal margins. They may be unilateral as well as bilateral and premalignant. Potential causes include excessive drinking and smoking and exposure to smoke-filled environments. The voice may be hoarse.

- **Some vocal fold changes are due to endocrine variations or disorders.** Vocal fold thickening may be caused by hypothyroidism or lowered estrogen and progesterone in women during menstruation. A lower or higher than the normal pitch and general hoarseness may be the main vocal characteristics. Menopause in women may be associated with a lowering of the vocal pitch.

- **Infectious (acute) laryngitis is inflammation of the larynx.** A nonspecific condition, inflammation may be due to viral infection (e.g., the common cold). Often associated with dry and sore throat, hoarseness is a common voice problem.

- **Leukoplakia are patchy, white lesions.** They tend to occur on the superior surface of the vocal folds and under the tongue. Leukoplakia may be precancerous, leading eventually to squamous cell carcinoma. Excessive and prolonged smoking and exposure to harmful chemicals may be the cause of these lesions. Hoarseness, diplophonia, and reduced vocal intensity are the vocal characteristics associated with leukoplakia.

- **Papilloma are mostly found in children, but may be present in adults.** These mulberry- or wart-like growths on the vocal folds and related structures may obstruct the airway, and therefore, be life threatening. The human papilloma virus is the cause of these growths and result in shortness of breath, vocal hoarseness, and infrequent aphonia.

- **Polyps are soft and fluid-filled lesions.** They are found on the anterior and middle one-third portion of vocal fold edges (the same typical site of vocal nodules). Typically found in adults, not children, they tend to be unilateral. Polyps may be broad-based *sessile* or narrowly based *pedunculated* (a small balloon with a narrow stem). If they are large enough, pedunculated polyps may obstruct the airway. Onset may be acute and the growth may be rapid. A single episode of vocal abuse may cause them, and frequent throat clearing may exacerbate them. Diplophonia, sudden voice breaks, and hoarseness may be the voice symptoms.

- **Reinke's edema is diffuse swelling in Reinke's space.** This typically bilateral edema consists of gelatinous material and may advance into enlarged fluid-filled bag-like structures (called polypoid degeneration). Smoking and chronic vocal abuse are thought to be the causes. The voice problems include hoarseness and low pitch (because of increased mass of the folds).

- **Sulcus vocalis is a longitudinal and narrow depression on the vocal folds.** These unilateral or bilateral grooves that develop along the vocal fold edges may be congenital in children and acquired in adults. A unilateral bowing or scar of the folds may accompany the sulci. Causes of sulcus vocalis are unclear and its diagnosis and treatment are difficult. The vocal symptoms include decreased vocal intensity, periodic aphonia, hoarseness, and a strained vocal quality.

- **Traumatic (chronic) laryngitis is mostly due to vocal abuse.** The vocal folds may be reddened, swollen, and thickened. Yelling, screaming, cheering, effortful phonation, excessive talking, frequent throat clearing and coughing, and forceful singing are among the frequent causes of laryngeal (phono) trauma. Smoke, dust, and toxic fume inhalation are contributing factors. Speaking with inappropriate pitch and loudness also are known to produce phonotrauma. A hoarse and low-pitched voice is the main vocal feature.

- **Vocal nodules are common vocal fold lesions.** They typically are bilateral, whitish, benign, callous-like growths on the midpoint of the vocal fold edges, although the site of growth may vary. In some cases, multiple nodules may develop. Nodule development is associated with vocal abuse and misuse (including frequent yelling and screaming, hard glottal attacks, excessive talking, and singing in abusive ways) over a period of time. Alcohol abuse and frequent throat clearing also are associated factors. Because they prevent optimal approximation of the folds, nodules cause breathiness, lower pitch, and hoarseness. The voice may sound like it lacks proper resonance. The patient may experience vocal fatigue toward the end of the day.

- **Webbing, often congenital, may be acquired.** They are a thin and web-like, small or large tissue growth that spreads across the vocal folds. The growth is often found at the anterior commissure where the two folds come together. Acquired webbing in adults is due to trauma to the medial edges of the folds. The symptoms include severe dysphonia and possible respiratory distress (shortness of breath).

- **Laryngeal trauma may be due to external factors.** This is in contrast to phono- or laryngeal trauma due to vocal abuse or misuse. Externally induced injury to laryngeal structures may be a medical emergency, requiring immediate medical or surgical treatment. Causes of external laryngeal trauma are of three kinds. First, the larynx may be injured due to automobile accidents, assault and gunshot wounds, attempted strangulation, and similar causes. Second, the larynx may be injured because of burning. Inhalation of hot smoke in burning buildings, gas inhalation, automobile exhaust inhalation when trapped in a closed space, and harmful chemical ingestion in industrial accidents or during an attempted suicide may burn the larynx. Third, the larynx may be injured during surgical procedures. Tracheostomy and long-term use of intubation may cause vocal fold irritation, edema, webbing, granuloma, and vocal fold paralysis.

- **Stomach acid reflux may cause vocal changes.** When the stomach juices flow back into the esophagus, the disorder is called the *gastroesophageal reflux disease (GERD)*. When the acid flow reaches the pharyngeal and laryngeal areas, the disorder is called the *laryngopharyngeal reflux* (LPR). Reflux may be responsible for nonspecific laryngeal disorders in certain patients served by otolaryngologists.

LPR tends to occur during daytime when the patient is mostly upright, whereas GERD occurs in the night when the patient is supine. In LPR, the stomach acids cause irritation and inflation of the laryngeal mucosa. Additional symptoms include globus pharyngeas (a lump-in-the throat feeling), excess mucus, chronic cough, and habitual throat clearing. Such other clinical conditions as contact ulcers, laryngitis, and subglottic stenosis have been linked to LPR. Heartburn and indigestion may or may not be present. Dysphonia may not be present in all patients with LPR, but when present, it may be mild to severe. Up to 55% of patients with hoarse voice may have LPR (Ylitalo, 2007).

Neurological Pathologies

Neurological diseases that impair the neural control of vocal folds are a common cause of voice disorders in the elderly population. Some neurological disorders may cause vocal fold paralysis, as noted in a previous section. Other neurological disorders, especially the neurodegenerative diseases, may affect swallowing and all aspects of speech production, including respiration, phonation, articulation, and prosody. A result of such widespread effects, found in many patients with neurological diseases, is dysarthria—a motor speech disorder. Both the central and peripheral nervous system may be affected (Duffy, 2005; Freed, 2000).

A wide range of neurological conditions can affect voice. Only a few major ones are highlighted here. Furthermore, description of dysarthria will be brief in this section because Chapter 5 provides more details about dysarthria and associated speech and voice problems.

- **Vocal fold paralysis may be unilateral or bilateral.** Both types may be associated with various disorders of communication, including voice problems.
    - *Unilateral vocal fold paralysis is often caused by damage to the recurrent laryngeal nerve (RLN).* Surgical accidents (including thoracic surgical accidents) are a major cause of damage to the RLN, affecting the laryngeal adductor muscles, especially the lateral cricoarytenoid muscle. Voice disorders include breathiness, hoarseness, monotone, intermittent diplophonia, pitch breaks, and reduced vocal intensity. Aphonia may be an infrequent symptom. These voice problems may be a part of flaccid dysarthria.
    - *Bilateral vocal fold paralysis produces more serious effects.* When both the folds are paralyzed, the airway may remain open, causing serious dysphagia. Damage to the descending motor tracts and the brainstem, caused by various diseases and trauma cause bilateral vocal fold paralysis. The paralysis may be of the abductory or adductory type. Both have serious consequences. As noted earlier, the patient's survival and feeding, not voice, are the main medical concerns.
- **Voice disorders are a part of neurological diseases that cause several forms of dysarthria.** A variety of neurological diseases and clinical conditions, including vascular problems, strokes, tumors, trauma, degenerative neurological diseases produce a complex motor speech disorder called *dysarthria* with specific

voice problems. There are seven types of dysarthria, each with a constellation of respiratory, phonatory, articulatory, and prosodic features. Voice disorders found in various types of dysarthria depend on the type of dysarthria, but generally include strained-strangled voice, pitch breaks, low pitch, harshness, monoloudness, excess loudness variations, weak voice, hyper- or hyponasality, nasal emission, breathiness, harshness, hoarseness, monopitch and monoloudness, voice tremors, and voice arrests.

Assessment of voice disorders in patients with neurological disorders is a part of the motor speech assessment. Therefore, the clinicians are referred to Chapters 5 and 6 for details.

Patterns of Vocal Behaviors

Vocal behavior patterns affect the health of the vocal folds. Several vocal behaviors are related to voice disorders because of their negative effects on the structure or function of the laryngeal mechanism. For instance, vocally abusive behaviors create such laryngeal structural changes as nodules or polyps, and account for voice disorders in many individuals. Speaking with an inappropriate vocal pitch, on the other hand, may not produce any tissue change. In this section, we describe vocal behaviors that are related to voice problems, whether they are traditionally classified as organic or functional.

- **Vocally abusive behaviors may induce laryngeal tissue change.** Such behaviors are a common cause of laryngeal damage and the resulting voice disorders.

- **Some inappropriate vocal behaviors are called *vocal misuse*.** Speaking at the upper end of the normal pitch range is an example of vocal misuse.

- **Some patterns of vocal behaviors may be a reaction to stressful situations.** Although the role of stress is recognized in the voice literature, the resulting voice disorders are often described as *psychogenic* or *conversion reactions*, a psychoanalytic or Freudian explanation lacking in experimental evidence. Considering such voice disorders in a behavioral context will help identify variables that are responsible, and therefore, could be modified to treat the client. Aphonia in the absence of organic or neurological impairments is the most frequently cited psychogenic voice disorder or conversion reaction. Some individuals may be genetically predisposed to react with a vocal disorder when under stress; once such a reaction is established, it may be maintained by positive or negative reinforcement, as noted previously.

- **Certain vocal behaviors may persist beyond their typical age range.** For instance, puberphonia in a postpubescent male is persistence of childhood vocal pitch. This persistence may be due to positive social reinforcement or negative reinforcement derived from the avoidance of socially embarrassing pitch breaks. Aphonia following a required vocal rest also may be a persistence of reinforced vocal behavior. An assessment of the sources and types of reinforcement maintaining the voice disorder is likely to help plan an effective treatment program.

Overview of the Assessment Process

Assessment of voice may precede or follow a medical evaluation of the patient. Because of the many serious and life-threatening medical conditions (e.g., cancer of the larynx) that are associated with voice disorders, it is essential to have medical consultation done before a final voice diagnosis is made and a voice treatment plan is established. If the patient has not been seen by a medical specialist (usually the otolaryngologist), the SLP should make a referral and wait for the report before initiating voice therapy.

Assessment of voice is a multidimensional activity. Both clinical judgments and instrumental assessments may be necessary. All aspects of voice production need to be assessed. Depending on coexisting disorders (e.g., neurological diseases and associated dysarthria), assessment may involve other aspects of speech production, including respiration, articulation, and prosodic features.

Assessment begins with a carefully recorded case history. The client may fill out a case history form and mail it to the clinician. The next step is a detailed interview of the client to get additional information, obtain clarification, and answer questions about the planned assessment. Chapter 18 provides an *Assessment of Voice: Interview Protocol* for the clinician's use.

A hearing screening and an orofacial examination may follow the interview. Protocols for these common procedures to assessing all disorders of communication are given in Chapter 2. The clinician may then audio- or videorecord a conversational speech for later analysis. Throughout the assessment period, the clinician may observe the client's general and vocal behaviors to evaluate the presence of neuromotor problems and potential behavioral disorders (such as anxiety or stress reactions). Most importantly, the clinician will be carefully listening to the client's voice to make judgments about its loudness, pitch, vocal qualities, any tension associated with phonation, excessive or extremely limited nasal resonance, and so forth.

Clinical Assessment of Voice

Clinical assessment is done with various kinds of voice and speech tasks but without the help of any instrumentation. It is typically called *perceptual evaluation* of voice, a term that unnecessarily introduces the hypothetical concept of *perception*. *Clinical assessment* consists of listening to a client's voice and making certain judgments that support a diagnosis and description of a voice disorder. Often some kind of a rating scale may be used to judge the severity of different aspects of dysphonias.

Clinical judgments play a significant role in assessing voice disorders, even though questions about their validity and reliability persist (Aronson & Bless, 2009). Currently, clinicians who do not have access to expensive instruments to measure vocal parameters may depend entirely on their clinical judgments to diagnose voice disorders. Clinicians who do use electronic instruments need to make a clinical assessment as well. It is essential to combine instrumental assessment with clinical assessment because the same pathologies (e.g., nodules or polyps) revealed by instruments (viewed through endoscopes) may produce differential effects on voice across clients. In addition, instruments may show differences in acoustic signals (e.g., spectrographic tracings of normal and hoarse voice), but the clinician still has to judge the voice production for adequacy, normalcy, and clinical significance of any deviations noted.

Observations of General and Vocal Behaviors

Throughout the assessment period, the clinician may carefully observe and take note of the client's general and vocal behaviors. The clinician is especially interested in answering several questions that will help evaluate how the client produces his or her voice:

- **Does the client exhibit general bodily tension?** Tensed posture of the client and any observed tension in the neck, jaw, and chest may be noted.

- **Are there signs of neurologic involvement?** Tics, tremor, rigidity, flaccidity, paresis, or paralysis may be present. The face may be expressionless (mask-like). Speech intelligibility and emotional expression in speech may be impaired. The flow of speech may be jerky, effortful, and dysfluent.

- **Does the client speak with adequate mouth opening?** The client may be speaking with less than the optimum mouth opening, affecting oral resonance.

- **Does the client speak very loudly or softly?** The client's loudness may vary unpredictably, a sign of neurological involvement (and dysarthria). If the client speaks very softly or whispers, neurological or behavioral factors may be at play.

- **Does the client speak excessively?** Perhaps the client begins to talk incessantly as soon as the clinician begins the interview. He or she may anticipate questions and goes on to answer, instead of waiting for the questions. Perhaps the client gives unduly extended responses.

- **Is there frequent throat clearing and coughing?** These are additional signs of vocal abuse.

- **How does the client initiate speech sounds?** The client may initiate speech sounds softly and gently or forcefully. The clinician may hear hard glottal attacks as the client initiates speech.

- **Does the client have signs of allergy or cold?** The client may frequently sneeze, sniff, blow the nose, and so forth.

Clinical Assessment of Breath Support for Voice Production

Impaired breath support for phonation is a factor that affects voice. Breath support may be assessed instrumentally, although clinical assessment is commonly done as well. The clinician may take note of the type of breathing that seems to be dominant in the client and record his or her observations on the *Adult Voice Evaluation Protocol* given in Chapter 18.

- **Is thoracic breathing dominant?** This type of breathing is the most typical and normal and includes an observable expansion of the chest.

- **Is calvicular breathing dominant?** In this type of breathing, there is an observable elevation of the shoulders. An inefficient manner of breathing, this type may be associated with muscular tension affecting voice. Its clinical significance, however, has been questioned (Stemple et al., 2010).

- **Is diaphragmatic or abdominal breathing dominant?** In this type of breathing, diaphragmatic contraction and abdominal expansion may be evident during inhalation. Upper chest movement may be minimal. Healthy and efficient, this type is often found in professional singers and speakers (Boone et al., 2010).

- **What is the maximum phonation duration?** The clinician may assess this by having the client to take a deep breath and produce /a/, comfortably sustained as long as possible on three trials. The clinician may compare the client's performance with the norms (Ptacek, Sander, Maloney, & Jackson, 1966), taking into consideration individual differences that are significant; the measures are in seconds:

  ○ Roughly, the maximum mean phonation duration is 28 for young adults and 13 for the elderly (Boone et al., 2010).

  ○ Males in the age range of 18–39 years: Mean of about 25 (SD 6.70), but may be as long as 30; the mean for females in the same age range is 20.90 (SD 5.70), but may be as long as 26.

  ○ Males in the age range of 68 to 89: Mean of 18.10 (SD 6.60), but may be as long as 25; the mean for females in the age range of 66 to 93 is 14.20 (SD 5.60), but may be as long as 20 (Andrews, 2006). Unusually high airflow will result in shorter and unusually low airflow will result in longer (maximum) phonation durations (Kent, 1994).

- **What is the s/z ratio?** The clinician may ask the client to sustain the production first of /s/ and then of /z/ for as long as possible on three alternating trials. The longest of the three trials for each sound is taken into consideration. Dividing the longest /s/ by the longest /z/, the clinician calculates the s/z ratio. A ratio of about 1.00 is typical, implying that the /s/ and /z/ durations are roughly equal. Growth on the vocal folds (e.g., nodules) reduce the duration of the voiced /z/ while not affecting the voiced /s/. Greater than 1:4 is an abnormal s/z ratio, suggesting vocal fold pathology, especially mass variations that prevent normal approximation of the two folds (Boone et al., 2010).

- **How many words per breath?** Although there are no precise norms, short phrases (fewer words per breath) indicate impaired breath support for phonation and speech production. It is thought that speakers should produce 12 or more words per breath (Haynes & Pindzola, 2004). Short phrases with significantly fewer words may be found in clients with neurological problems.

Clinical Assessment of Vocal Pitch

A higher or lower than the normal pitch and unexpected variability in pitch may be found in voice disorders of several etiologies. The clinician may assess the following aspects of pitch and record the results on the *Adult Voice Evaluation Protocol* given in Chapter 18:

- **The habitual pitch may be assessed by several methods.** Using a piano or a pitch pipe, the clinician can match the client's pitch as he or she counts from

1 to 10, reads aloud a printed passage, engages in conversational pitch, or produces a prolonged /a/. The clinician also may play back audiorecorded models of adult male and female voice samples (production of vowels prolonged for about 3 seconds) and ask the client to match the pitch. The client may be asked to say "mmmhhumm" in response to a question that is answered *yes* and "hhmm-mmm" in response to a question answered *no*. The pitch of the "mmm" is thought to be the client's most desirable (habitual) pitch. The clinician may compare the client's habitual pitch with the norms given in Table 17–1.

- **The client's pitch range should be established.** The client may be asked to count from 1 to 25 while progressively lowering the pitch until the lowest pitch is recorded. The client may be asked to produce the /i/ with rising pitch until the highest pitch (a falsetto) is reached. The client also may be asked to "step up" and "step down" the musical scale to observe the range.

- **Clinical assessment of pitch should be compared to instrumental assessment.** When both clinical and instrumental assessment of pitch are made, the clinician may compare the results of the two procedures.

Clinical Assessment of Vocal Loudness

Clinical assessment of vocal loudness is less precise than the assessment of pitch. Vocal loudness varies across speaking situations and tasks. Nonetheless, the clinician may use several procedures to make the following kinds of judgments and record the results on the *Adult Voice Evaluation Protocol* given in Chapter 18:

- **Interviewing the family members is a good starting point.** Family members may agree that the client's vocal loudness is adequate, inadequate, or unpredictably (inappropriately) variable.

Table 17–1. Typical (average) Vocal Fundamental Frequencies in Males and Females in the Age Range of 20 to 90

Age	Male	Female
20–29	120	224
30–39	112	196
40–49	107	189
50–59	118	199
60–69	112	200
70–79	132	196
80–90	146	202

Note: Generally adult males have a mean fundamental frequency of 124 Hz and females 227 Hz. Based on studies reported by Hollien & Shipp (1972) and Stoicheff (1981).

- **Listening to the client's speech throughout the assessment period is essential.** The clinician may judge whether loudness of voice is normal, too soft, or too loud.

- **Variation in loudness needs to be noted.** The clinician may judge whether the client maintains a comfortable (normal) loudness level throughout the assessment period. The clinician may take note of variations in loudness as typical or unpredictable.

- **Specific tasks are useful in assessing loudness.** The clinician may ask the client to vary loudness to assess the range of loudness the client is capable of. The client may be asked to whisper, speak softly, speak as loudly as possible, and shout. Asking the patient to count from 1 to 20, gradually increasing the intensity as counting is continued will also reveal the different loudness levels the client can produce.

- **The results of clinical and instrumental assessments should be compared.** When both clinical and instrumental assessment of loudness are made, the clinician may compare the results of the two procedures.

- **Evaluate the client's vocal loudness against the typical:**
  - typical speech intensity level: 60 dB SPL at about 1 meter
  - maximum speech intensity level: 100 to 110 dB SPL at about 1 meter
  - minimum speech (not whispered) intensity level: 40 dB SPL

Clinical Assessment of Vocal Quality

Clinical assessment of vocal quality is essential in evaluating voice in almost all clients with voice disorders. Vocal quality is impaired in both behavioral and neurological disorders that affect voice. The clinician should carefully listen to the voice throughout the assessment and take note of quality deviations. The clinician may use the *Adult Voice Evaluation Protocol* given in Chapter 18 to record his or her observations:

- **The degree of vocal fold tension may be inferred from the vocal quality.** The clinician may note whether the client phonates with excessive laryngeal tension (hyperfunction) or with too little tension. If the voice sounds strained, tight, and effortful, the clinician may infer excessive tension and medial compression of the folds. If the voice sounds breathy or weak, inadequate approximation is inferred.

- **Audible air leakage during speech suggests breathiness of voice.** Less than optimal approximation of the folds due to various organic pathologies or a learned pattern of vocal behavior may be inferred from breathiness.

- **Harshness of voice suggests aperiodicity of vocal fold vibrations.** A harsh vocal quality may be one of the initial impressions a clinician gains at the beginning of assessment. The clinician may find the voice unpleasant, rough, or strident. The clinician should also take note of hard glottal attacks, excessive vocal effort, and abrupt initiation of sound.

- **Hoarseness is a combination of breathiness and harshness.** The clinician should listen for air leakage during phonation, vocal roughness, and a grating or husky voice to judge the presence of hoarseness. The laryngeal tension and hyperfunction may also be noted in clients with hoarse voice.

Clinical Assessment of Resonance

Resonance disorders may be assessed clinically or instrumentally. Clinical assessment includes judgments of hypernasality, hyponasality, and assimilative nasality. The clinician may use the *Resonance Assessment Protocol* given in Chapter 18 to make a thorough clinical assessment of hypernasality, hyponasality, nasal emission, and assimilative nasality. The clinician then may use the *Adult Voice Evaluation Protocol* in Chapter 18 to make summative statements about resonance.

- **Hypernasality or hyponasality often may be assessed simultaneously.** The clinician may use the following procedures to assess the two types of nasal resonance problems:
  - *Hyper- or hyponasality is best judged in connected speech.* Connected speech reveals the presence or absence of nasal resonance better than single word productions. Throughout the interview of the client, the clinician may take note of the extent of nasal resonance.
  - *Nasal resonance may be judged in oral reading.* An oral reading sample may be recorded to judge the degree of nasal resonance. A rating scale may be used to record the results.
  - *Specific speech tasks help evaluate nasal resonance.* Production of phrases or sentences with no nasal sounds in them may reveal a nasal snort, suggestive of inappropriate nasal resonance. The clinician also may have the client produce "maybe-baby-maybe-baby" (Boone et al. 2010). If *baby* within the phrase sounds like *maybe*, the client has hypernasality; if *maybe* in the phrase sounds like *baby*, the client has hyponasality. The client who cannot hum properly also has hyponasality. Finally, the clinician may occlude and release the client's nose when he or she produces phrases loaded with nasal sounds. Hyponasality is indicated when the occluded and unoccluded productions sound the same.
  - *Sustained phonations of vowels /i/ and /u/ are helpful.* As the client produces the vowels, the clinician alternately occludes and releases the client's nostrils. Hypernasality is suspected if the voice changes.
  - *Counting 60 to 100 will differentially reveal nasal and oral resonance.* The 60 series will reveal nasal emission due to frequent /s/ productions; 70 series will reveal assimilation nasality; the 80 series should reveal normal or near normal nasal resonance; the 90 series should sound normal if the client is hypernasal. A /d/ for /n/ substitution would suggest hyponasality.
- **Nasal emission may be assessed by the production of pressure consonants.** Nasal emission is due to inadequate velopharyngeal closure that causes hypernasality.
  - *Counting the numbers in the 60 series will reveal nasal emission.* Repeated productions of /s/—a pressure consonant—in the series will reveal nasal emission.
  - *Phrases loaded with pressure consonants are especially useful.* The clinician may construct phrases loaded with English pressure consonants and have the client produce them.

○ *Nasal emission may be heard or otherwise evaluated.* The clinician may hold a small hand mirror or a shiny spoon under the nose while administering the specific speech tasks. Fogging of the object under the nose suggests nasal emission (as well as hypernasality).

- **Assimilative nasality may be assessed by specific words, phrases, and sentences.** In all tasks, the clinician listens for nasal resonance on oral sounds that precede or follow the nasal sounds:

  ○ *Counting numbers in the 70 series will reveal assimilative nasality.* The frequent occurrence of /n/ in the series will help assess assimilative (assimilated) nasality.

  ○ *Selected word productions will reveal assimilative nasality.* The clinician may construct words that contain a nasal sound in the initial or final positions (e.g., *nice* and *now*; *Ben* and *him*) and ask the client to produce them. Words with a nasal sound in the initial as well as final position (e.g., *moon* and *noun*) also will be good to use.

The clinician may use the *Resonance Assessment Protocol* given in Chapter 18. Accessing the protocol on the CD, the clinician may modify it to suit the individual client.

Assessment of Vocally Abusive Behaviors

Assessment of vocally abusive behaviors that cause organic tissue changes in vocal folds is essential to design an effective treatment program for many clients with voice disorders. Unless these behaviors are assessed and later modified in treatment, the voice disorders may not be successfully eliminated, even with surgical treatment. Therefore, the clinician may assess the presence of several kinds of vocally abusive behaviors.

- **Clinical interview is a typical method to assess vocally abusive behaviors.** Some initial information may be gathered through case history if it is especially designed for voice clients. Typically, the clinician questions the client about the presence and frequency of a wide range of vocally abusive behaviors including:

  ○ *Loud and excessive talking is a basic problem.* The clinician may investigate whether the client engages in excessive talking during upper respiratory illness or menstruation. Other behaviors to be assessed include excessively loud voice; overly argumentative behavior; frequent shouting, screaming, cheering, and throat clearing; habitual name shouting; and hard and abusive laughing

  ○ *Any vocal misuse needs to be assessed.* This includes habitual talking in inappropriate pitch or talking with excessive laryngeal tension.

  ○ *Occupational voice use should be evaluated.* The client may be questioned about abuse or misuse of voice in occupational settings (e.g., teaching, preaching, sports coaching, singing, aerobic instruction, pep club activities); working and talking in noisy conditions (e.g., bars and sports arenas, construction sites); and working in smoke-filled rooms.

  ○ *Smoking and exposure to second-hand smoke are important to assess.* In addition, alcohol abuse and a combination of smoking and excessive drinking need to be evaluated.

A checklist of vocal abuse and misuse is efficient. The clinician may use the *Vocal Abuse and Misuse Assessment Protocol* given in Chapter 18 and access it on the accompanying CD to individualize it.

Instrumental Assessment of Voice

A variety of computerized instruments are now available to measure various vocal parameters that are clinically related to disorders of voice. Although not all clinicians have access to these instruments, the computer-based programs to analyze speech and voice are becoming more affordable. Various instruments allow for aerodynamic, acoustic, electromyographic, and electroglottographic analysis of speech and voice production. Added to these are the imaging techniques that help evaluate the laryngeal structures and their health.

Aerodynamic Assessment

Several instruments help make aerodynamic assessment. Clinicians can measure such aerodynamic variables as airflow rates, tranglottic airflow, subglottic air pressure, supraglottic pressure, glottal impedance, glottal resistance, and vital capacity. Some of the commonly available instruments include the following:

- **Pneumotachograph helps make most airflow measures.** A divided air mask may be used to separately measure oral and nasal airflow during speech production. A *pneumograph* may be used to measure thoracic and abdominal movements caused by respiration. *The phonatory Aerodynamic System* is a computerized pneumotachographic system developed by KayPENTAX Corporation. It helps assess phonatory flow rate, vital capacity, derived subglottal pressure, glottal resistance, and several other voice parameters.

- **Spirometers help measure inspired and expired air from the lungs.** Although they help measure air volume and lung capacity, spirometers do not allow speech production as the client should blow air into the instrument through a tube.

- **The Nagashima Phonatory Function Analyzer helps measure aerodynamic parameters.** A clinician may use this instrument to make acoustic as well as multiple aerodynamic analysis, including airflow rates and total volume of expired air. The instrument is capable of making simultaneous measurement of phonation and airflow, revealing interaction between voice production and aerodynamic variables.

- **The norms for laryngeal airflow rates are available.** The clinician may compare the client's flow rate with the norms (Kent, 1994):
  - For adult speakers, the normal flow rate is between 100 and 150 cc/sec (ml/sec).
  - For patients with laryngeal pathology (e.g., vocal fold paralysis), the flow rate may increase up to 400 cc/sec, resulting in breathiness.
  - The clinician may consult the manual of specific instruments used to measure different aerodynamic measures for other normative information.

Acoustic Analysis

A direct instrumental analysis of phonation and speech production, acoustic analysis is done to diagnose normal and disordered phonation. The measures include fundamental, average, minimal, and maximal frequency (pitch) and intensity (loudness) of vocal fold vibration. Maximal phonation time, average percentage of jitter and shimmer, harmonics-to-noise ratio, and average s/z ratios also may be analyzed. More or less sophisticated instruments that help make an acoustic analysis of voice and speech include:

- **Piano or an electronic keyboard is a simple means of pitch assessment.** A pitch pipe also may be useful. The client is asked to produce tones that are matched to these instruments. The adult male voice is around B2 (123 Hz) and the adult female voice is around A3 (220 Hz).

- **A sound level meter is a simple instrument to measure vocal intensity.** Analog and digital versions of sound level meters may be found in some electronic stores. Held at a distance of 50 cm from the speaker, a sound level meter may be used to measure vocal intensity from about 40 to 130 dB SPL.

- **Computerized instruments may be used in assessment as well as treatment.** Several such instruments are available for a thorough assessment of the acoustic properties of voice and speech. A more commonly used and comprehensive instrument is the Computerized Speech Lab (CSL) from KayPENTAX. It offers a multidimensional voice profile and helps measure 33 vocal parameters, including real-time pitch, the voice-range profile, jitter, shimmer, and harmonics-to-noise ratio. Several other instruments that the clinician might use include the Visi-Pitch III by Kay Elemetrics Corp., Dr. Speech by Tiger Electronics, and Speech Studio by Lryngograph Ltd. Most computerized instruments may be used to set treatment goals and positive reinforcement for achieving them.

Electroglottography

Electroglottography (EGG) is a method to measure patterns of vocal fold approximations. It requires the placing of one electrode on each side of the thyroid cartilage, at the level of the vocal folds. As the client phonates, this noninvasive procedure generates distinct waveforms that correspond to such clinically judged voice qualities as breathiness and hoarseness. Commonly available instruments include:

- **Electroglottograph by KayPENTAX interfaces with the CSL.** When interfaced, the CSL and the electroglottograph in combination is an efficient method of making instrumental assessment of various aspects of voice production.

- **Other instruments are available.** These include the Electroglottograph EG2-PC by Glottal Enterprises and the Digital Laryngograph by Laryngograph Ltd.

Laryngeal Visualization and Imaging

Techniques that help visualize the laryngeal structures provide a direct method of assessing the health of the vocal folds. Tissue changes and related pathologies may be directly viewed and evaluated with various imaging and visualization techniques. The position of the American Speech-Language-Hearing Association (2004, 2007) is that speech-language pathologists who have received appropriate training may use instruments to visualize the laryngeal structures. Although a diagnosis of laryngeal pathology is the responsibility of laryngologists, well-trained speech-language pathologists may use laryngeal visualization and imaging techniques in their teaching, research, and treatment (American Speech-Language-Hearing Association, 2007). *Laryngoscopy* is a general term that refers to the viewing of the larynx and includes several specific instrumental procedures:

- **A laryngeal mirror is a simple yet commonly used instrument.** It is a method of indirect laryngoscopy because the larynx is not viewed directly, but as a reflection on a small mirror, which is mounted at an angle on a thin handle. The mirror is placed in the oropharynx, angled downward to reflect back the image of the laryngeal structures.

- **A rigid endoscope is inserted through the oral cavity and oropharynx.** The rigid tube (scope) projects downward a high-intensity light to offer a view of the larynx. Because of its placement in the oral cavity, the client is not able to articulate speech during the examination, although the folds may be examined during coughing, laughing, and phonation of vowels.

- **The flexible endoscope is inserted nasally.** The nasal insertion of the flexible tube allows for speech production. When placed above the velum, the scope helps evaluate the velopharyngeal mechanism. When passed farther down into the oropharynx or lower, it helps visualize the larynx and the related structures.

- **The stroboscopy uses flashes of light.** Used in conjunction with a rigid or flexible endoscope, the strobe intermittently illuminates the vocal folds at a rate that is slower than the rate at which the folds vibrate. The result is that the clinician can see the vocal fold movement in slow motion. The Digital Videostroboscopy System by KayPENTAX is a commonly used instrument.

Quality of Life Assessment

A voice disorder can affect an individual's personal, social, and occupational life. It might limit social communication, negatively affect occupational choices or access, and impair interpersonal relations. A client's quality of life (QOL) is affected by the degree to which the voice disorder is a handicap. Therefore, it is important to assess the degree to which a client's voice disorder is a handicap and the extent to which the disorder degrades the QOL (Benninger, Gardner, & Jacobson, 2005).

The quality of life and the degree to which the disorder poses a handicap is measured through questionnaires. Among others, the following may be administered to voice clients:

- **The Voice Handicap Index (VHI) is a 30-item rating scale.** It is a means for the client to self-rate on a 5-point rating scale (0 = *Never* to 5 = *Always*). It includes three sections, each with 10 items to rate the emotional (E), functional (F), and physical (P) nature of the handicap. The emotional items include such statements as *My voice problem upsets me* and *I am ashamed of my voice problem.*

The functional items include such statements as *I tend to avoid groups of people because of my voice* and *My voice problem causes me to lose income*. The physical items include such statements as *I run out of air when I talk* and *I use a great deal of effort to talk* (Jacobson et al., 1997).

- **Voice-Related Quality of Life Measure (V-RQOL) is brief.** It contains only 10 items the client rates on a 5-point rating scale (1 = *None, not a problem* to 5 = *Problem is as "bad as it can be"*). The client is asked to rate such statements as *I sometimes get depressed (because of my voice)* and *I have become less outgoing (because of my voice)* (Hogikyan & Sethuraman, 1999).

- **Some questionnaires target specific groups.** For instance, the *Singing Voice Handicap Index* (SVHI) is especially designed for singers whose voice disorder may interfere with their professional lives (Cohen et al.t, 2007).

In Chapter 18, we offer a *Voice Handicap Assessment Protocol* and a *Voice Quality of Life Assessment Protocol*. The clinician may access both on the CD and individualize it for her or his use.

Assessment of Voice in Ethnoculturally Diverse Adults

In assessing voice disorders in ethnoculturally diverse individuals, clinicians should consider how the client and his or her cultural milieu view the disorder, its effects, and its treatment. An understanding of the client's cultural and language background will help make a valid assessment. Knowledge of a few empirical facts about voice disorders across ethnoculturally varied groups of people helps prepare the clinician to make a culturally appropriate assessment (Holland & DeJarnette, 2002). It should be noted that research studies are limited, and many are unreplicated. Clinicians should watch for new and replicated evidence that may or may not support earlier evidence:

- **Diseases that cause voice disorders are differentially distributed in ethnocultural groups.** The clinician should be aware of the previously summarized information on how diseases that cause voice disorders differentially affect varied populations.

- **Assessment of vital capacity may need to consider the ethnocultural background.** African American men and women may have smaller vital capacities than the whites (Williams, 1975).

- **Mean fundamental frequency for African-American males may be lower than the general norm.** In assessing this variable, the clinician should consider that the normal (modal) fundamental frequency may be 110.15 Hz for African American males and 193.10 Hz for females (as compared respectively to 116.65 Hz for white men and 217.00 Hz for white women) (Hudson & Holbrook, 1981).

- **Listeners may judge the race and age of a speaker correctly.** One variable that might help judge the race is the tendency of African Americans to produce more glottal fry than whites. Older African Americans also may be judged younger than they are (see Holland & DeJarnette, 2002, for studies).

It should be noted that not all minority groups have been studied for differences in their vocal characteristics. The clinician should make a client- and culture-specific assessment with no stereotypic assumptions.

Postassessment Counseling

The clinician concludes the assessment session with postassessment counseling. The clinician shares the assessment information with the client, accompanying family members, and other caregivers. Subsequent to the postassessment counseling, the clinician makes an analysis of information obtained from the case history and interview, reports from other specialists, clinical assessment results, instrumental evaluations, and results of questionnaires or other tests. Integrating the information collected from all sources and means, the clinician writes a diagnostic report. See Chapter 1 for details on the analysis and integration of assessment data and clinical report writing.

During the postassessment counseling, the clinician makes a diagnosis, offers recommendations, and suggests a prognosis. The clinician also answers questions from the client and the family members about the disorder and the planned clinical services.

Make a Tentative Diagnosis

Although a final analysis of assessment results has not been made, the clinician nonetheless will have come to tentative but generally valid clinical conclusions at the end of the assessment session. The clinician can make statements about the nature of the voice disorder, its prognosis, and treatment options. The clinician might describe the client's voice characteristics (e.g., deviant pitch, loudness, quality, and resonance) that justify the diagnosis. The clinician also might point out potential causes that led to the voice disorder. For instance, the clinician might relate the client's vocally abusive behaviors to the vocal nodules and the resulting vocal hoarseness.

Make Recommendations

The clinician may recommend voice treatment. Whether the client has had a medical evaluation for the voice problem or the SLP is the first professional to be consulted will determine the immediate course of action, however. The client with a voice disorder but has no other complicating medical conditions needs to be referred to a laryngologist if no prior laryngeal consultation has taken place. A client with possible neurological involvement should be referred to a neurologist. Other professionals, including an audiologist, a psychologist, or a psychiatrist may need to be consulted before starting voice therapy. The clinician may schedule voice treatment when the laryngologist or other medical specialists recommend it.

Suggest a Prognosis

Improved voice production typically follows effective voice therapy (Aronson, 2009; Boone et al., 2010; Stemple et al., 2010). When combined with behavior modification, therapy is usually successful in treating voice disorders due to vocal abuse. Successful voice treatment may help avoid laryngeal surgery in many cases. Therefore, with effective treatment, prognosis is generally good for improved voice.

Several other factors, however, may affect the rate of improvement, even with effective therapy. The type and the severity of the disorder need to be considered. For instance, severe spasmodic dysphonia has not been especially responsive to voice treatment. Prognosis may be guarded for voice disorders associated with degenerative neurological diseases that cause speech and voice problems (as in several types of dysarthria). Other variables that affect prognosis include the motivation of the client and family members and resources to support prolonged therapy, if needed.

Answer the Client's Questions

Not only the client, but also his or her spouse or other family members will have several questions about voice disorders and their treatment. They deserve honest and scientifically justified answers. Some commonly encountered questions and their answers are described here; but the clinician should be ready for other questions. Clients with complicated medical conditions will have additional questions specific to those conditions. The clinician also needs to modify the terms to suit the educational level of the client and the accompanying family members.

What causes voice disorders in adults? Voice disorders have many causes. In some individuals, they are due to vocal abuse or misuse. [*The clinician provides an explanation of vocal abuse and misuse, give examples.*] Excessive and loud talking, for example, can cause vocal nodules or polyps, and hoarseness of voice.

In other individuals, voice may be affected because of cancer of the vocal folds. Treatment in such cases is medical, followed by voice therapy. Several neurological diseases that affect the vocal fold functioning are known to cause voice disorders along with other types of communication problems. For example, Parkinson's disease can cause speech and voice disorders. [*The clinician addresses the client's specific type of voice disorder and gives more details.*]

How long does it take to treat a voice disorder effectively? It depends on the type of the disorder. Some take more time than others. Some may need medical attention before or during voice therapy; this tends to extend the treatment time. The progress will be faster if we start the treatment soon and we are consistent than if we delayed it or have frequent interruptions. We offer treatment twice a week. [*If not, the clinician gives the actual schedule.*] If you work at home on our assignments and the family members offer support, the progress will be even better. As you can guess, more severe problems and a problem with additional medical complications will take more time. [*The clinician expands the answer to give additional information relevant to the client's voice disorder.*]

What are some of the treatment options? Voice treatment varies, depending on the type of disorder. We use a combination of effective procedures. For instance, if the voice disorder is caused by nodules which are in turn caused by vocal abuse, our main task is to change such abusive behaviors. Whether medical treatment is combined or not, our treatment is mostly concerned with teaching the client to use his or voice effectively and in a healthy manner. We want to reduce the kinds of actions that are not helpful in maintaining a good voice. Sometimes we may use computerized instruments that help produce good voice. [*The clinician expands the answer to give more treatment information relevant to the client's voice disorder.*]

When do we start treatment? It is better to start treatment as soon as possible. The sooner we start, the better the outcome. [*The clinician gives additional information, depending on whether the client needs to be referred to other specialists before starting treatment; also, depending on the service setting, the clinician tells when and how the treatment might begin.*]

References

American Speech-Language-Hearing Association. (2004). *Vocal tract visualization and imaging* [Position Statement]. Rockville, MD: Author. Available from http://www.asha.org/policy

American Speech-Language-Hearing Association. (2007). *Scope of practice in speech-language pathology* [Scope of Practice]. Rockville, MD: Author. Available from http://www.asha.org/policy

Andrews, M. L. (2006). *Manual of voice treatment: Pediatrics through geriatrics* (3rd ed.). Clifton Park, NY: Thompson Delmar Learning.

Aronson, A. E., & Bless, D. M. (2009). *Clinical voice disorders* (4th ed.). New York, NY: Thieme.

Benninger, M. S., Gardner, G. M., & Jacobson, B. H. (2005). New dimensions in measuring voice treatment outcome and quality of life. In R. T. Sataloff (Ed.), *Clinical assessment of voice* (pp. 149–155). San Diego, CA: Plural.

Blumin, J. H., & Berke, G. S. (2007). Spasmodic dysphonia. In A. L. Merati & S. A. Bielamowicz (Eds.), *Textbook of voice disorders* (pp. 179–190). San Diego, CA: Plural.

Boone, D. R., McFarlane, S. C., Von Berg, S. L., & Zraick, R. L. (2010). *The voice and voice therapy* (8th ed.). Boston, MA: Pearson Education.

Case, J. L. (2002). *Clinical management of voice disorders* (4th ed.). Austin, TX: Pro-Ed.

Cohen, S. M., Jacobson, B. H., Garrett, C. G., Noordzi, J. P, Stewart, M. G., Attia, A., . . . Cleveland, T. F. (2007). Creation and validation of the Singing Voice Handicap Index. *Annals of Otology, Rhinology & Laryngology, 116,* 402–406.

Deem, J. F., & Miller, L. (2000). *Manual of voice therapy* (2nd ed.). Austin, TX: Pro-Ed.

Duffy, J. R. (2005). *Motor speech disorders: Substrates, differential diagnosis, and management* (2nd ed.). St. Louis, MO: Elsevier Mosby.

Eckel, F. C., & Boone, D. R. (1981). The s/z ratio as an indicator of laryngeal pathology. *Journal of Speech and Hearing Disorders, 46,* 147–150.

Freed, D. (2000). *Motor speech disorders: Diagnosis and treatment.* Clifton Park, NY: Cengage Delmar.

Haynes, W. O., & Pindzola, R. H. (2004). *Diagnosis and evaluation in speech-language pathology* (6th ed.). Boston, MA: Pearson Education.

Herrington-Hall, B. L., Lee, L., Stemple, J. C., Niemi, K. R., & McHome, M. M. (1988). Descriptions of laryngeal pathologies by age, sex, and occupation in a treating-seeking sample. *Journal of Speech and Hearing Disorders, 53,* 57–64.

Holland, R. W., & DeJarnette, G. (2002). Voice & voice disorders. In D. Battle (Ed.), *Communication disorders in multicultural populations* (3rd ed., pp. 299–333). Boston, MA: Butterworth-Heinemann.

Hogikyan, N. D., & Sethuraman, G. (1999). Validation of an instrument to measure voice-related quality of life (V-RQOL). *Journal of Voice, 13,* 557–569.

Hollien, H., & Shipp, T. (1972). Speaking fundamental frequency and chronological age in males. *Journal of Speech and Hearing Research, 15,* 155-159.

Hudson, A. L., & Holbrook, A. (1981). A study of the reading fundamental frequency of young African American adults. *Journal of Speech and Hearing Research, 24*, 197–201.

Jacobson, B., Johnson, A., Grywalski, C., Silbergleit, A., Jacobson, G., & Benninger, M. (1997). The Voice Handicap Index (VHI): Development and validation. *American Journal of Speech-Language Pathology, 6*, 66–70.

Kent, R. (1994). *Reference manual for communication sciences and disorders*. Austin, TX: Pro-Ed.

Kent, R. (1997). *The speech sciences*. San Diego, CA: Singular.

Ptacek, P. H., Sander, E. K., Maloney, W. H., & Jackson, C. C. R. (1966). Phonatory and related changes with advanced age. *Journal of Speech and Hearing Research, 9*, 353–360

Raphael, L. J., Borden, G. J., and Harris, K. S. (2007). *Speech science primer* (5th ed.). Baltimore, MD: Lippincott, Williams & Wilkins.

Roy, N., Stemple, J., Merrill, R. M., & Thomas, L. (2007). Epidemiology of voice disorders in the elderly: Preliminary findings. *Laryngoscope, 117*(4), 228–633.

Roy, N., Merrill, R. M., Gray, S. D., & Smith, E. M. (2005, November). Voice disorders in the general population: Prevalence, risk factors, and occupational impact. *Laryngoscope, 115*(11), 1988–1995.

Roy, N., Merrill, R. N., Thibeault, S., Gray, S. D., & Smith, E. M. (2004, June). Voice disorders in teachers and the general population: Effects on work performance, attendance, and future career choices. *Journal of Speech, Language, Hearing Research, 47*(3), 542–551.

Roy, N., Merrill, R. M., Thibeault, S., Parsa, R. A., Gray, S. D., & Smith, E. M. (2004). Prevalence of voice disorders in teachers and general population. *Journal of Speech, Language, and Hearing Research, 47*, 281–293.

Roy, N., Weinrich, B., Gray, S. D., Tanner, C., & Stemple, J. (2003). Three treatments for teachers with voice disorders: A randomized clinical trial. *Journal of Speech, Language, and Hearing Research, 46*, 670–688.

Sapienza, C., & Hoffman-Ruddy, B. (2009). *Voice disorders*. San Diego, CA: Plural.

Stemple, J., Glaze, L., & Klaben, B. (2010). *Clinical voice pathology: Theory and management* (4th ed.). San Diego, CA: Plural.

Stoicheff, M. L. (1981). Speaking fundamental frequency characteristics of nonsmoking female adults. *Journal of Speech and Hearing Research, 24*, 437–441.

Titze, J. R., Lemke, J., & Montequin, D. (1997). Voice as an occupational tool of trade. *Journal of Voice, 11*, 254–259.

Verdolini, K., & Ramig, L. O. (2001). Review: Occupational risks for voice problems. *Logopedics, Phoniatrics, Vocology, 26*(1): 37–46.

Wilson, D. K. (1987). Voice problems of children (3rd ed.). Baltimore, MD: Paul H. Brooks.

Williams, R. A. (1975). *Textbook of black-related diseases*. New York, NY: McGraw-Hill.

Ylitalo, R. (2007). Reflux and the larynx. In A. L. Merati, & S. A. Bielamowicz (Eds.), *Textbook of voice disorders* (pp. 215–224). San Diego, CA: Plural.

CHAPTER 18

Assessment of Voice: Protocols

Overview of Voice Protocols

Assessment protocols provided in this chapter help assess voice disorders in adults in an efficient manner. The protocols offer ready-made formats that clinicians can use in structuring their client and family interviews and assessing various parameters of voice and its disorders.

The protocols offered in this chapter also are available on the accompanying CD. The clinician may print the needed protocols in evaluating his or her clients. The clinician may combine these protocols in suitable ways to facilitate the evaluation of an adult's voice disorders.

In assessing adults with multiple disorders, the clinician may combine these protocols with protocols from other chapters. For example, the clinician may combine the voice assessment protocols with dysarthria assessment protocols (Chapter 6) or fluency assessment protocols (Chapter 16).

The protocols given in this chapter are specific to voice disorders in adults. To complete the assessment on a given client, the clinician should combine these disorder-specific protocols with the common assessment protocols given in Chapter 2:

- The Adult Case History
- Orofacial Examination and Hearing Screening Protocol
- Diadochokinetic Assessment Protocol for Adults
- Adult Assessment Report Outline

Assessment of Voice: Interview Protocol

Name _____ DOB _____ Date _____ Clinician _____

Individualize this protocol on the CD and print it for your use. 💿

Preparation

- Review the guidelines given under *The Initial Clinical Interview* in Chapter 1.
- Arrange for comfortable seating and lighting.
- Audio- or videorecord the interview.
- Initially interview the client alone and then have the accompanying person join the interview.
- Review the case history ahead of time and take note of areas you want to explore during the interview.

Introduction

☐ Introduce yourself. Describe the assessment plan and tell the client the time it will take.

Example: "Hello Mr./Mrs. [*client's name*]. My name is [*your name*]. I am the speech-language pathologist who will be assessing you today. I would like to start by reviewing the case history and asking you a few questions. After we finish talking, I will work with you. Today's assessment should take about [*estimate the amount of time you plan to spend*]."

Interview Questions

The questions are generally directed toward the adult client. When interviewing the client and the accompanying person together, it is essential to pose the same, but reworded, question to the accompanying person. A few examples are shown within the brackets; the clinician may use this strategy whenever necessary.

- What is your main concern regarding your voice? [What do you think is his (her) main problem?]
- How would you describe your voice problem? [How would you describe her (his) voice problem?]
- When did you first notice that your voice was different? [When did you notice that his (her) voice was different?]
- Has your voice changed over time? If so, how?
- Have you seen your family doctor about your voice?

(continues)

Assessment of Voice: Interview Protocol (continued)

- Did your family doctor refer you to an ear, nose, and throat specialist?

- What did the doctor(s) tell you?

- Have you seen a speech-language pathologist before? What was the advice?

- Did you follow the advice? Have you received voice therapy before?

- Would you describe your voice therapy procedure? For how long did you receive therapy and what were the results?

- Besides a voice problem, are you concerned with any other aspects of your speech?

- How would you describe those other problems of speech? [How would you describe his (her) overall speech?]

- Are there times when your voice is better or worse? For example, is it better in the morning than in the evening? [Do you also think her (his) voice varies throughout the day?]

- Have you ever lost your voice completely? How long did it last?

- Do you believe that your voice problem is affecting your social interactions? Would you describe how?

- Do you think that your voice problem is affecting your job performance? How is it affected?

- Has anyone else in your family ever experienced a voice problem?

- Does anyone in your family have difficulty hearing?

- Do you smoke? How many cigarettes do you smoke each day? Does any other person living in your home smoke? Are you exposed to second-hand smoke in your workplace, home, or any other place you frequently visit?

- Do you participate in sports? Which ones? How often?

- Do you attend sports events? How often?

- Do you tend to cheer loudly when you are watching games and sports?

- Do you have to speak much in your job? How often and what periods of time do you speak?

- Are you on the phone a lot?

- Do you sing? What kind of singing do you do?

- Do you have asthma? Do you frequently get upper respiratory infections?

- Do you have reflux (GERD or LPR)? [provide a brief explanation of these problems, as needed]

- Have you seen any specialists for the reflux problem? Who and when? What were their recommendations? How have you followed up on them? What were the results?

- Do you experience frequent or chronic allergies or colds?

- Have you had a history of ear infections? For how long? Do you still have them?

- Have you ever had a hearing test? When and where? What were the results and recommendations? Did you follow up on them?

- Do you have any other chronic health conditions or concerns?

- Are you currently on any medications?

- It looks like I have most of the information I wanted from you. Do you have any questions for me at this point?

- Thank you for your information. It will be helpful in my assessment. I will now work with you to better understand your voice problem. When we are done, we will discuss our findings.

Review the case history again and ask additional questions if needed.

Adult Voice Evaluation Protocol

Name _____ DOB _____ Date _____ Clinician _____

Individualize this protocol on the CD and print it for your use. 💿

Voice Parameter	Clinical Evaluation		
Hard glottal attacks	☐ none	☐ some	☐ excessive
Hyperfunctional voice (tensed)	☐ none	☐ occasional	☐ frequent
Hypofunctional voice (lax, weak)	☐ none	☐ occasional	☐ frequent
Voice breaks	☐ none	☐ occasional	☐ frequent
Vocal tremors	☐ none	☐ some	☐ excessive
Breath support	☐ adequate	☐ somewhat inadequate	☐ inadequate
Loudness	☐ too soft	☐ normal	☐ too loud
Loudness variations	☐ too few	☐ normal	☐ excessive
Pitch	☐ too low	☐ normal	☐ too high
Diplophonia	☐ none	☐ occasional	☐ frequent
Pitch breaks	☐ none	☐ occasional	☐ frequent
Pitch inflections	☐ monopitch	☐ normal	☐ uncontrolled
Quality	☐ normal	☐ deviant	
Breathiness	☐ none	☐ occasional	☐ excessive
Harshness	☐ none	☐ occasional	☐ excessive
Hoarseness	☐ none	☐ occasional	☐ excessive
Strained/strangled voice	☐ none	☐ occasional	☐ excessive
Resonance	☐ normal	☐ deviant	
Oral	☐ limited	☐ normal	
Nasal	☐ hyponasal	☐ normal	☐ hypernasal
Muscle tension (face, neck, and shoulders)	☐ lax	☐ normal	☐ excessive
Body posture (during speech)	☐ appropriate		☐ inappropriate

Comments and Diagnostic Summary:

Clinician: _____ Date: _____

Resonance Assessment Protocol

Name _____ DOB _____ Date _____ Clinician _____

Individualize this protocol on the CD and print it for your use. 💿

Hypernasality

1. ☐ *Alternate nose holding technique*
    - have the client say /u/ -or- alternate /a/-/i/-/a/-/i/
    - alternate between occluding and releasing the client's nostrils

      Results: ☐ the client's voice changed (suspect hypernasality)
      ☐ the client's voice did not change (hypernasality is not indicated)

2. ☐ *Non-nasal words and phrases*
    - have the client recite non-nasal words and phrases (Boone, McFarlane, Von Berg, & Zraick, 2010)
      - This horse eats grass.
      - I saw the teacher at church.
      - Sister Suzie sat by a thistle.

      Results: ☐ excessive nasal pressure is felt, or a nasal snort is heard (suspect hypernasality)

3. *"Maybe-baby"* (Boone et al., 2010)
    - have the client recite "maybe-baby-maybe-baby . . . "

      Results: ☐ it sounds like "maybe-maybe-maybe . . . "
      (suspect hypernasality)
      ☐ it sounds like "baby-baby-baby-baby . . . "
      (suspect hyponasality)

4. *Count from 60 to 100* (adapted from Mason & Grandstaff, 1971)
    - have the client count from 60 to 100 and judge as indicated:
      - 60 to 69 = listen for VPI and nasal emission secondary to frequent /s/ productions
      - 70 to 79 = listen for assimilation nasality secondary to the recurring /n/ phoneme
      - 80 to 89 = listen for normal or near normal resonance and articulation
      - 90 to 99 = listen for substitutions of /d/ for /n/, suggestive of hyponasality

      Results: ☐ nasal emission/VPI   ☐ assimilation nasality
      ☐ hyponasality   ☐ normal resonance

(continues)

Resonance Assessment Protocol (continued)

Nasal Emission

1. ☐ *Counting from 60 to 79* (see Hypernasality task #4)

2. ☐ *Production of pressure consonants*
    - have the client recite phrases loaded with pressure consonants, such as those listed later (See Assimilation Nasality and VPI, task #5)

    Result: ☐ production of these phrases resulted in increased nasal emission

Hyponasality

1. ☐ *"Maybe-baby-maybe-baby"* (see Hypernasality task #3)

2. ☐ *Count from 90 to 99* (see Hypernasality task #4)

3. ☐ *"Humming"*

    Result: ☐ impaired humming (suggests hyponasality)

4. ☐ *Nasally loaded words and phrases* (Boone, 1993)
    - have the client produce phrases that are loaded with nasals as you occlude and release the nose (see list in *Assimilation Nasality,* task #4)

    Result: ☐ the occluded and unoccluded productions sound the same (hyponasality is present)

Assimilation Nasality and Velopharyngeal Insufficiency

1. ☐ *Count from 60 to 80* (see Hypernasality task #4)

2. ☐ *"Suzy-suzy-suzy-suzy . . . "* This task can be used to determine if the client's hypernasality is the result of a physical etiology or if it is functional
    - have the client recite "suzy-suzy-suzy . . . " as you occlude the nares
    - suddenly release the nares

    Results: ☐ the client immediately reverts back to the hypernasal pattern (it is likely the result of a physical, organic etiology such as VPI)

    ☐ the client has one or more normal productions before reverting to the hypernasal pattern (it is likely functional)

3. ☐ *Modified tongue anchor procedure* (Fox & Johns, 1970)
    - Tell the client to "puff up your cheeks like this" and model the behavior. Practice until the client is able to do it.
    - Tell the client to stick out the tongue. Hold the tongue tip with a piece of sterile gauze.
    - While you are holding the tongue, tell the client to puff up his or her cheeks again. At the same time, occlude the client's nares.

- Tell the client to continue holding the air in his or her mouth. Release the nose.
- As the nostrils are released, listen for nasal emission.

  Results: ☐ nasal emission occurs (the velopharyngeal seal is considered inadequate)

  ☐ no nasal emission occurs (the velopharyngeal seal is considered adequate)

- Repeat this procedure several times to verify your observations.

4. ☐ *For assimilation nasality recite phrases that have a combination of nasal and non-nasal sounds*

- have the client recite the words, phrases, and sentences; the combination of nasal and non-nasal sounds in these phrases will exaggerate the presence of assimilation nasality, making it easier to identify:

Words	Phrases	Sentences
knees	another night	Mike wants more noodles.
now	no more	Mommy made lemon jam.
money	more money	Jenny made me mad.
moon	man on the moon	No more singing tonight.
my	Mickey Mouse	Make noise with a drum.

  Result: ☐ assimilation nasality is present no assimilation nasality noted

5. ☐ *Pressure consonants*

- Have the client produce words, phrases, and sentences that contain pressure consonants (/p/, /b/, /t/, /d/, /k/, /g/, /s/, /z/, /f/, /v/, /ʃ/, /ʒ/, /tʃ/, /dʒ/, /ð/, and /θ/) that stress a weak velopharyngeal system and reveal hypernasality or nasal emission:

Words	Phrases	Sentences
pepper	black pepper	Pass the pepper.
baby	baby bib	The baby bib is blue.
tickle	teddy bear	Tickle the teddy bear.
daddy	daddy digging	Daddy dug a deep ditch.
cake	birthday cake	Don't kick the birthday cake.
goat	big goat	Give the goat a big hug.
feather	soft feather	Find a soft feather.
vest	blue vest	The blue vest is size five.
Suzie	Suzie sews	Suzie sews zippers.
shoe	dishwasher	The shoe is in the dishwasher.
cheese	cheese sandwich	Chew the cheese sandwich.
third	third bath	Her third bath was on Thursday.
they	their father	They saw their father the other day.

  Result: ☐ hypernasality or nasal emission noted (possible VPI)

Vocal Abuse and Misuse Assessment Protocol

Name _____ DOB _____ Date _____ Clinician _____

Individualize this protocol on the CD and print it for your use.

Instructions: Please rate each item according to the rating scale specified. Please write any comments you may have about the amount or the frequency of actions you rate. Let me know if you need an explanation of an action.

Rating: 0 = *never*   1 = *occasionally*   2 = *frequently*   3 = *always*

Rating	Actions you engage in	Your comments
	Yelling, screaming	
	Arguing with colleagues and friends	
	Daily excessive talking	
	Talking with inappropriate pitch	
	Talking with inappropriate loudness	
	Loud cheering and talking at sports events	
	Talking with muscular tension	
	Excessive talking on the telephone	
	Talking in the car	
	Talking in a noisy environment	
	Talking in a smoky environment	
	Abusive singing	
	Participation in plays, debate club, public speaking, or sports coaching	
	Grunting during exercise or lifting	
	Tensed or forceful manner of starting voice production (hard glottal attacks)	
	Crying or loud laughing	
	Smoking	
	Frequent or excessive coughing	
	Frequent or excessive throat clearing	
	Breathing through the mouth	
	Talking with inadequate breath support	

Rating	Actions you engage in	Your comments
	Exposure to environmental irritants	
	Exposure to second-hand smoke	
	Upper respiratory infections	
	Asthma attacks	
Consumption of		
	Dairy products	
	Caffeine products (coffee, tea, soft drinks)	
	Mint products (gum, mints, candy)	
	Tomato-based products	
	Citrus products	
	Spicy foods	
	Alcohol	
Clinician's summative statement:		

Voice Handicap Assessment Protocol

Name _____ DOB _____ Date _____ Clinician _____

Individualize this protocol on the CD and print it for your use. 💿

Have the client fill out this questionnaire. Go over the answers to get details or clarifications.

Rating: 0 = *never*   1 = *occasionally*   2 = *frequently*   3 = *always*

#	Your Rating	How your voice problem affects your life	Your explanations or details
1.		People ask me to speak loudly because they can't hear me.	
2.		People ask me to repeat what I say.	
3.		Since the onset of my voice problem, I am making fewer phone calls.	
4.		I am often frustrated because of my voice doesn't sound normal.	
5.		Sometimes I feel depressed because of my voice problem.	
6.		My voice makes me feel tense and anxious in social situations.	
7.		Since the onset of my voice problem, I have been avoiding social interactions.	
8.		Because of my voice problem, I have been avoiding interactions with people at work.	
9.		My voice prevents me from getting the job I want.	
10.		I speak less with friends and relatives because of my voice problem.	
11.		Speaking takes much effort because of my voice problem.	
12.		People react negatively to my voice.	
13.		I feel that some people avoid talking to me for an extended period of time.	

#	Your Rating	How your voice problem affects your life	Your explanations or details
14.		I think that my voice problem is an occupational and personal handicap.	
15.		I talk much less in the evening because of my vocal fatigue.	
Clinician's summative comments:			

Voice Quality of Life Assessment Protocol

Name _____ DOB _____ Date _____ Clinician _____

Individualize this protocol on the CD and print it for your use. 💿

Administer this to the client. Give an example of how the client should read and respond.

"I would like to know how your voice problem has affected your life. I would like you to read the item in this manner: *With my voice in social situations, I am . . . Satisfied, Somewhat Satisfied, Somewhat Dissatisfied,* or *Dissatisfied,* and then place a check mark in one of the columns for your answer."

With my voice	*I am*				
	Satisfied	Somewhat satisfied	Somewhat dissatisfied	Dissatisfied	N/A
in social situations					
over the phone					
at home					
at my workplace					
while talking to my supervisors					
when I am with my friends					
during my speech to a group					
toward the end of the day					
during job interviews					
as I talk to strangers					
when I talk to members of the opposite sex					
in expressing my feelings and opinions					
when I talk to my neighbors					

With my	I am				
	Satisfied	Somewhat satisfied	Somewhat dissatisfied	Dissatisfied	N/A
own reaction to my voice					
enjoyment of life					
feelings and thoughts about myself					
level of self-confidence					
own enjoyment of personal relationships					
educational achievements					
job performance					
job advancement					
feelings and thoughts about myself					
level of self-confidence					
general quality of life					

References

Boone, D. R. (1993). *The Boone voice program for children* (2nd ed.). Austin, TX: Pro-Ed.

Boone, D. R., McFarlane, S. C., Von Berg, S. L., & Zraick, R. L. (2010). *The voice and voice therapy* (8th ed.). Boston, MA: Pearson Education.

Fox, D. R., & Johns, D. (1970). Predicting velopharyngeal closure with a modified tongue-anchor technique. *Journal of Speech and Hearing Disorders, 35,* 248–251.

Mason, R., & Grandstaff, H. (1971). Evaluating the velopharyngeal mechanism in hypernasal speech. *Language, Speech, and Hearing Services in Schools, 4,* 1–10.

Index